IMPULSIVITY

IMPULSIVITY
Theory, Assessment, and Treatment

EDITED BY

CHRISTOPHER D. WEBSTER

AND

MARGARET A. JACKSON

Foreword by John Monahan

THE GUILFORD PRESS
New York London

© 1997 The Guilford Press
A Division of Guilford Publications, Inc.
72 Spring Street, New York, NY 10012

Printed in the United States of America

This book is printed on acid-free paper.

Last digit is print number: 9 8 7 6 5 4 3 2 1

Library of Congress Cataloging-in-Publication Data

Impulsivity: theory, assessment, and treatment / edited by
   Christopher D. Webster and Margaret A. Jackson; foreword
   by John Monahan
      p. cm.
   Includes bibliographical references and index.
   ISBN 1-57230-225-9
   1. Impulsive personality. 2. Impulse control disorders. 3.
Violence—Forecasting. I. Webster, Christopher D., 1936–   .
II. Jackson, Margaret A.
RC569.5.I46I49   1997
616.85′84—dc21   97-20961
                                                          CIP

Contributors

R. Michael Bagby, PhD, Clarke Institute of Psychiatry, Toronto, Ontario; Department of Psychology, University of Toronto, Toronto, Ontario

Douglas P. Boer, PhD, Correctional Service of Canada, Pacific Region, Abbotsford, British Columbia; Department of Psychology, Simon Fraser University, Burnaby, British Columbia

Marilyn L. Bowman, PhD, Department of Psychology, Simon Fraser University, Burnaby, British Columbia

J. Maxwell Clark, BA, Department of Psychology, Simon Fraser University, Burnaby, British Columbia

E. Michael Coles, PhD, Department of Psychology, Simon Fraser University, Burnaby, British Columbia

G. Neil Conacher, MB, ChB, MRCPsych, FRCP(C), Kingston Psychiatric Hospital, Kingston, Ontario; Department of Psychiatry, Queen's University, Kingston, Ontario

Donald V. Coscina, PhD, Department of Psychology, Wayne State University, Detroit, Michigan; Clarke Institute of Psychiatry, Toronto, Ontario

Rebecca J. Dempster, BA, Department of Psychology, Simon Fraser University, Burnaby, British Columbia

Kevin Douglas, MA, Department of Psychology, Simon Fraser University, Burnaby, British Columbia

Donald G. Dutton, PhD, Department of Psychology, University of British Columbia, Vancouver, British Columbia

Derek Eaves, MB, ChB, FRCPsych, FRCP(C), Forensic Psychiatric Services Commission of British Columbia, Vancouver, British Columbia; Department of Psychiatry, University of British Columbia, Vancouver, British Columbia; Department of Psychology and School of Criminology, Simon Fraser University, Burnaby, British Columbia

Claudine M. Gauthier, BA, Correctional Service of Canada, Pacific Region, Abbotsford, British Columbia

Grant T. Harris, PhD, Department of Psychology, Mental Health Centre, Penetanguishene, Ontario; Department of Psychology, Queen's University, Kingston, Ontario

Stephen D. Hart, PhD, Department of Psychology, Simon Fraser University, Burnaby, British Columbia

Stephen J. Hucker, MB, BS, FRCPsych, FRCP(C), Departments of Psychiatry and Psychology, Queen's University, Kingston, Ontario

Jeremy Jackson, PhD, Department of Psychology, Simon Fraser University, Burnaby, British Columbia

Margaret A. Jackson, PhD, School of Criminology, Simon Fraser University, Burnaby, British Columbia

P. Randall Kropp, PhD, Forensic Psychiatric Services Commission of British Columbia, Vancouver, British Columbia; Department of Psychology, Simon Fraser University, Burnaby, British Columbia

Robert Menzies, PhD, School of Criminology, Simon Fraser University, Burnaby, British Columbia

James R. P. Ogloff, JD, PhD, Department of Psychology, Simon Fraser University, Burnaby, British Columbia

James D. A. Parker, PhD, Department of Psychology, Trent University, Peterborough, Ontario

Natalie H. Polvi, MA, Correctional Service of Canada, Pacific Region, Abbotsford, British Columbia; Department of Psychology, Simon Fraser University, Burnaby, British Columbia

Marnie E. Rice, PhD, Research Department, Mental Health Centre, Penetanguishene, Ontario; Department of Psychology, Queen's University, Kingston, Ontario; Department of Psychology, McMaster Univerity, Hamilton, Ontario

Lee Ryan, PhD, Department of Psychology, University of California, San Diego, California

Steven Taylor, PhD, Department of Psychiatry, University of British Columbia, Vancouver, British Columbia

George Tien, PhD, Forensic Psychiatric Services Commission of British Columbia, Vancouver, British Columbia; Department of Psychology, Simon Fraser University, Burnaby, British Columbia

Christopher D. Webster, PhD, FRSC, Department of Psychology, Simon Fraser University, Burnaby, British Columbia; Department of Psychiatry, University of British Columbia, Vancouver, British Columbia; Department of Psychiatry and Centre of Criminology, University of Toronto, Toronto, Ontario

Derek Wilson, MA, Forensic Psychiatric Services Commission of British Columbia, Vancouver, British Columbia

Robin J. Wilson, PhD, Correctional Service of Canada, Ontario Region, Toronto, Ontario

Judy Zaparniuk, MA, Department of Psychiatry, University of British Columbia, Vancouver, British Columbia

Foreword

As the century draws to a close, "impulsivity" is emerging as a master construct in many areas of behavioral science. In the past 20 years, the *Social Science Citation Index* informs us, some 650 articles have appeared with impulsivity in the title. The World Wide Web lists over 700 current web page matches with the term "impulsivity." These printed and electronic references have a remarkable range of application. Many are to attention-deficit/hyperactivity disorder or to aggression. Others refer to a wide variety of biological correlates of impulsivity. Still others deal with how to attempt practical regulation of impulsive behaviors that imperil the financial and/or physical security of individuals (e.g., impulsive shopping and seemingly irrepressible urges to mutilate the body; topics mentioned in Chapter 11 of this book). The references in the citation index and the World Wide Web also drive home the point that the general impulsivity construct is becoming key in that it directs our attention to the whole area of decision making. Explorations on the web made me realize that my own safety as an air passenger lies in the hands of pilots trained according to the motto "Not so fast. Think first." Although it is a comfort to know that, beyond mottos, the FAA and other such organizations have "judgment training programs" for employees charged with taking responsibility for our lives, there can be no doubt whatever that impulsivity as a construct offers excellent opportunity to examine matters with impact on our daily life (a point acknowledged in Chapter 1 of this book).

Although this book is not limited to issues in the assessment and prediction of violence, it does place considerable emphasis on the topic, which has been one of my major preoccupations over the past several years. As is made clear in Chapters 10 and 11, impulsivity is implicated in a wide range of formally defined mental disorders. Even more important, or so it seems to me, is that the construct features very consistently in the day-to-day decision-making activities of clinicians. That impulsivity is a key aspect in the clinical risk assessment of violence has been abundantly clear at least since the work of Segal, Watson, Goldfinger, and Averbuck (1988). These researchers studied assessment of violence risk by clinicians as it relates to specific symptoms of mental disorder. What they found from their research in five psychiatric emergency rooms in California is that there is a strong correspondence between perceptions of impulse control and perceptions of dangerousness. Impulsivity is a term the clinicians associated with grave disability. More than any other dimension of mental disorder, impulsivity was linked to danger to self and danger to others. Indeed, so strong was the association found in the study by Segal et al. (1988), that persons appearing at the emergency rooms were apt not to be considered dangerous *unless* their disturbed behaviors and judgments were perceived to be due to deficiencies in impulse control. In the words of the researchers, "it would appear that clinicians, in the same process by which they decide whether poor judgment or disorganized or bizarre behavior results from disorders of thought, mood, perception, orientation, or memory, also attempt to assess the origins of any impairment in impulse control" (p. 757). It therefore appears that not only is impulsivity comingled with dangerousness in legal contexts (Chapter 4) but the same likely holds true in routine mental health, forensic, and correctional practice. A more definite acknowledgment of this state of affairs, one implied by the present book, may do much to prompt new research inquiries and perhaps may even improve the practical assessment of the risk of violence.

Christopher D. Webster and Margaret A. Jackson have brought together an exceptional group of scholars to address a broad range of issues arising from the concept of impulsivity. From biopsychology to deconstruction, these issues are systematically and thoroughly examined. It is difficult to imagine how anyone could study, assess, or treat impulsivity in the future without frequent reference to this state-of-the-art compendium.

It is hard not to notice that the cast who produced this extraordinary work is virtually all-Canadian. This is merely one more illustration, as if one were needed, of the remarkably strong international presence of Canada in forensic psychology and psychiatry, a presence out of all proportion to relative population size, not to mention relative crime rate. Indeed, I sometimes have had the impression that half of all Canadians work in the field of mental health law. Then it occurs to me that I have a biased sample: it is only half of the Canadians that I know personally who are working in mental health law. But even so, the Canadian prominence in the field is clear. And as this superb book amply demonstrates, the rest of us in North America and throughout the world are deeply in Canada's debt.

JOHN MONAHAN, PHD
Doherty Professor of Law and
Professor of Psychology and Legal Medicine
University of Virginia School of Law

REFERENCE

Segal, S. P., Watson, M. A., Goldfinger, S. M., & Averbuck, D. S. (1988). Civil commitment in the psychiatric emergency room: 11 mental disorder indicators and three dangerousness criteria. *Archives of General Psychiatry, 45,* 753–758.

Acknowledgments

As is usual in enterprises of this sort, we, the editors, have many people to thank for the fact that it reached fruition. Principal among those who deserve acknowledgment of our appreciation are, of course, the contributors to the book. As well, we are indebted to many other colleagues who offered their expertise in conferences on impulsivity held at the Clarke Institute of Psychiatry (1991) and at Simon Fraser University (1994). The former was organized by Ms. Rosemary Scaglione, the latter by Ms. Beverley Davino. Particular thanks are due to Professor Paul Garfinkel, President of the Clarke Institute of Psychiatry and Chair of the Department of Psychiatry, University of Toronto. It was Paul who had the vision of an Impulsivity Program for the Clarke Institute and who allowed one of us (C. D. W.), to bring it into existence. At Simon Fraser University we are grateful to the Dean of Arts, Professor Evan Alderson, for encouraging collaboration between the Department of Psychology and the School of Criminology, and for providing much-needed financial assistance. That assistance, in part, allowed us to secure the expert services of Dr. Monique Layton, whose firm editorial hand did much to enhance the readability and coherence of the book. Helpful assistance was also provided by Ms. Erika Ford under the Work Study Program of Simon Fraser University. Ms. Aileen Sams stepped in near the end to organize and finalize the chapters for us; we appreciate her cheerful assistance. Finally, we thank Robert Egert, Carolyn Graham, Allie London, Rochelle Serwator, Marie Sprayberry, William Meyer, and Seymour Weingarten of the Guilford Press for expert advice and for being so thoughtful about the preparation of this book.

Contents

III. PRACTICE: ASSESSMENT

IV. PRACTICE: TREATMENT

Introduction

MARGARET A. JACKSON
CHRISTOPHER D. WEBSTER

The chapters in this volume were written in response to a conference on "Impulsivity: New Directions in Research and Clinical Practice," held at the Harbour Centre campus of Simon Fraser University (SFU) in May 1994. The conference was sponsored by the Department of Psychology and the School of Criminology at SFU, and was also supported by the Departments of Psychology and Psychiatry at the University of British Columbia, the Forensic Psychiatric Services Commission of British Columbia, and Riverview Hospital. The conference focused on the concept of impulsivity from a variety of perspectives, all of which are represented in this text. This type of multidisciplinary approach is consistent with our own continuing interest in the development of the area of clinical criminology (Ben-Aron, Hucker, & Webster, 1985; Hilton, Jackson, & Webster, 1990), from which the concept of impulsivity is derived.

In a previous edited text (Hilton et al., 1990), we indicated our belief that clinical criminology has a certain utility and convenience in pointing directions for future clinical and research efforts within the mental health, criminal justice, correctional, and other related systems. Five foundations for the area were articulated; these form the underlying bases for the present text on impulsivity.

We first proposed that properly trained clinicians and other practitioners working with disturbed individuals not only should have a firm grasp of the clinical realities of the individual case, but should be informed by actuarial realities derived from statistical information. This allows for balanced decision making, whether about assessment, treatment, or supervision. Such an approach creates a pressure to develop devices and procedures that are more refined, valid, and reliable than those presently available.

The second foundation is knowledge about the wider policy climate in which these procedures take place. Clinicians and practitioners need to know about the actual state of the prisons and mental hospitals in which their clients reside, as well as the manner in which they are treated within. What are the effects of these institutions on the clients? What factors in societal, economic, social, or other domains influence how disturbed individuals are dealt with and cared for? Mental health workers can be remarkably uninformed about the "true" rather than the intended effects of standard assessment and treatment procedure—a point sometimes made with admirable clarity by persons who have the ability and courage to write of their experiences in both receiving and offering care.

The interdisciplinary base noted above forms the third foundation. Disciplinary territoriality often does not serve the best interests of a client. Professional tensions—among social workers, psychiatrists, police, medical personnel, and so on—need to be transcended in order for services to be provided effectively and humanely. It is important for individuals working with disturbed and disruptive people to be able to communicate and cooperate easily with one another. This applies within interdisciplinary teams and between agencies and government offices.

Ethical and moral considerations form the basis of the fourth foundation. All individuals involved in the care of disturbed people—psychiatrists, psychologists, nurses, correctional officers, social workers, parole officers, child care workers, and others—need to be aware of their own biases when making assessments or other judgments about these clients. They are, after all, often in a position of power over clients, and thus they need to monitor their personal feelings about their clients carefully and continually. Opinions of colleagues can often improve in this process. It is hard to sustain healthy attitudes when working over the long haul with demanding and disruptive people who may commit highly violent crimes, or inflict serious injuries on themselves, without much warning.

Finally, the last foundation consists of the notion that we need to develop a positive attitude about working with impulsive people. As Donald West suggests in a 1985 text on clinical criminology, "Current criminological thinking sees little scope for the application of depth psychology to the average criminal and little credibility in theories that set criminals apart from the rest of humanity or suggest that they are in some way defective, maladjusted or suitable cases for treatment" (quoted in Ben-Aron et al., 1985, p. 2). The idea behind clinical criminology is to prevent harm and, wherever possible, to help would-be perpetrators overcome their impulses toward deviant acts and repetitive antisocial behavior. More generally, the aim is to improve the quality of all our lives.

With the grounding described above as our beginning, we move in the present text to a consideration of the specific concept of impulsivity. As Derek Eaves, George Tien, and Derek Wilson indicate in Chapter 21, "The concept of impulsivity is one that can be viewed from many different perspectives; as a consequence, it has been defined in a number of ways, not all of which are consistent with one another. . . . Instances of impulsivity, or the behaviors associated with impulsivity, have been identified as part of the constellation of symptoms in many psychiatric disorders" (p. 409).

To a large extent, progress in science is forwarded by constructs, ideas, and formulations. Such constructs do not necessarily remain static; they evolve or shift over time. New findings and opinions work themselves into the existing fabric and change the nature of the fabric as they do. Scientific constructs usually have the effect (at least for a time) of guiding research in a field and pulling observations together, and they possess explanatory power. The construct of impulsivity, although it may be hard to define concretely, has held a place of prominence in both psychiatry and psychology for some time and has become increasingly important over the past decade.

As a guiding construct in psychiatry, psychology, and the allied mental health disciplines, impulsivity should accomplish several ends, which we hope to elucidate in the text to follow. It should (1) provide a language that can be held by both researchers and clinicians, (2) offer information and opinions that should be helpful to members of a variety of disciplines, (3) permit definitions of terms, and (4) encourage verification of ideas and procedures through observational or experimental tests. In this respect, one goal of the text is to stress the commonalities among the impulse-control disorders and related disorders in the (DSM-IV; American Psychiatric Association, 1994), and to suggest general approaches to treatment, management, and therapy.

DSM-IV ORGANIZATION

Much of psychiatry depends on categorization, on diagnostic systems. Conditions are evident or they are not; patients do or do not meet the criteria for a disorder. The DSM-IV not only provides more explicit criteria for most disorders than heretofore, but brings the impulsivity construct to the fore by devoting a whole section to the so-called "impulse-control disorders not elsewhere classified." It focuses attention on five specific conditions: (1) intermittent explosive disorder, (2) kleptomania, (3) pyromania, (4) pathological gambling, and (5) trichotillomania (hair pulling). These five disorders would not appear to have much in common on the surface. Yet DSM-IV would have it that they are bound together, in that in all five conditions, the sufferer typically experiences an increase in tension before the act and a decrease after it. There is an implication that persons suffering from impulse-control disorders are driven to act irrationally and perhaps irresponsibly. These matters are considered by Stephen J. Hucker in Chapter 11. On the other hand, the point is made by E. Michael Coles in Chapter 10 that the notion of impulsivity, though centrally constructed in the disorders above, is still in need of tighter clarification and definition.

WORK ON SCALES FOR ASSESSING IMPULSIVITY

Psychology has always stressed the normality in distribution of entities like intelligence. It is not that some people have or do not have it; rather, the challenge lies in figuring out precisely how much they do have. To psychologists, most constructs are best conceived of as dimensional. The challenge then becomes one of finding scales or tests to measure the existence of impulsivity and similar constructs.

Impulsivity, as it turns out, is a central element in many well-established personality tests. Although there is much dispute about what different kinds of impulsivity may be measured in these various devices, and although it is recognized that some kinds of impulsivity are dysfunctional while other kinds are functional (Eysenck, 1993, p. 59), there seems every reason to believe that the overall construct can be captured by a more precise definition than is presently available or accepted. In one recent study, for example, we were able to isolate from psychometrically obtained scores two fairly distinct components (Parker, Bagby, & Webster, 1993). Our general point is that there is an expanding role for psychometric work. We need instruments that are strongly theoretically grounded, and we need data both from "normal" and from clinical and correctional populations. These issues are dealt with in this book by James D. A. Parker and R. Michael Bagby (Chapter 8) and by Judy Zaparniuk and Steven Taylor (Chapter 9).

BIOMEDICAL ADVANCES

It has been known for some time that stimulant drugs such as methylphenidate are helpful in modifying the impulsive behavior of children (e.g., Garfinkel, Webster, & Sloman, 1981). Despite these and other such incontrovertible findings, there remain doubts about the function of monoaminergic systems in humans. The measures of metabolites in cerebrospinal fluid, urine, plasma, and the like are indirect; they require an assumption that levels of the metabolites correspond to the general neural activity of particular neurotransmitters. With these limitations in mind, it is, of interest that impulsive adults have been found to possess relatively low platelet monoamine oxidase activity (Zuckerman, 1991). This appears to be especially true in the case of aggressive and antisocial persons, or "thrill seekers." Many studies have implicated other neural substances in violent and impulsive offenders (e.g., Virkkunen, 1985). In addition, there have been important attempts to develop impulsivity models from animal-based research (e.g., Gorenstein & Newman, 1980, Flora & Dietze, 1993). Although "it seems unlikely that impulsive behavior is reflective of any single aspect of brain organization . . . it seems reasonable to expect that structural and functional characteristics of the monoaminergic pathways would be relevant to the occurrence of impulsive behavior, because they influence dynamic aspects of brain organization" (Daruna & Barnes, 1993, p. 32). Donald V. Coscina addresses these and other matters in Chapter 6 of the present volume.

LEGAL DEFINITION

The case of Lorena Bobbitt in the United States excited a good deal of interest in the "irresistible impulse" defense. But the notion of impulse control is important in much North American criminal law at a workaday level. It is, for example, implicated in Section 16 of the *Criminal Code of Canada*, which states that persons should not be held criminally responsible for their violent conduct if they were, at the time of commission, unable to appreciate "the nature and quality of the act" (quoted in Rodriques, 1996, p. 20). In a different spirit, individuals may be declared to be "dangerous offenders," and so made liable to indefinite detention, for "failure to control his sexual impulses" (Rodriques, 1996, p. 582).

Judges, it seems, are almost as interested as psychologists in what action an individual can or will take between the appearance of the stimulus and the execution of the response (Doob, 1990). Some believe that as time goes by, they will be listening to more and more arguments about the extent to which a person's behavior was or was not under reflective control (Davis, 1993). These and other related legal discussions are considered in this text by James R. P. Ogloff (Chapter 4).

THE PHENOMENOLOGY OF IMPULSIVE DISORDERS

There are two interesting observations to be made about impulsive disorders at the outset of this text. The first is the point that different individuals who are experiencing impulsive feelings tend to describe these feelings in much the same way, regardless of how they come to be manifested behaviorally. Second, it is clear that many individuals so afflicted act markedly impulsively in more than one domain (Kennedy & Grubin, 1990; Wishnie, 1977; Woodcock, 1986). It becomes evident that such people may be troubled by one type of disorder at one stage and may reappear at a later stage with another. Both these observations lend further support to our argument that the construct of impulsivity underlies many disorders. Given this possibility, our examination and treatment of the individuals themselves, as well as our further academic study of the disorders, can benefit from this consideration of impulsivity as a unifying construct.

TREATMENT POSSIBILITIES

Although it is generally acknowledged that highly impulsive people are hard to help (Butz & Austen, 1993), some ideas about how best to try to help them are slowly beginning to develop. One thing that makes treating highly impulsive people so discouraging is that they are apt to terminate therapy very abruptly. Another is that they can be very personally intrusive and demanding of therapists. It has been argued that impulsivity is itself a good starting topic for therapy (Butz & Austen, 1993, p. 326). It may be, too, that a therapist, in having diagnosed an impulsive disorder, can win the confidence of the client during the early stages of work together. As already noted, impulsive disorders often do not come singly, and the impulsivity construct can be valuable in providing an anchor. McCown and Johnson (1993), for example, stress the value of "inoculating" families at the outset to the notion that the clients are likely to terminate. We know that it is often hard to "get it right" during the early stages of almost any therapy, and that clients are apt to leave unhappy and disillusioned. Imparting this information to impulsive patients may help forestall their departure. Relapse prevention techniques have come to the fore in the last decade. These are based on simple, easy-to-teach principles, and appear to be applicable to persons suffering from a wide range of impulsive disorders. The same can be said for the use of specific behavioral control techniques, such as differential reinforcement of low-rate schedules (Gordon, 1979).

There seems good reason for searching for commonalities among the DSM-IV-specified impulse-control disorders, and also broadening research to include related conditions (McElroy, Hudson, Pope, Keck, & Aizley, 1992). This search should be continued simultaneously and synergistically at biological, psychometric, behavioral, phenomenological, and even cultural levels (McCown & Johnson, 1993, pp. xvii–xxi). We hope that the present text assists in that exercise and further advances the concept of impulsivity as a tool for integration of these ideas.

To set the text in a contemporary framework, and to explain why it is relevant to be discussing issues of impulsive behavior in a wider context of meaning, it should be noted at the start that the public's preoccupation with crime has resulted in increasing pressures on the criminal justice system to deal harshly with criminals. These concerns have often been triggered by high-profile cases in which offenders, while either on parole or on supervised release, have committed seemingly impulsive violent crimes. The costs of processing offenders keep increasing, but because members of the public fear serious crime, they are not very supportive of the cost-saving early release of these individuals into the community. In the United States, some states have "three strikes and you're out" laws, as well as legislation aimed specifically at sexual predators; in Canada, public sentiment is certainly moving toward the advocation of longer sentences for violent offenders. At the same time, there is also correctional and clinical interest in what can be done with offenders and forensic psychiatric patients to render them less of a risk to society upon release.

In this regard, two U.S. authors, Roth and Moore (1995), have recently noted that a problem-solving approach to the crime issue has been gaining public prominence, in response to the doubts raised about the effectiveness of traditional reactive forms of dealing with violent offenders. They observe, for example, that problem-oriented policing has become popular. Such a policing style involves the crafting of "simple, low-cost, common-sense" solutions to specific problems. Underlying each "call for service" (p. 1), there is a particular problem to be solved. The rationale behind problem-oriented policing is that the best police response is the one that attempts to understand and "fix" the problem proactively, so that violence will not recur. This is in contrast to the prevailing tendency simply to respond to each incident as a separate and unrelated one—with the result that future violent behavior is more or less assured.

The second movement Roth and Moore (1995) discuss is the treatment of violence as a public health problem. Violence, they argue, "is a threat to a community's health as well as to its social order" (p. 4). Medical personnel are often in a position to make assessments of both victims and offenders. Epidemiological methods can be useful in measuring overall levels and patterns of violence, and in identifying factors correlated with the risk of violence. Both of these approaches require decision making or problem solving based upon an assessment of each individual case as it exists within a constellation of individual and societal factors.

Traditional approaches to violent behavior, however, have separated those two factors in the development of response strategies. Being trained as psychologists, we ourselves initially became aware of the first approach—that is, the belief that the individual offender is the problem that needs to be addressed through individual treatment, in order to alter future behavior. Another facet to this approach is the emphasis placed on means to predict such behavior. After further training in the field of criminology, we became influenced by the second approach in explaining and dealing with violent behavior. This approach examines the "root causes" of criminality. Attention is paid to the effect of social ills, such as poverty and power imbalances in society, on criminal behavior.

It seems that contemporary problem-solving approaches are attempting a merger in thinking about how to deal with violent behavior. Both problem-oriented policing and public health models of response recognize that violence may be preventable not only by changing the individual's behavior, but by changing his or her physical and social environments as well (Roth & Moore, 1995, p. 5). The policy and programming implications of this approach are quite remarkable. In the case of public health, for example, success in reducing *unintentional* injuries led epidemiologists to imagine that they could be equally successful with *intentional* injuries. Public information campaigns, requirements that consumer products be made safer, and lobbying for preventive measures (e.g., laws mandating seat belts) were some of the policy and programming techniques employed.

What has not been examined to any great extent at this point is the translation of these two contemporary approaches into a predictive scheme—one based on the fact that both individual characteristics and the individual's environmental characteristics somehow interact to result in the violent or unacceptable behavior. How is it possible to predict what will happen in the individual case? Following from that, if it is somehow possible to predict an individual's violence potential through the identification of individual and environmental predictive factors, what methods can be developed or already exist to address that potential? Contributors to this book address these concerns (e.g., Stephen D. Hart in several chapters, Donald G. Dutton in Chapter 2).

The public health model appears a good one to explore and expand, through a linking to recent developments in the forensic clinical field. The latter area of research, as will be seen in the text following, has greatly expanded. There are now assessment guides for a wide variety of problem areas, such as suicide, domestic assault, and sexual offending. What seems to be needed is the integration of these efforts into a model of operation. The public health approach certainly appears to be a useful one. Assessment is key to any problem-solving exercise that attempts to search for preventive interventions to impulsive behavior. The epidemiological identification of patterns of violence and of factors correlated with the risk of violence is not sufficient without a systematic method for assessing those correspondences in individual cases. Thus clinical instruments derived from the experience of actually working with these individuals can be merged with the public health approach, as a components in dealing with the problem in a holistic manner. The section in the text on management of these individuals (e.g., Chapter 21 by Eaves et al.) undertakes preliminary discussion along this line of thinking. If individual and societal factors associated with the risk of violent behavior can be identified and assessed in the individual case, as has been attempted in many of the instruments laid out in this text, it will still require the cooperation of many agencies in the field to assist in the understanding and resolution of the problem—not only for assistance to the individual in terms of care and control, but also in terms of society's interests.

Part I of this book, "Perspectives," focuses on paradigmatic and theoretical issues. Clinical, legal, social, psychological, criminological, sociological, and even cybernautical perspectives are presented, with the intention of setting out the contours of the construct as articulated within each perspective. Yet with this broadening of the construct, we, as editors, see reason also to "rein it in." Robert Menzies, in Chapter 3, accumulates arguments against the unthinking use of the construct. He warns that although it has become a popular concept, impulsivity cannot be expected to account for all problems associated with the varied behaviors it encompasses.

In Part II of the text, "Foundations," the underlying assumptions of the construct are drawn out. From the biopsychology of impulsivity to specific disorders of impulsivity, this section begins to tease out the nature of the construct as seen in the clinical setting. Part III shifts the focus to assessment issues. The main features of this section are descriptions and discussions of various instruments that have been developed for the assessment of troubling impulsive behaviors. Some of these instruments were created specifically for the present text. Whether the behaviors in question are associated with violence to others, violence to self, paraphilias, or psychopathy, it is important to have valid, standardized methods for determining the presence of impulsivity—both for the fair treatment of individuals, and for the training of professionals who have to make such assessments.

Finally, in Part IV, actual treatment issues are discussed. In addition to a consideration of current pharmacological and clinical interventions for impulsivity, recent management approaches that seem appropriate for this specialized problem are presented. The final chapter attempts to drive home the point that people who act impulsively and disruptively are to be found in all avenues of society, and that the points made in the earlier chapters of the book seem to be pertinent to a wide range of problems to be found in almost all social organizations. We emphasize that there are few simple solutions to the kinds of complex problems impulsivity presents, legally, biologically, and in other ways.

REFERENCES

American Psychiatric Association. (1994). *Diagnostic and statistical manual of mental disorders* (4th ed.). Washington, DC: Author.

Ben-Aron, M. H., Hucker, S. J., & Webster, C. D. (Eds.). (1985). *Clinical criminology: The assessment and treatment of criminal behavior.* Toronto: Clarke Institute of Psychiatry.

Butz, M., & Austen, S. (1993). Management of the adult impulsive client: Identification, timing, and methods of treatment. In W. G. McCown, J. L. Johnson, & M. B. Shure (Eds.), *The impulsive client: Theory, research, and treatment* (pp. 323–344). Washington, DC: American Psychological Association.

Daruna, J. H., & Barnes, P. A. (1993). A neurodevelopmental view of impulsivity. In W. G. McCown, J. L. Johnson, & M. B. Shure (Eds.), *The impulsive client: Theory, research, and treatment* (pp. 23–37). Washington, DC: American Psychological Association.

Davis, S. (1993). Changes in the Criminal Code provisions for mentally disordered offenders and their implication for Canadian psychiatry. *Canadian Journal of Psychiatry, 38,* 1–5.

Doob, L. (1990). *Hesitation: Impulsivity and reflection.* New York: Greenwood Press.

Eysenck, H. J. (1993). The nature of impulsivity. In W. G. McCown, J. L. Johnson, & M. B. Shure (Eds.), *The impulsive client: Theory, research, and treatment* (pp. 57–69). Washington, DC: American Psychological Association.

Flora, S. R., & Dietze, M. A. (1993). Caffeine and impulsiveness in rats. *Bulletin of the Psychonomic Society, 31,* 39–41.

Garfinkel, B. D., Webster, C. D., & Sloman, L. (1981). Responses to methylphenidate and varied doses of caffeine in children with attention deficit disorder. *Canadian Journal of Psychiatry, 26,* 399–401.

Gordon, M. (1979). The assessment of impulsivity and mediating behavior in hyperactive and non-hyperactive boys. *Journal of Abnormal Child Psychology, 7*(3), 317–326.

Gorenstein, E. E., & Newman, J. P. (1980). Disinhibitory psychopathology: A new perspective and model for research. *Psychological Review, 87,* 301–315.

Hilton, Z., Jackson, M. A., & Webster, C. D. (Eds.). (1990). *Clinical criminology: Theory, research and practice.* Toronto: Canadian Scholars' Press.

Kennedy, H. G., & Grubin, D. H. (1990). Hot-headed or impulsive. *British Journal of Addictions, 85,* 639–643.

McCown, W. G., & Johnson, J. L. (1993). *Therapy with treatment resistant families: A consultation–crisis intervention model.* Binghamton, NY: Haworth Press.

McElroy, S. L., Hudson, J. L., Pope, H. G., Keck, P. E., & Aizley, H. C. (1992). The DSM-III-R impulse-control disorders not elsewhere classified: Clinical characteristics and relationship to other psychiatric disorders. *American Journal of Psychiatry, 149,* 318–327.

Parker, J. D. A., Bagby, R. M., & Webster, C. D. (1993). Domain of the impulsivity construct: A factor analytic investigation. *Personality and Individual Differences, 15,* 267–274.

Rodriques, G. (Ed.). (1996). *Pocket criminal code.* Toronto: Carswell.

Roth, J., & Moore, M. (1995). *Reducing violent crimes and intentional injuries.* Washington, DC: National Institute of Justice, U.S. Department of Justice.

Virkkunen, M. (1985). Urinary free cortisol secretion in habitually violent offenders. *Acta Psychiatrica Scandinavica, 72,* 40–44.

Wishnie, H. (1977). *The impulsive personality: Understanding people with destructive character disorders* New York: Plenum Press.

Woodcock, J. H. (1986). A neuropsychiatric approach to impulse disorders. *Psychiatric clinics of North America, 9,* 341–352.

Zuckerman, M. (1991). *Psychobiology of personality.* Cambridge, England: Cambridge University Press.

I

PERSPECTIVES

CELEBRANT: Will you persevere in resisting evil and, whenever you fall into sin, repent and return to the Lord?

PEOPLE: I will, with God's help.

—The celebration of Holy Baptism, in *The Book of Alternative Services of the Anglican Church of Canada* (1983, p. 159)

He wasnay feeling so hot. Before he had been good. Now he wasnay. There was things out his control. There was things in his control but there were other things out, they were out his control, he had put them out his control.

—JAMES KELMAN, *How Late It Was, How Late* (1994, p. 7)

In what abyss of non-feeling did Dolly dwell? She made careful placements of affection, always ready to be withdrawn in a fit of indignation. Her world was loveless, and she craved love as others crave sugar, and for the same reason: to replace a sudden lack, of which she would be abruptly and fearfully aware.

—ANITA BROOKNER, *Dolly* (1995, p. 159)

"Isn't this everyone's Point of View?" asked Tock, looking around curiously.

"Of course not," replied Alec, sitting himself down on nothing. "It's only mine, and you certainly can't always look at things from someone else's Point of View. For instance, from here that looks like a bucket of water," he said, pointing to a bucket of water; "but from an ant's point of view, it's a vast ocean, from an elephant's just a cool drink, and to a fish, of course, it's home. So, you see, the way you look at things depends a great deal on where you look at them from. . . . "

—NORTON JUSTER, *The Phantom Tollbooth* (1988, pp. 107–108)

1

A Clinical Perspective on Impulsivity

CHRISTOPHER D. WEBSTER
MARGARET A. JACKSON

The actions of most people make sense most of the time. Although we may not always approve of what politicians, public figures, colleagues, or even members of our own families may do from time to time, it is usually possible to discern some kind of logic or guiding principle. "Common sense" seems quite sufficient to explain why a leader of one country would want to invade another, why a criminal might want to rob a bank, or why a sister has refused to speak to her brother for the past 10 years. When common sense runs out, there is always the possibility of invoking contemporary psychological and psychiatric explanations. Such theories hold the prospect of enlarging our understanding of experiences and behaviors that fall outside the ordinary public ken. Courses on these and related topics abound in colleges and universities, and doubtless they play a vital role in integrating new knowledge of the human condition into traditionally held beliefs. Psychologists and criminologists devote their lives to amassing statistically based information to help us deal with the rational side of humankind. Their efforts, though not without their own limitations, can be helpful in everyday decision making (e.g., Laudan, 1994).

Although it is comforting to know that most human conduct of an "ordinary" kind is understandable, or at least potentially explainable, in terms of lay or reasonably accessible scientific knowledge, we are puzzled, as was Freud, by conduct that at times is seemingly irrational, apparently senseless, and utterly self-defeating. This book centers on the use of "impulsivity," which remains a rather obscure and difficult construct despite the efforts of some scientists (e.g., Barratt, 1994; Parker, Bagby, & Webster, 1993). The notion does, though, have a certain elasticity that makes it useful, at least for present purposes. Our task in this book is a difficult one: to help explain why some people engage repeatedly—and seemingly without due consideration—in conduct that may result in financial and social ruin, along with serious emotional and physical harm to themselves and/or to other people. Psychiatry and psychology have of late made liberal use of impulsivity and related concepts by implicating them in a broad range of conditions, as well as grouping some of them as specific disorders of impulse control (see the *Diagnostic and Statistical Manual of Mental Disorders,* fourth edition [DSM-IV]; American Psychiatric Association, 1994). However, there remains an absence of ideas on how best to understand and approach "driven" impulsive conduct, recent publications notwithstanding (Baumeister, Heatherton, & Tice, 1994; Dolan & Coid, 1993; Franzini & Grossberg, 1995; Hare, 1993; Hollander & Stein, 1995; Lykken, 1995; McCown, Johnson, & Shure, 1993; Raine, 1993).

We would like to be able, just as Dostoyevsky would have liked to be able, to explain why a person gambles compulsively or fritters away the family's finances on shopping binges. It would be helpful to know why an otherwise law-abiding man apparently cannot resist his urges to watch surreptitiously while women undress in the privacy of their homes, especially considering the possible consequences to him of being discovered. Certainly, it would be of immense assistance to know why some persons quite literally drink themselves to death, especially in cases where, at least on the surface, there is no apparent reason for such self-destruction. In a slightly different vein, it would be of great importance to be able to understand better why some individuals inhibit themselves from acting in their apparent own interests, when by taking a few obvious and simple steps they could seemingly eliminate constant sources of worry and distress.

It would be very helpful to prepare would-be helpers to work with impulsive people. This is not a simple task, for the very reason that impulsive, bizarre, and highly unacceptable conduct is as much a problem between people as it is within a person. Those who would wish to assist soon learn that the behavior of a highly impulsive person often entails marked deviations from accepted social standards. It is not that impulsive people do not follow rules—only that the rules may be idiosyncratic ones. To an extent, the challenge for the assessor or therapist is to elucidate those rules in the hope that, with patience, forbearance, and (when needed) firmness, impulsive people can be helped to learn new types of conduct or to curtail old ones. Yet, because impulsive people often have "boundary problems," it becomes easy for therapists, counselors, and others to lose their own psychological and moral moorings (Bolen, 1994). In short, it pays to be aware of the riskiness of this type of work.

The main purpose of this first chapter, as already noted, is to give the reader an appreciation of what we mean by "impulsivity" and "impulse-driven conduct." This is done despite the fact that several other contributors to the book themselves wrestle with the task of defining impulsivity. We also wish to draw attention to the scope of this volume, which is in some respects quite broad and in others quite limited. Below, we mention briefly a few definitions provided by the dictionary; they anchor the text to some degree. After this, we offer a view of impulsivity-related disorders from a clinical perspective. Here we try to describe, largely without resource to the DSM-IV, the kinds of attitudes and behaviors that appear characteristic of impulsive people. We attempt to drive home the point that there seem to be important commonalities among these conditions, despite the fact that the surface manifestations appear markedly different (i.e., as in some instances of drug abuse, excessive drinking, pyromania, paraphilia, etc.). Finally, we present and discuss a diagram that helps position impulsive individuals in relation to other types of persons.

DEFINITIONS FROM DRUG STORES AND DICTIONARIES

A product called Impulse is currently obtainable in drug stores. The can informs the would-be purchaser that Impulse is a "body spray," a "gentle deodorant and a light high-quality fragrance." Above the word "Impulse" on the container, there is a stylized butterfly in blissful upward flight; below it, as a kind of "subtitle," appears a second and presumably related phrase, "Free Spirit." Buyers in need of a lift or a freeing of spirits will be pleased by the label's promise: "Use it all over your body anytime and you'll feel refreshed, revitalized and confident." The fine print tones this broad claim down slightly by indicating that users should not dampen Impulse's restorative and confidence-building powers through too liberal application to particular "intimate areas" of the body. Still, all in all, Impulse looks like a good bet for those who wish to reduce their own physical and social repugnance and to set out on a new and exciting life. Perhaps, as responsible editors, we should have tested the stuff on our own persons in order to provide our readers with "empirical findings." Maybe it works. If it does—and this is not beyond the bounds of possibility for the simple reason that suggestion can play a role—we would not be faced with the ambitious task of assembling a book on "impulsivity"; we would be enjoying life. We would be the sort of "free spirits" we deserve to be.

The makers of Impulse knew what they were doing when they created their product. Whether or not they consulted the *Concise Oxford*

Dictionary (1995, p. 684) is not of course known, but if they did they would have learned that the word "impulse" and its relatives, "impulsion" and "impulsive," have a variety of meanings in everyday language. The word "impulse" captures a great deal of what the manufacturers were aiming at. There is the connotation of impelling or pushing. Proper application of the spray will give people that little extra shove—that inclination to push, to strike out in a new and different way. The term reaches into physics, where it means "an indefinitely large force acting for a very short time but producing a finite change of momentum," as in the blow of a hammer. Impulse gets things happening. There is also a connection with biology; in this context, we learn, the word means "a wave of excitation in a nerve." Impulse, our spray product, implies not just excitation in one nerve, but a generalized sparking action all over the body. At a more psychological level, the dictionary offers "a sudden desire or tendency to act without reflection." Impulse, the spray, will get rid of restraining inhibitions, will loosen the strings that bind. The *Concise Oxford Dictionary* gives as an example "impulse buying," which means "the unpremeditated buying of goods as a result of a whim or impulse." In this last example, we finally begin to come around to the notion understood by most of us because of harsh personal experience—namely, that it can sometimes be a big mistake to give in to our impulses. We learn (or at least most of us do) that unless some urges are controlled, we can soon be without money, self-respect, or freedom of movement. We may now have a good suit hanging in the closet, but no cash for dinner or for our children's much-needed shoes. We may have "decided" to stay late at the office party, but in today's clouded light, we may doubt whether it was actually wise to have done so.

This book is about people who, for one reason or another, appear to be even less able than most to control certain critical impulses. It is about "irrational" and seemingly self-defeating action. The book places little stress on the positive aspects of being impulsive at the right time in the right place. It would take us too far afield to try to document what lies behind heroic deeds undertaken with little or no reflection (though it is worth noting that persons in the military can be trained to act more or less reflexively, often in pursuit of other people's objectives). Similarly, we have no space to consider how seemingly impulsive and generous acts can transform impossible situations. It is only necessary for the reader to keep in mind, as we pick our way through the negative aspects of impulsivity, that the concept is also associated with all manner of positive and admirable qualities.

In the various chapters of the book, our contributors write about defining and measuring impulsivity in proper detail. Here, it is only necessary to give a broad indication of the kinds of concepts that attach or are applied to "impulsivity." This book centers on the kinds of everyday actions that most of us take to gain pleasure, but that when overdone, can yield pain. For some people, smoking starts as a pleasant distraction, becomes utterly "necessary," and may end with severe health complications or even early death. As viewed by others, this "vice" makes no sense. It is illogical, and would-be helpers are puzzled, in view of the grave consequences, as to why the smokers persist with such a self-destructive habit. Or those who wish to help may sit powerless as they watch some friends, relatives, colleagues, and clients allow themselves to become addicted to food, alcohol, drugs, or strange sexual proclivities. These behaviors likewise make little sense, and they end quite often in financial ruin, family discord, imprisonment, and the graveyard.

In certain respects, this book is about the old-fashioned idea of "vice." Here again the dictionary is of assistance. The *Concise Oxford Dictionary*, (1995, p. 1560) tells us that vice is "evil or grossly immoral conduct; depravity" involving prostitution, drugs, and the like. It can mean "an immoral or dissolute habit or practice" and "a defect or weakness of character." Although the word "vise," describing the tool, derives from a root different from that of "vice," it too possesses an instructive meaning. An object is clamped between the jaws of a vise so that it cannot move while it is being worked on. From this may stem the phrase "in the grip of vice," which seems rather close to addiction. Some people do indeed seem to be so firmly under the influence of a habit, compulsion, single fixed idea, mental disorder, or personality disorder that they can no longer act with any appreciable degree of independence. Or, should they free themselves from the jaws of one vice, they can "inexplicably" fall prey to another. People may be treated for an eating disorder, often successfully, only to take up drinking. When individuals are studied in some detail, it often transpires that they act in markedly impulsive ways in more than one domain (Kennedy & Grubin, 1990; McElroy, Hudson, Pope, Keck, & Aizley, 1992). It seems that there is quite often (especially given the penalties involved) a curiously illogical, senseless, and self-destructive aspect to these actions.

A CLINICAL PERSPECTIVE ON IMPULSIVE PEOPLE

One of us (C. D. W.), in partnership with another contributor to this volume (Stepehn J. Hucker), established a clinic for impulsive people a few years ago on a trial basis. A colleague, Rosemary Scaglione, coordinated the activities of this clinic, which operated one morning a week. We were anxious to assess people who had had little or no previous experience with psychiatrists, psychologists, or other mental health or criminal justice officials. The people we interviewed suffered from a variety of conditions—eating disorders, explosive temper outbursts, compulsive gambling, pointless stealing, urges to be voyeuristic, excessive drinking, and so on. What struck us later as we went over the files was that the fact that the actual "presenting problem" did not seem to be the feature of importance. Indeed, we learned that many of these persons were driven to act impulsively in more than one area at the same time (i.e., they drank and watched other people undress, or they gambled and could not stop smoking). Or, alternatively, they had in the past overcome being a slave to one addiction or impulse, only to become subject to another. From our meetings with these persons, we came to experience something of the intensity with which they were driven to act. Here are some of the things they said:

> "To be on the wire is life; the rest is waiting" (pathological gambler).
> "I have control through fear of the law" (kleptomania patient).
> "There's something exciting about watching a woman doing something private, something that is not supposed to be seen, and when it comes to this thing, I'm crazy!" (voyeur).
> "I would feel less restless and more comfortable if the devil was on my side. He would do me favors if I set fires" (fire setter).
> "I feel a void there, an emptiness you wouldn't believe, and I just have to fill it" (eating-disordered patient).
> "There is something artistic about gambling. It's like playing a violin . . . when it works right, it's like a symphony" (pathological gambler).
> "At the time I did it, I felt nothing. . . . I rarely think about the actions I do" (kleptomania patient).
> "I didn't mean to kill the cat. Something just went off. . . . I was very mad; it was enough to drive anyone to kill" (explosive patient).

At about the time we were establishing our clinic, we came across a 1977 text by the psychiatrist Howard Wishnie, entitled *The Impulsive Personality: Understanding People with Destructive Character Disorders*. The book is based on Wishnie's work with addicts at the National Institute of Mental Health's Clinical Research Center in Lexington, Kentucky, as well as his subsequent work in an outpatient clinic for drug abusers. We cannot here summarize Wishnie's text. Instead, we have performed for our readers the task of extracting from his text some of the salient characteristics of impulsive people as he saw them. Although Wishnie himself did not create the list we offer below (and reproduce in the Impulsivity Checklist [ICL], which constitutes the Appendix to this chapter), we found it helpful in describing the kinds of persons we saw in our own impulsivity clinic. We have taken from his work, and our own experience, 20 items. We consider impulsive people to be well described by five overarching categories: interpersonal dysfunction (item 1); lack of plans (item 5); esteem of self is distorted (item 9); rage, anger, and hostility (item 13); and taxing irresponsibility (item 17). Readers will note that the full 20 items are arranged below and in the Appendix so as to provide a mnemonic device: The first letters of the items spell out the phrase "IMPULSIVE CHARAC[H]TERS" (we trust that readers will forgive us the extra

H!). We consider the impulsive person to be well described by the following terms:

1. Interpersonal dysfunction
2. Manipulative
3. Perception of others as all good/all bad
4. Unformed relations/distrustful
5. Lack of plans
6. Self-protection against change
7. Immediate gratification
8. Volatile lifestyle/chaotic
9. Esteem of self is distorted
10. Causes of actions unknown
11. Hopelessness/self-destructiveness
12. Acts to avoid feeling
13. Rage, anger, and hostility
14. Aggressiveness to family/friends/others
15. Criticism not tolerated
16. High explosivity
17. Taxing irresponsibility
18. Entitled
19. Rejection of norms
20. Sidestepping of anxiety/discomfort

Readers will realize that our 20-item checklist is provided here solely for purposes of exposition; it is no more than a sketch of a scheme that could conceivably be developed. Were that to be attempted, it would be necessary to pay attention to definition and refinement of the items, along with collection of normative data. However, such an attempt to develop a clinically centered device might be worth the effort: As the contributors to this volume make clear, the bulk of measurement work on the impulsivity construct to date has been done from the point of view of personality theories (see Parker & Bagby, Chapter 8, this volume).

The draft items outlined here could eventually be scored on a scale from 0 to 2, and we have provided a format for doing so in the ICL as given in the Appendix. Hare (1991) has found it almost ideal to evaluate psychopathy (a concept evidently related to impulsivity) by means of such a scale: 0 indicates that a factor is definitely not apparent, 2 means that it is in certain evidence, and 1 is meant to show that there is some but not complete support for the existence of the particular factor in the case at hand. It could well be that a properly developed ICL or similar vehicle may make it be possible to describe different kinds of impulsive people more clearly than at present (e.g., ones who score 1 or 2 on almost all items, thereby gaining high total scores, vs. individuals who, though perhaps correctly viewed as impulsive, score high on one or two items only). As noted above, all this is speculation only; the work has not yet been done.

With these reservations in mind, we now attempt a brief sketch of a typical impulsive person who might be seen in a clinic such as the one we established experimentally some years ago. Many of our comments are drawn from the earlier work of Wishnie (1977; see also Wishnie & Nevis-Olesen, 1979), mentioned previously. (Direct quotations below are from Wishnie's 1977 book unless otherwise indicated. Copyright 1977 by Plenum Press. Reprinted by permission.)

1. Interpersonal Dysfunction

According to Wishnie, many of his drug-abusing men had strong desires for personally satisfying relationships with others, and at the same time feared that such possibilities might develop. In his words, "Many addicts avoid significant relationships because they perceive themselves as internally weak and inadequate. The addict fears that he will lose his identity by merging or blending with the other person's 'stronger' character" (p. 42). Because such people have deep-seated doubts about their own worth, they are inclined to put any and all relationships to extreme, perhaps impossible, tests. There is a therapeutic implication here, in that it makes little sense to attempt to help persons induce change in themselves unless and until strict objectives and limits have been established.

2. Manipulative

Impulsive people are commonly inclined to deceive others, to distort information, to make false claims, to persuade others into bad deals, to falsify statements, to promise more than is needed, and the like. When most people are accused of being manipulative, they see it as an unpleasant reflection on them. This is not necessarily so with the impulsive person. As Wishnie puts it, "To the impulse-ridden person, [being manipulative] is the skill upon which he bases his hope of success. It is the major tool of his life's trade. He prides himself on his ability to use and improve his skill of 'conning' " (p. 44).

3. Perceptions of Others as All Good/All Bad

Impulsive people often have a difficult time avoiding seeing others in an unduly positive or unduly negative light. Young children also perceive others this way, but gradually come to see that both good and bad qualities can and do exist in the same person. This process is quite possibly interrupted early in persons whose parents are chaotic and unreliable. It can be a difficult problem to overcome in therapy, since such a client may try initially to place the therapist on an unrealistically high pedestal. After the first perceived slip, the therapist can be quickly and permanently dismissed. Wishnie notes that an impulsive person is constantly seeking perfect parental attributes in others. When these other people fail, as they almost inevitably do, the impulsive person "reexperiences the initial loss and panics. When he runs out of energy and can no longer pursue the lost parent, drugs may temporarily allay the disappointment and depression" (p. 92).

4. Unformed Relations/Distrustful

Wishnic suggests that "patients distrust everyone, including their comrades. They view the world as an unsafe environment in which others are always trying to take them off guard and use them" (p. 156). Such distrust comes about in part because supposed helpers often come from backgrounds different from the impulsive person. Moreover, therapists make patients and prisoners anxious when they expect them to change long-held attitudes.

5. Lack of Plans

It is common when talking to some impulsive people to hear them make large statements about what they intend to achieve in the future. They will announce ambitions to achieve a commercial pilot's license, to complete a PhD degree, to marry and have children. In Wishnie's experience, as in our own, these chats have a "dreamlike quality" about them (p. 57). Impulsive people's ability to create and sustain plans that stretch into the future is often very limited and easily disrupted. They tend to be indecisive and lacking in motivation. As Wishnie says, "There seems to be no use to anything. They seem to be stuck in time, unable to move forward with their own lives. They live in a state of existential paralysis" (p. 69).

6. Self-Protection against Change

The defense mechanisms play, deservedly, a crucial role in psychoanalytic theory as applied to neurotic and ordinary persons. Impulsive people tend to rely on a particular set of defenses. These enable them to avoid (at least temporarily) feelings of failure, worthlessness, and emptiness. Badly thought-out activities and misuse of alcohol and drugs help mask feelings. In individual or group therapy, such individuals may seek engagement in pointless argument or may withdraw as a means of avoiding taking concrete steps or making definite plans. Wishnie points out, helpfully, that therapists also do not usually like to experience too much discomfort. He argues, though, that "the discomfort is mutual, but is a necessary part of change" (p. 50).

7. Immediate Gratification

For an impulsive person, it is necessary that demands be met right away, since he or she has no expectation that matters will be better in the future. As Wishnie puts it, "The concept of the coming months and years is vague, and the focus is only on the present. The past is often too painful to review" (p. 58). If demands are not met, there may be a strong and excessive response.

8. Volatile Lifestyle/Chaotic

According to Wishnie, an impulsive person views his or her life as a series of piecemeal happenings: "All events are treated as separate and unrelated. Any similarity between today's crisis, last week's, or last year's is seen as coincidence" (p. 55). Such a person can present each week with a new problem—one that is supposedly completely outside his or her control. Fate is invoked, and fate is not on the side of the affected individual. The notions of choice and of responsibility for decisions made tend to be foreign and threatening. Yet, with patience and without moralizing, some persons can be helped to see the similarity among their maladaptive patterns of thought and action.

9. Esteem of Self Is Distorted

Wishnie (1977) suggests that those with "destructive personalities usually evidence little that they value about themselves" (p. 40). This is often not immediately apparent, though, because such people try hard to cover this lack with excessive bravado and willingness to take risks. The tendency to act may veil their deep self-doubts. Wishnie reminds us, "Many such life-and-death struggles have developed over a book of matches, a place in line, or a game of pool" (p. 41). Absence of self-esteem can in some cases be linked to marked deficiencies in education and the like.

Wishnie argues that depression is a core problem for many persons with disabling impulsivity. His view—one that remains current (see, e.g., National Advisory Mental Health Council, 1996)—is that this is established in many cases in childhood. Such people do not receive adequate parental attention and come to the view that they are worthless. In Wishnie's words, "If a child fails to receive adequate love and affection, which include reasonable expectations and limits, he painfully assumes that there is something wrong or bad within himself" (p. 79). One of the difficulties is that institutions like prisons seem poised to fill the emotional gap for such people, in the sense that they provide constraint for impulses, a means of relieving guilt through the application of punishment, and some acknowledgment of personal importance through supervision. It goes without saying that these services do little to equip such a person for life in the community. According to Wishnie, some impulsive people appear to make the following assumptions about themselves: "(1) 'There is something *irrevocably* wrong about me.' (2) 'I am different and separate from others.' (3) 'I am therefore unlovable.' (4) 'My parents were right in not caring for me' " (p. 80, emphasis in original).

Distortion in self-esteem can also be in the direction of overvaluing the self, as the National Advisory Mental Health Council (1996) notes:

> Researchers have discovered as well that, among a group of unpopular children, those deemed aggressive had relatively inflated self-esteem and overestimated their attributes and abilities in academics, appearance, athletics, and peer relations. . . . Children who are aggressive and unpopular are at increased risk for behavioral problems and juvenile delinquency. . . . (p. 26)

10. Causes of Action Unknown

As suggested above in connection with item 8, impulsive people tend to be weak on personal awareness. They seldom reflect on their own difficulties and shortcomings because of the anxiety and discomfort these induce. Wishnie observes that it is easier for them to account for their conduct by pointing to factors that seemingly lie outside their control. As Wishnie says of the character-disordered person, "He tends to explain his behavior solely in terms of superficial and external circumstances" (p. 155).

11. Hopelessness/Self-Destructiveness

Many impulsive people, at least according to the way we are trying to define them in this chapter, view themselves as incapable of change. They see no possibility of giving up an ideal of bodily thinness, the "high" that comes with a win at a gambling table, the pleasurable dullness that some drugs can induce, and so on. As Wishnie puts it, impulsive people can come to believe that "to invest energy in the process of change would be foolish and wasteful" (p. 16). It can be is easy for a therapist to collude with this notion, to endorse the hopelessness.

Self-destructive acts, which characterize impulsive people, appear to yield passing relief from the internal pressures created by feelings of worthlessness. It makes little difference what form the self-destruction takes (setting fires, compulsive gambling, temper outbursts, self-slashing, binge eating, drug taking, etc.). Not uncommonly, the self-destructiveness is carried out as a way of inflicting pain on others. As Wishnie says, "The self-destructiveness always seems to be related to significant people in the patient's life. It does not matter whether they are present or absent. The patient carries them about internally all of the time" (p. 66).

12. Acts to Avoid Feeling

Highly impulsive people tend to seek relief from internal emotional discomfort through prompt, rash, ill-considered acts. However, such acts may not be as impulsive or impetuous as they might at first appear to be. This is because, to some extent, such individuals learn to cut off painful feelings and to replace them with rage-related thoughts and actions. Although the exact form of the eventual response may not be known, it is very likely that there has been rehearsal of a considerable range of violent acts. These verbal and physical acts at once shut down any tendency toward reflection and provide momentary relief. If this idea is stretched a little, it helps explain why some people never achieve much emotional maturity. Wishnie says this of the male drug addict: "Because he cannot bear anxiety, sadness, anger, and humiliation, he resorts to activities that provide sufficient external stress so as to distract him from his own feelings" (pp. 52–53).

13. Rage, Anger, and Hostility

Wishnie makes the obvious point that most of us learn to repress dangerous and frightening impulses, and that it takes us years to do so. What do we do then, he asks, "when we are confronted with people who act on feelings that we contain" (p. 145)? He notes in answer to the question that it is not in the least unnatural to be frightened and alarmed when some patients or prisoners divulge their fantasies or the details of their past actions. Yet it remains clinically vital to be able to investigate the source of these feelings and the context in which they arise. Wishnie reminds us, too, that "not all violence is shown in gross behavior. Tone of voice, appearance, eye contact, and manner of interaction can convey a menacing quality" (p. 148).

14. Aggressive to Family/Friends/Others

Once again, highly impulsive people tend to view themselves as unfortunate victims of social programs, flawed legal decisions, inadequate parents, and so on. They portray themselves as being at the whim of fate. They feel that there is no point in planning because they hold no power over events. All they can hope for is some passing pleasure. When this pleasure does turn up, it is rarely as satisfying as they have hoped. Wishnie says, "Their chronic anger and desperation are seen in their lashing-out at friends, family, and society" (p. xvi). The desperation may have its roots in psychotic illness.

15. Criticism Not Tolerated

As already noted in connection with item 9, persons with severe problems of impulse control tend to have very low levels of self-esteem. When they are attacked, they have little to fall back on. Their responses to criticisms tend to be exaggerated and needlessly abrupt or even violent. It is important for them to counterattack or preempt attack by finding deficiencies in other people or in institutions. Only by doing so are they able to defend the notion that there is no possibility of change in attitude or conduct on their part. As Wishnie points out, knowing this helps in treatment, because "the capacity of the staff to review their own performance critically and make appropriate changes is a vital factor" (p. 57).

16. High Explosivity

It is highly common for impulsive people to show reactions that are out of all proportion to what might be usual or reasonable. When thwarted or challenged, they tend to retaliate quickly and without reflection. Actions may be seemingly without meaning. This is their way of protecting themselves from unpleasant facts and experiences. As Wishnie notes, "Under increased pressure, the individual may use alcohol, other substances, or distracting behavior to reinforce the defenses. Under excessive pressure or in acute situations, the primitive explosion occurs. Such people are walking bombs" (p. 160).

17. Taxing Irresponsibility

Wishnie (1977) establishes the idea that it is hard for the layperson to understand why impulsive people commit destructive acts against others or against themselves (p. 37). By comparison, it is easier to comprehend the plight of individuals who suffer from anxiety disorders (e.g., panic disorder). Such persons usually adopt the patient status willingly and seek appropriate help, which not uncommonly includes the taking of corrective medication. The same might be said about individuals who are floridly psychotic. In this instance, it is easy (too easy, perhaps) to invoke derangement in mental processes to explain just about any act imaginable. The difficulty in devising similar explanations for impulsive people, as Wishnie observes, is that such people for the most part "can speak rationally and persuasively" (p. 37). They are not easy to "excuse" on psychiatric or psychological grounds. At least on early acquaintance in therapy, it seems that they ought to be able to "get a grip on themselves." At times it seems that their irresponsibility to friends, family, and society is designed largely to tax the patience and forbearance of those around them—the would-be helpers.

18. Entitled

It is common for impulsive people to exhibit outrage when their demands are denied. They come to expect that staff members and institutions will cater to their every whim. It is their right, so they claim, to be served. The same holds true of family members, who not infrequently support and reinforce these wholly unacceptable demands. Groups of patients can come to see themselves as privileged and take unto themselves powers that they have not been granted. Wishnie remarks of a typical male patient: "Minimal provocation entitles him to a maximum response. It is someone else's responsibility to provide for his needs. His only role is that of the wrongly deprived individual who has earned the right to some form of restitution" (p. 60).

Impulsive people tend to be constantly "on the move" in their search for others who will accept them completely and put them at ease. Alcohol and drugs may help in the short run. Yet, as noted in connection with item 1, most fear genuine intimacy because of the danger of becoming lost in another person's stronger psychological framework. This does not mean that an impulsive person does not aspire to a perfect relationship; indeed, most do. The difficulty is that the other person is expected to be all-giving, all-wise, and all-sacrificing. Such standards are hard to meet, and it is common for therapists' commitment and understanding to be frequently tested. Wishnie makes the point that it is imperative, in trying to assist impulsive people, to set out limits in advance:

> Many counselors who do not define the motives and goals of treatment become involved in running to courts, judges, social workers, and clinics in a perpetual round of efforts to stop the maladaptive and self-destructive behavior or to protect the addict from the consequences of his behavior. The failure to define initial goals only supports the addict's wish and expectation of finding the perfect all-giving person. (p. 43)

19. Rejection of Norms

Impulsive people often feel entitled to obtain what they want by whatever means lie at hand. They will argue that this is what everyone does most of the time. Such an idea is supported through reference to stories reported daily in the mass media concerning the misdeeds of doctors, politicians, lawyers, and so on. Since everyone else is acting immorally and irresponsibly, so the argument goes, why should the impulsive person be held to entirely unreasonable standards? Indeed, Wishnie notes that they can turn the point to their advantage by invoking the idea that " 'Everyone is a con man. They're just fooling themselves. In fact, I am more honest than those hypocrites' " (p. 32).

20. Sidestepping of Anxiety/Discomfort

To an impulsive person, it is the therapist who is supposed to be doing the work. All the person has to do is lay out the problem. The clinician or counselor is expected to find a complete solution that will take away immediately any further physical or emotional discomfort. If it is physical pain, then large amounts of strong medications must be prescribed; if it is a problem with living, then officials must be prevailed upon to solve it. The idea that the person might be able to participate actively in reducing the magnitude of his or her difficulty is often, at least initially, quite foreign. Such a person seems not to have learned to appreciate that discomfort is a fact of life—one that cannot, and indeed should not, be altogether eliminated. Wishnie's patients "demonstrated little ability to put up with physical pain, emotional frustration, depression or anxiety. They demanded immediate relief, which had to come from someone else" (p. 61).

Comments

An obvious criticism of the ICL as described above and presented in the Appendix is that it is based on attributions made by clinical and correctional staff members about particular kinds of people. It does not take much account of the very large literature on impulsivity and reflectivity as measured in normal populations (e.g., Doob, 1990). Yet impulsivity—if gauged merely by the extent to which it is invoked in DSM-IV, to say nothing of its daily use in clinical conferences of all types—remains one of a dozen or so key ideas in contemporary psychiatry and psychology. The fact that it is hard to define and measure via standard psychological tests (see, e.g., Oas, 1985; Parker & Bagby, Chapter 8, this volume) does not obviate its importance. As Barratt (1994) puts it, "from a clinical viewpoint, we still think there is a cognitive impulsiveness factor" (p. 68). Helpfully, he goes on to say this: "The reason it is difficult to measure relates to the inferential nature of cognition. A basic question involves the extent to which persons can assess *their own* cognitive functions, especially if they are impulsive" (p. 68, emphasis in original). Our point is that it may prove advantageous to emulate Wishnie (1977) by approaching impulsivity largely from a practical perspective in clinical criminology.

A SEVEN-TYPE DESCRIPTIVE SCHEME

Even by this stage of the present text, it should be evident that although impulsivity possesses attractive features as a psychological construct, impulsive disorders are not easily defined. One reason for this is that they are "expression[s] of moral values of the reigning culture, which are constantly changing" (Zinberg, 1979, p. 27). Another is that highly impulsive actions are found not only in people with major mental and personality disorders, but occur at times in "normal" people. A Venn diagram may help clarify the matter (Figure 1.1).

In Figure 1.1, we start with three main groups: (1) normal people; (2) persons with major mental illness (e.g., schizophrenia or mood disorders); and (3) individuals with strong antisocial and psychopathic tendencies. It goes without saying that those in category 1 live mainly unfettered in society; those in category 2 have experience in mental hospitals; and those in category 3 wind up periodically in prison. Persons in category 4 span categories 1 and 2 and may be defined as "eccentric." Some in this category will receive assistance from psychiatric outpatient and other social and welfare services. Persons in category 5 are sometimes called "delinquent." Often they wind up on bail or on probation, meaning that they are neither imprisoned nor fully free in society. Persons in category 6 are what we would refer to as "mentally disordered offenders." At different times, or at the same time, they will display features of both frank mental disorder and serious criminality. They tend to move back and forth between prisons and secure mental hospitals. Hans Toch (1982) has referred to such people as "disturbed disruptive inmates," and, in light of their frequent transfers between hospitals and prisons, calls

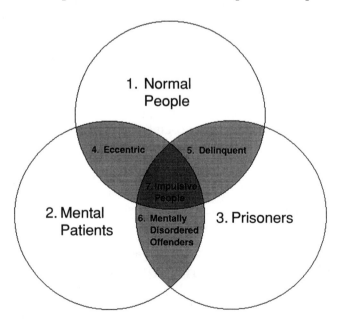

FIGURE 1.1. Venn diagram illustrating a division of the general population into seven major types. Adapted from Webster, Menzies, and Jackson (1982, p. 88). Copyright 1982 by Butterworths. Adapted by permission.

attention to the fact that the main treatment they receive is "bus therapy." People in category 7 form the core of the group on which this book is focused. They may exhibit features of seeming normality, may at times be quite mentally ill, and may also find themselves periodically involved in serious violent crime. Some pass consistently as ordinary citizens, because they are able to mask their condition and keep their crimes or risky undertakings from detection. It goes without saying that the possession of money and other resources makes this much easier for some than for others.

CONCLUDING COMMENT

Much of the substance of this chapter, as we have acknowledged, we owe to Dr. Howard Wishnie's work published 2 decades ago. Since Dr. Wishnie was kind enough to comment on a draft of this chapter, it seems appropriate to give him the last word. While agreeing that we have managed to distill some of his main ideas, he would wish to emphasize just two main points. The first is that "impulsive actions occur when projective defenses that ward off recognition of a deep self-loathing fail. The individual externalizes this annihilatory sense of self as if it is an external attack" (personal communication, 1997). The second is that, on the basis of continued clinical experience with a wide range of people with impulsive character disorder, there is every reason to remain "convinced of the treatability of many of them." However, he continues, "prevention—pre- and perinatal care for mothers, adequate child nutrition, stable early childhood developmental experiences, early diagnosis of learning disorders and attention-deficit/hyperactivity disorder—would be preferable."

REFERENCES

American Psychiatric Association. (1994). *Diagnostic and statistical manual of mental disorders* (4th ed.). Washington, DC: Author.

Barratt, E. S. (1994). Impulsiveness and aggression. In J. Monahan & H. J. Steadman (Eds.), *Violence and mental disorder: Developments in risk assessment* (pp. 61–79). Chicago: University of Chicago Press.

Baumeister, R. F., Heatherton, T. F., & Tice, D. M. (1994). *Losing control: How and why people fail at self regulation*. San Diego: Academic Press.

Bolen, D. E. (1994). *Stupid crimes: A novel*. Toronto: Vintage Books.

Concise Oxford dictionary (9th ed.). (1995). New York: Oxford University Press.

Dolan, B., & Coid, J. (1993). *Psychopathic and antisocial personality disorders: Treatment and research issues*. London: Gaskell.

Doob, L. W. (1990). *Hesitation, impulsivity and reflection*. New York: Greenwood Press.

Franzini, L. R., & Grossberg, J. M. (1995). *Eccentric and bizarre behaviors.* New York: Wiley.

Hare, R. D. (1991). *Manual for the Hare Psychopathy Checklist—Revised.* Toronto: Multi-Health Systems.

Hare, R. D. (1993). *Without conscience: The disturbing world of the psychopaths among us.* New York: Pocket Books.

Hollander, E., & Stein, D. J. (Eds.). (1995). *Impulsivity and aggresion.* Chichester, England: Wiley.

Kennedy, H. G., & Grubin, D. H. (1990). Hot headed or impulsive. *British Journal of Addictions, 85,* 639–643.

Laudan, L. (1994). *The book of risks: Fascinating facts about the chances we take every day.* New York: Wiley.

Lykken, D. T. (1995). *The antisocial personalities.* Hillsdale, NJ: Erlbaum.

McCown, W. G., Johnson, J. L., & Shure, M. B. (Eds.). (1993). *The impulsive client: Theory, research, and treatment.* Washington, DC: American Psychological Association.

McElroy, S. L., Hudson, J. I., Pope, H. G., Keck, P. E., & Aizley, H. C. (1992). The DSM-III-R impulse-control disorders not elsewhere classified: Clinical characteristics and relationship to other psychiatric disorders. *American Journal of Psychiatry, 149,* 318–327.

National Advisory Mental Health Council. (1996). Basic behavioral science research for mental health: Vulnerability and resilience. *American Psychologist, 51,* 22–28.

Oas, P. (1985). The psychological assessment of impulsivity: A review. *Journal of Psychoeducational Assessment, 3,* 141–156.

Parker, J. D. A., Bagby, R. M., & Webster, C. D. (1993). Domain of the impulsivity construct: A factor analytic investigation. *Personality and Individual Differences, 15,* 267–274.

Raine, A. (1993). *The psychopathology of crime: Criminal behavior as a clinical disorder.* San Diego: Academic Press.

Stone, A. A. (1976). *Mental health and law: A system in transition.* New York: Jason Aronson.

Toch, H. (1982). The disturbed disruptive inmate: Where does the bus stop? *Journal of Psychiatry and Law, 10,* 327–349.

Webster, C. D., Menzies, R. J., & Jackson, M. A. (1982). *Clinical assessment before trial: Legal issues and mental disorder.* Toronto: Butterworths.

Wishnie, H. (1977). *The impulsive personality: Understanding people with destructive character disorders.* New York: Plenum Press.

Wishnie, H. (1997). Personal communication.

Wishnie, H., & Nevis-Olesen, J. (Eds.). (1979). *Working with the impulsive person.* New York: Plenum Press.

Zinberg, N. E. (1979). Determinants of impulsive behavior: Toward an integration of social and psychological factors. In H. A. Wishnie & J. Nevis-Olesen (Eds.), *Working with the impulsive person* (pp. 19–30). New York: Plenum Press.

Impulsivity Checklist (ICL)

Item		Score		
		0	1	2
1.	INTERPERSONAL DYSFUNCTION			
2.	Manipulative			
3.	Perception of others as all good/all bad			
4.	Unformed relations/distrustful			
5.	LACK OF PLANS			
6.	Self-protecting against change			
7.	Immediate gratification			
8.	Volatile lifestyle/chaotic			
9.	ESTEEM OF SELF IS DISTORTED			
10.	Causes of action unknown			
11.	Hopelessness/self-destructiveness			
12.	Acts to avoid feeling			
13.	RAGE, ANGER, AND HOSTILITY			
14.	Aggressive to family/friends/others			
15.	Criticism not tolerated			
16.	High explosivity			
17.	TAXING IRRESPONSIBILITY			
18.	Entitled			
19.	Rejection of norms			
20.	Sidestepping of anxiety/discomfort			
Totals				
Overall Score				**/40**

Note. Based on the ideas of Wishnie (1997). Copyright 1996 by Christopher D. Webster. Reprinted by permission.

2

A Social Psychological Perspective on Impulsivity/Intimate Violence

DONALD G. DUTTON

As recently as the 1970s, academic texts divided aggression into two categories: "normal" aggression, which was believed to be directed toward either a stranger or an enemy, and "intimate violence," which was seen as abnormal, the act of madmen. Like the cursed monster created by Dr. Frankenstein and given the brain of a criminal by his assistant, men who abuse their wives or were believed by medical science to commit violence because of an aberrant neural structure that generates disordered impulses. In 1977 I went to an international conference of psychiatrists and criminal lawyers, and noticed that some research papers were to be presented on wife assault. These papers, much to my disappointment, focused exclusively on neurological "causes" of wife assault. This complex action—filled with symbolism and rich meanings of the woman as lover/savior/mother/betrayer, and awash with obsessions, revulsions, tensions, jealousy, anger, and rage—was being reduced to a perturbation in the limbic system, the part of the brain believed to control emotions. In effect, these psychiatrists were claiming that disturbances in a neural structure such as the temporal lobe could cause wife assault.

An example of this line of thought was an article first published in the medical journal *The Practitioner* in 1976 (Elliott, 1976/1977). Its author, Frank Elliott, was a psychiatrist at the Pennsylvania Hospital. The article describes something called the "episodic dyscontrol syndrome"—a term coined first by the famous Karl Menninger, founder of the clinic named after him. Menninger had originally described episodic dyscontrol as an unconscious bodily reaction to chronic stress (Menninger, Mayman, & Pruyser, 1962). It referred to episodes in which a person suddenly and inexplicably goes out of control, literally runs amok. It was thought to be beyond rational "ego" control and to be explosive in nature. In this sense it was believed to stand out as a different level of reaction to stress, compared to the other types of stress adaptation, such as anxiety, neurotic symptoms, and psychosis. Episodic dyscontrol is currently listed in the *Diagnostic and Statistical Manual of Mental Disorders,* fourth edition (DSM-IV; American Psychiatric Association, 1994) as one of the impulse-control disorders; there, it is called "intermittent explosive disorder" (IED) and given the official code number of 312.34. The diagnostic criteria include several separate instances of loss of control of aggressive impulses, resulting in serious acts of assault or property destruction; the degree of aggression expressed is hugely disproportionate to any psychological or social factor that might have precipitated it. The episodes also do not occur during the course of a psychotic disorder or other disorders (e.g., antisocial personality disorder). In other words, the person is not psychotic or otherwise mentally disordered, but can burst out in a rage that is entirely out of proportion to whatever preceded it.

TWO CASE EXAMPLES

The following two case histories of wife assaulters highlight some of the features of IED, as well as related treatment and criminal justice issues. As one examines real-life cases, the difficulties and complexities of dealing with such individuals became quite apparent.

> A man I will call Robert was referred to our treatment group while his wife, Carol, was still hospitalized for injuries sustained through his beating (Dutton, 1995). He was, as they say, "average-looking"— medium height, medium build, brown hair. He wore blue jeans, a denim shirt, and heavy work boots. He was in his early 20s and a deep sea diver by profession. He looked tense, rocking back and forth in his chair, clenching and unclenching his fists repeatedly, and staring at the floor as if he was trying to burn a hole in it with his eyes. He avoided all eye contact and seemed, whenever asked a question, to be on the verge of tears. He made the other 10 men in the group nervous, even though they all had problems with anger and violence too. (In fact, 8 of the 10 had been sent for treatment by court order after having been found guilty of wife assault.) I asked Robert how he was feeling at that moment; he shrugged and said, "I don't know, not really anything. . . . Nothing, I guess." I asked the other men in the group how they experienced him, and they told him

he looked scared, depressed, and upset. They also told him that he made them nervous and edgy. He was surprised to hear this.

It took about 3 weeks before Robert could talk about the violence that had led to his being in the group. The trouble started at his wife's office party. About 30 people were drinking and chatting when, according to Robert, Carol disappeared (i.e., he could not find her in a large, unfamiliar house). After 10–15 minutes he did see her and insisted that they leave the party. I asked him what he was feeling at this point. "Nothing," he said after a pause. They drove home; she went to bed, and he began to watch television.

Robert's next memory was of seeing Carol lying in a pool of blood on the floor of their bedroom. He called her relatives and the police. The police report said that when asked what happened, he replied, "I must have hit her." He pleaded guilty in court, saying only that "I must have done it." When I asked him about the time period between watching television and seeing Carol covered in blood, he drew a blank. He said he believed he must have hit her, but he couldn't remember doing it.

At that time, I believed that shame had clouded Robert's memory. Now I know that something else was going on—a type of dissociative rage state with enormous physical arousal. Once he was back in his "normal" state, he really could not remember what had happened; the memory never got stored.

Carol remembered, though. "I was asleep when he grabbed me. He pulled off the covers and then yanked me out of bed by my hair. The light was on in the bedroom and I could see his face. . . . It was terrifying." His expression was grossly distorted: His mouth was pulled down at both corners "like a fish mouth," his teeth were clenched, his jaw protruded, his nostrils flared, and his eyes "were sort of blank." He started to punch her with a closed fist, first on her stomach and side, then in her face. She could hear him yelling, "You bitch, you cunt, you slut, you fucking whore!" Then she lost consciousness. She had a broken nose, a broken jaw, two chipped teeth, and bruised ribs. It was 2 months before she could go back to work.

Carol's mother told her office that she had been in a car accident. Only her mother and father, her sister, and two female friends knew what had really happened. Robert did not want to tell anybody.

In treatment, Robert eventually revealed his belief that his wife was having an affair, and that when she "disappeared" at the party she was having sex somewhere with a male coworker. (She was talking to two female coworkers on an outside balcony.) When we asked him where he imagined this to be happening in a crowded party, he said, "I don't know—in a car or something."

He also claimed that he would have what he called "red-outs," when he got angry and could not remember what happened after that. It was like "drowning in a red tide."

Two months into treatment, Robert phoned me in a panic: "I'm about to kill my wife!" He had returned from an out-of-town business trip to find "a key with a man's name on it." He "knew" his wife was having an affair and became enraged. Fortunately, he had learned enough by this time to recognize imminent high-risk situations for his rage.

When he came to see me, Robert was shaking and distracted. I asked to see the evidence; he showed me the key. I recognized the name on it immediately—it was the largest key manufacturer in town. I told him this, but he did not believe me. I got the telephone book, opened it to the Yellow Pages, and showed him. He appeared to calm down. I asked him whether he could see how he jumped to conclusions about Carol's imagined infidelity. He said, "Yes," but he seemed distant, distracted, as if some inner voice was competing successfully for his attention. I spent another hour soothing him. I got him to do some deep relaxation exercises, and made him promise he would not go home until he was completely in control. I suggested that he spend the night with a male friend. He thought that was a good idea.

Robert left, but he drove directly to his house and his wife. A shouting match ensued but no violence, except that he smashed into a wall while screeching out of the driveway. Only then did he go to the friend's house. It took him 3 days to calm down completely.

Was this a case of IED? Although Robert may have felt some vague discomfort during his wife's office party, he did not act aggressively while at the party or even express his discomfort to his wife. Also, although his beliefs about her having an affair were delusional, he was not in any way psychotic. He did not have hallucinations, and he was in touch with reality as experienced by other people. He was entirely capable of carrying out his job as a deep sea diver—surely a dangerous occupation for a psychotic person. In addition, he did not appear to be psychopathic. He did not get into fights with people other than his wife, and he was not irresponsible. He had not had numerous jobs, relationships with women, or run-ins with the law. He was not emotionally shallow. In fact, he showed much remorse for what he had done, even calling the police on himself. In other words, Robert may have qualified for a diagnosis of IED. But does that diagnosis "explain" his behavior? Does it explain, for example, why his violence was always directed toward his wife and always occurred in private? I think not.

Recently I was phoned by a man in great distress, whom I will call Sam. He was a construction foreman, and although he was known on the job as demanding and irritable, he had had no major problems with the men he worked with. The previous week he had been at his golf club with his wife, casually drinking with some friends. He and his wife returned home and began making dinner. That was the last thing he remembered before waking in the middle of the night with the house trashed and his wife gone. He had a vague sense that he had caused the problem, but could not remember anything. His wife phoned him at work the next day and agreed to meet him, but only in a public place.

Then and there, she told him she was afraid of him and was leaving. She told him how he had "gone off out of the blue" about the dinner's being cooked a certain way. He had screamed at her, pushed her, and (as she fled) threw the frying pan with steaks in it at her, hitting the wall. I talked to her alone first. She described Sam as moody and irritable but not abusive; however, there had been about three occasions when "he became someone else" and exploded. This one was the last straw for her.

Sam met the diagnostic criteria for IED. The only constant he could recall was that these bouts only occurred when he had been drinking. He now insisted that he would swear off alcohol. He fully believed his wife's account of his violence, but maintained that he could not remember it. His childhood had not been particularly happy; he had a great hatred for his mother who had taken a lover while his father was bedridden with illness. It was notable that all his bouts of IED were directed at his wife.

A CRITIQUE OF PSYCHIATRIC/NEUROLOGICAL EXPLANATIONS FOR INTIMATE VIOLENCE

Elliott (1976/1877) believed that episodes such as those Robert and Sam experienced are caused by a neurological disorder—literally, some electric microstorm in the brain. He speculated that the site of this disorder might be the limbic system, an "ancient" part of the brain situated in the brainstem, down underneath the cerebral hemispheres. The limbic system is called "ancient" because it is believed to have developed far back in humanity's evolution. It contains structures with fascinating names, such as the amygdala, the hippocampus, and the temporal lobe. Together, these areas are believed to constitute the "seat of emotion," and microelectrode stimulation of the amygdala in animals produces rage or pleasure, depending on the exact location of the implant. Some locations will cause monkeys to press a bar repeatedly to keep the stimulation turned on. They press until they literally drop from exhaustion. Other locations cause monkeys to bare their teeth and attack.

Almost every psychology student has sat through the riveting film of the Spanish neuropsychologist Jose Delgado, dressed like a matador and being charged by a bull. The bull, however, had received a microimplant that Delgado could activate by remote control. When Delgado flipped the switch in a small control box, the bull stopped in its tracks. Obviously, electrical activity in this area can have extensive effects on behavior associated with aggression. One kind of internally generated electrical activity in the brain is an epileptic seizure. Hence, authors such as Elliott (1976/1977) speculated that this kind of epilepsy might be the cause of uncontrollable aggression.

Elliott believed temporal lobe epilepsy to be the most common "organic" condition associated with explosive rage. Temporal lobe epilepsy, in turn, can be caused by any early trauma such as "an anoxic incident in early infancy" (i.e., the infant's air supply is cut off) or "traumatic scars" (Elliott, 1976/1977, p. 102). Elliott did not speculate as to how these traumatic scars might be inflicted. He did not explicitly connect temporal lobe epilepsy to being a victim of physical abuse, although in the years to come this type of experience would become a strong risk factor for adult abusiveness in men. The excellent cross generational studies by Egeland (1993) and his colleagues found a "transmission rate" of maltreatment from one generation to the next of 40% (meaning that 40% of adults who maltreated their children were themselves maltreated as children), and psychologists Rosenbaum and Hoge (1989) would found 61% of men assessed for outpatient treatment for wife assault had themselves received prior head injuries. The suggested causal pathway was as follows: Early trauma (e.g., blows to the head) causes temporal lobe epilepsy, which in turn causes IED. Is head trauma leading to temporal lobe epilepsy the source of these outbursts?

I must add that my own clinical experience has been that many men come into our treatment group who do have the obvious "soft signs" of neurological disorder. These sometimes include pronounced nystagmus (jerky or saccadic eye movement) and attention deficits.

> One man, whom I will call Mark, had all these signs plus an IQ level in the dull-normal range. He was a huge beefy man with the reflective ability of an 8-year-old. He had had a horribly conflicted relationship with his mother and was now living with a woman 20 years his senior, who was also his boss. We did not like his chances, but decided we had to try something. He reoffended within a few weeks of starting treatment. We asked him whether he knew he was getting angry. He said, "Yes." We asked him why he did not take a "time out" to calm down. It was clear that he was only taking in very limited amounts of information, and that his deficits were probably more than we could handle in the treatment group. He became the worst failure in the history of the group, with six repeat offenses in the decade after treatment. I have seen other men who also seemed to me to have neurological damage. But they also had, in every case, a rageful and conflicted relationship with their mothers. The neurology, by itself, was only part of the story.

Metabolic disorders can also cause explosive rage. Elliott (1976/1977) described a case of matricide triggered by hypoglycemia in a man who had suffered brain damage at birth or infancy. Elliott went on to describe the features of dyscontrol as being episodes of intense rage "triggered by trivial irritations and accompanied by verbal or physical violence" (p. 104). The individual usually has a "warm, pleasant personality" but may have "a history of traffic accidents resulting from aggressive driving" (p. 105). More recent psychiatric explanations have maintained this focus. A study by Felthous, Bryant, Wingerter, and Barratt (1991) is typical. The authors found a group of 15 men (out of 443 studied) whom they diagnosed as having IED. The typical victim of their outbursts was "a spouse, lover, or boyfriend/girlfriend." In study after study, these neurological explanations seem to avoid the obvious—namely, that something about intimate relationships generates the violence, which only occurs in the context of intimacy and typically in private. How, then, is it uncontrollable?

The literary example provided by Elliott (1977) unintentionally underscores this problem with the concept of IED. He described the character of Jacques in Emile Zola's novel *La Bête Humaine* as "a man with the symptoms of temporal lobe epilepsy who could not always control an urge to kill women who attracted him" (Elliott, 1976/1977, p. 105). How does a neurological disorder lead one to attack only attractive women? Or, to restate the earlier question, why would Robert and Sam only attack their wives and only in private? Clearly, some higher-order process of mental association between the meaning of the target person to the perpetrator and the context of the violence must direct and influence the act of violence. In a case of intimate violence, what does the man's wife or partner mean to him? What symbolic baggage does this man carry from his earlier days that gives shape to this meaning? Is there something special about intimacy that alters the meaning of the other person?

Tics can be differentially expressed in different contexts. The best example is Tourette's syndrome, a tic disorder or impulse-related disorder that manifests itself in uncontrollable cursing (coprolalia) and/or involuntary mimicry of others (echolalia). Oliver Sacks (1995) has written a marvelous description of a surgeon in British Columbia who suffers from Tourette's syndrome and manifests its expressions every day, but never while he is operating. Is this not then an example of an impulse-related disorder expressed only in specific circumstances? Yes, but a tic is a relatively unintegrated response sequence, compared to the complexity of abusiveness. The tic utterance is not specifically aimed at whoever is present. Many abusive men, on the other hand, express abuse only toward intimate others. The behavioral sequence is person-specific and complex, including a chained sequence of verbal and physical actions. The contents are designed to hurt an intimate other and are based on knowledge of that individual's weaknesses. Whether the situational specificity of a tic disorder (which does have a neurological basis) could also apply to neurologically induced complex action patterns seems to be dubious.

The insufficiency of the activation of neural mechanisms as an explanation for more molar behavior was demonstrated in another classic study by Jose Delgado, reported by Bandura (1973). In this study, stimulation of an area of the temporal lobe in a dominant male monkey produced a rage response: teeth baring and attack. Stimulation of the same area in a subordinate monkey produced withdrawal, cowering, and huddling in the corner of the cage. To Bandura (1973), as a social psychologist, this finding of Delgado's suggested that direct stimulation of brain systems is never a direct cause of aggression and that aggression always has learned aspects to it. The "prepotent" or most used response at the time of the brain stimulation is the response evoked by the stimulation. That habitual response should change with the circumstances. For example, the dominant monkey had learned to attack; attack was at the top of its hierarchy of responses, the one most likely to be used when neural mechanisms were kicked into action by any triggering event. The subordinate monkey had learned that any attempt to attack would be met by severe punishment. Its response hierarchy was different; it had learned to supplicate. The dominant and subordinate monkeys made opposite responses to stimulation of the same brain area. The neural mechanism did not have functions that were permanently fixed, and the decision to attack or to curl into a ball or show the jugular vein (in an act of submission) seemed to be based in part on what expectations were generated at that time by being in a particular social status.

Years later, in a study on humans, I found that human emotional responses were likewise very much determined by differences in hierarchical status (Dutton, Webb, & Ryan, 1994; Strachan & Dutton, 1992). I measured the emotional reactions of people while they were listening to recordings of family arguments. Some of these people were assigned to low positions in a hierarchical group created for the experiment, whereas others were assigned to high-status positions. I created on-the-spot "bosses" and "underlings." People in these two positions experienced the same family arguments differently. In these human experiments, however, greater rage was associated with low status—the opposite of what the monkey studies found. In either case, however, status mattered. There was no direct line from a neural event to broader actions like rage. The context in which rage could be acted out influenced not only the choice of action but the very experience of emotion. The potentially angry persons not only had their choice of action shaped by the context, but also their actual emotion, whether they felt anger or anxiety more strongly.

The question left unanswered by early psychiatric/neurological explanations was this: How do we explain the direction of rage outward only in specific circumstances and to specific targets (e.g., Zola's character's murderous impulses toward attractive women) when the problem is attributed either to a neurological disorder or to an incompletely defined one such as IED? Why, for example, would the rage not be generalized to whatever targets are available—to, in effect, whoever is around at the time? Why would Felthous et al.'s (1991) perpetrators only direct their rage to someone with whom they were in an intimate relationship?

The assault of intimate others typically occurs under specific circumstances (at home, in private) and at specific times (upon one partner's return home or late at night). Episodic dyscontrol would lead us to expect random times for attacks that would be just as likely to occur in public as in private. The research data on intimate violence suggest that this is not at all a random act. Something more is going on. Something guides the direction or the focus of rage—something learned about male–female relationships.

SUBTYPES OF ABUSERS

I have predicated my critique of psychiatric/neurological explanations of intimate violence on the assumption that such abusiveness is relationship-specific. For many abusive men this is the case, whereas for other sub-types the violence seems to be expressed toward people in general. I have not so far addressed this issue of subtypes of abusers. Several reviews of subtypes have been written (Dutton, 1988; Holtzworth-Monroe & Stuart, 1994). Although the terminology may change from author to author, three categories of abusers are generally recognized: "psychopathic," "avoidant," and "borderline."

Of these three, the psychopathic batterers can be differentiated from the other categories as being generally violent and abusive. They are the only batterers whose violence and abuse are not relationship-specific. From descriptions by their wives or partners, these men appear to use violence instrumentally. Also, rather than being flooded by intense arousal states, psychopathic batterers appear to experience a paradoxical inner tranquility while acting out abusively (Jacobson, 1993). This auto-nomic suppression and the instrumental aspect of their violence appear to contradict notions that violence is impulsive. It appears, rather, to be a coolly sadistic form of control.

Avoidant batterers express relationship-specific violence and typi-cally do so after extended periods of suppressed anger. Locating avoidant men on a continuum of impulsivity–instrumentality is difficult. These men do not exhibit the cool cunning of the psychopathic batterers. Their violence is typically a response to long-stored negative affect, which is itself generated by their deficits in assertiveness.

Borderline batterers fall more, I believe, toward the impulsive end of the continuum. They respond to strong inner cues, usually of building tension, accompanied by negative ruminations about the intimate other as the source of their misery. As I have argued elsewhere, these aspects appear to have early origins (Dutton, 1994; Dutton, Starzomski, Saunders, & Bartholomew, 1994; Dutton, Starzomski, & van Ginkel, 1995). The tension may be a lifelong reaction to intermittently rewarding–punishing attachment, and it may be relieved by cathartic abusive outbursts. These men are impulsive in their abusiveness, sexuality, and substance use, but all three forms of acting out are intimacy-related. The promiscuity and substance abuse are typically related to perceived loss of the intimate other. The impulsivity occurs within parameters set by intimacy and attachment, and may in the future be described as a manifestation of an attachment disorder.

REFERENCES

American Psychiatric Association. (1994). *Diagnostic and statistical manual of mental disorders* (4th ed.). Washington, DC: Author.

Bandura, A. (1973). *Aggression: A social learning analysis.* Englewood Cliffs, NJ: Prentice-Hall.

Dutton, D. G. (1988). Profiling wife assaulters: Some evidence for a trimodal analysis. *Violence and Victims, 3*(1), 5–30.

Dutton, D. G. (1994). Origin and structure of the abusive personality. *Journal of Personality Disorders, 8*(3), 181–191.

Dutton, D. G. (1995). *The batterer: A psychological profile.* New York: HarperCollins.

Dutton, D. G., Starzomski, A., Saunders, K., & Bartholomew, K. (1994). Intimacy–anger and insecure attachment as precursors of abuse in intimate relationships. *Journal of Applied Social Psychology, 24*(15), 1367–1386.

Dutton, D. G., Starzomski, A., & van Ginkel, C. (1995). The role of shame and guilt in the intergenerational transmission of abusiveness. *Violence and Victims, 10*(2), 121–131.

Dutton, D. G., Webb, A., & Ryan, L. (1994). Gender differences in affective reactions to intimate conflict. *Canadian Journal of Behavioural Science, 26*(3), 353–363.

Egeland, B. (1993). A history of abuse is a risk factor for abusing the next generation. In R. J. Gelles & D. R. Loseke (Eds.), *Current controversies on family violence* (pp. 197–208). Newbury Park, CA: Sage.

Elliott, F. (1977). The neurology of explosive rage: The episodic dyscontrol syndrome. In M. Roy (Ed.), *Battered women: A psychosociological study of domestic violence* (pp. 98–109). New York: Van Nostrand Reinhold. (Original work published 1976)

Felthous, A. R., Bryant, S., Wingerter, C. B., & Barratt, E. (1991). The diagnosis of intermittent explosive disorder in violent men. *Bulletin of the American Academy of Psychiatry and the Law, 19*(1), 71–79.

Holtzworth-Monroe, A., & Stuart, G. L. (1994). Typologies of male batterers: Three subtypes and the differences among them. *Psychological Bulletin, 116*(3), 476–497.

Jacobson, N. (1993, October). *Domestic violence: What are the marriages like?* Paper presented at the annual meeting of the American Association for Marriage and Family Therapy, Anaheim, CA.

Menninger, K. A., Mayman, M., & Pruyser, P. W. (1962). *A manual for psychiatric case study* (2nd ed.). New York: Grune & Stratton.

Rosenbaum, A., & Hoge, S. (1989). Head injury and marital aggression. *American Journal of Psychiatry, 146*(8), 1048–1051.

Sacks, O. (1995). *An anthropologist on Mars.* New York: Knopf.

Strachan, K., & Dutton, D. G. (1992). The role of power and gender in anger responses to sexual jealousy. *Journal of Applied Social Psychology, 22*(22), 1721–1740.

3

A Sociological Perspective on Impulsivity: Some Cautionary Comments on the Genesis of a Clinical Construct

ROBERT MENZIES

Throughout the 1980s and 1990s, the mental health professions in developed societies have been enjoying an unprecedented surge of popularity and growth. Bolstered by the widespread revival of biological explanations of psychiatric disabilities, fueled by a new generation of psychoactive drugs and clinical interventions, and virtually unopposed in the wake of antipsychiatry's near-demise, the "psi sciences" have been extending into ever-widening spheres of public and private life. For many, these trends are a source of comfort and celebration—a testament to the remarkable domination of medical and psychological knowledge over the dark forces of human deviance, disorder, and danger (Andrews & Bonta, 1994; American Psychiatric Association [APA], 1994; Hodgins, 1993; Monahan & Steadman, 1994; Prins, 1990). For others, this latter-day explosion of new theories, institutions, languages, and practices is a deeply troubling development. To them it signifies less science's mastery of madness, and more the rise of influential new professions that command the power to define the limits of normality and to determine the life courses of those deemed unworthy or unwell (often with disastrous effects) on the basis of standards that are at best nebulous and suspect, and at worst arbitrary, biased, self-interested, and fictitious (Chunn & Menzies, 1990; Cohen, 1990, 1994; Coleman, 1984; Ingleby, 1981; Menzies, 1989).

But whatever the grind of one's own ideological lens—whether these new clinical regimes are cast as pillars of progress or as the stuff of Orwellian nightmares—there is no disputing the tumultuous changes with which they have been associated, or the powerful tremors that have been reverberating inside and beyond our myriad mental health institutions, agencies, and professions over the past 20 years. Psychiatry, psychology, and allied disciplines in the mid-1990s are profoundly distinct in structure, culture, and operation from their precursors of earlier decades. Arguably, the most striking of these transformations has occurred in the concrete, everyday practices of the professions themselves. Against the background of what we have elsewhere termed the "posttherapeutic" state (Menzies & Webster, 1994), it would appear that the very mission of clinical experts has been shifting systematically away from the traditional goals of treatment, rehabilitation, and cure, toward a more pragmatic (and perhaps more organizationally legitimate) emphasis on classification, management, regulation, and control (Brown, 1990; Castel, 1991; Menzies, 1989; Menzies, Chunn, & Webster, 1995).

Needless to say, this concentrated focus on the categorization of human mentality and pathology is by no means new, and the treatment imperative does of course live on (albeit in diluted and diversified form) in the words and deeds of most therapeutic professionals. Nonetheless, in my view, this current fixation upon the mandates of psychiatric classification is a hugely important and dramatic development; it may very well represent the most critical shift in clinical theory and practice that we have witnessed in the past half-century. Already it has affected the lives of authorities and subjects, practitioners and patients, throughout the mental health enterprise. And yet, not altogether surprisingly, the content and properties of these trends have yet to be explored in even a cursory fashion. Nor have their implications been adequately addressed in the clinical or social scientific literatures.

With these issues in mind, in this chapter I propose to take a somewhat different approach to the impulsivity concept from that adopted by most of the other authors in this book. First of all, from the outset I must confess to harboring a rather skeptical, if not wholly inimical, perspective on "impulsivity" as a clinical construct and diagnostic label. This chapter is therefore intended to insert an unabashedly critical and cautionary note into the general chorus of approval on behalf of impulsivity (and its categorical cousins) that has echoed from the literature to date (e.g., Eysenck & Eysenck, 1978; Hollander & Stein, 1995; McCown, Johnson, & Shure, 1993; Wishnie, 1977). Second, from a sociologist's vantage point, I am intrigued not only by the rise of impulsivity itself (without question a compelling topic on its own terms), but also by what it represents and how it is linked to the broader currents in clinical classification work that constitute the main subject of this chapter. Impulsivity is in some respects a paradigmatic example of the new psychiatric and psychological categories that have been burgeoning across myriad clinical domains in recent years. It is not yet a component of the official psychiatric nosology in its own right (although "impulse-control disorders" are very plainly in evidence—see below); however, impulsivity does cut across numerous other sectors, and it shares many of their attributes and limitations. Consequently, an analysis and critique of impulsivity as an idea and an ascription may be able to shed some light on the organization, theory, and methodology of mental health diagnostic work in the 1990s.

In the following two sections, I begin this process with an extended look—using various illustrations, and borrowing from the writings of various feminist and other critics—at the systems and practices of clinical classification that are currently predominant in psychiatric and psychological circles. My main concern is with explaining and appraising what I consider to be the vast overproduction of symbols, labels, classifications, genera, and other such bits and bytes of (purported) knowledge that take on value as commodities within the mental health marketplace. Next, I enlist some of these observations to address the impulsivity concept itself, by underscoring its connection to these wider trends and drawing parallels with some other recently introduced (and controversial) clinical constructs. Finally, the chapter concludes with a few guarded reflections on the politics and science of impulsivity itself, and with a call for circumspection and restraint in the use of such notions in both academic and diagnostic realms.

DSM AND THE "SELLING" OF PSYCHIATRIC DIAGNOSES

In their 1992 book, *The Selling of DSM: The Rhetoric of Science in Psychiatry*, Stuart A. Kirk and Herb Kutchins examine the role of diagnostic categories in the legitimation and empowerment of the clinical professions. Their historical study of the APA's *Diagnostic and Statistical Manual* (DSM) is unquestionably one of the most insightful books to have yet been written on the sociology of the definition, identification, and treatment of mental disorders. (The quotations in this section are from this book unless otherwise indicated. Copyright 1992 by Aldine de Gruyter. Reprinted by permission.)

Kirk and Kutchins look at what they characterize as the political struggle over DSM, and specifically the provocative chain of events leading up to and following the publication of its third edition (DSM-III) in 1980. They offer a meticulous, and rather alarming, assessment of the mechanisms and manipulations through which DSM has come to life. According to Kirk and Kutchins, this enormously influential diagnostic manual—by far the world's foremost barometer of disorder and wellness—has been forged in a crucible of pressure group lobbying, moral entrepreneurship, ideological bias, and cynical deals made in back rooms. The authors chronicle how, in the making and selling of DSM, certain constituencies (mainly white male middle-class psychiatrists) have been granted a privileged voice; those marginalized from the process have included the progressive Group for the Advancement of Psychiatry (GAP), along with women and visible-minority psychiatrists, clinical psychologists, and, most glaringly, psychiatric survivors/consumers/patients themselves.

Kirk and Kutchins unleash a quite stunning assessment of the clinical research and professional rhetoric involved in the campaign to promote this manual and its hundreds of categories. They characterize the events surrounding the rise of DSM-III in particular as a kind of public relations operation: The results of evaluation studies were carefully managed, and journal contents and conference proceedings were orchestrated, to present a one-sided version of the models and methods that its advocates embraced—and to deflect and defuse the condemnations issuing from both within and without the APA. At its heart, this story is about the power of professional people (mostly men) to make and sell ideas about sanity and madness, which then circulate through the public culture and infiltrate institutions and agencies far beyond their original source. As Kirk and Kutchins warn us,

> There are no restrictions, beyond public tolerance, on what the APA may claim as mental disorders. The validity or reliability of its claims is of little importance, as long as most psychiatrists consent to their use and no other interested parties create embarrassing public disputes. The constantly changing mix of diagnostic categories attests to this fluidity, in which many new categories were added to DSM-III and some categories of DSM-II ceased to exist. . . . There are no limits to these changes beyond the internal negotiations within the APA and the desire of the profession to avoid public ridicule. (pp. 185–186)

Furthermore, these authors observe a number of regularities in the methods and tactics deployed by the APA in its selling of DSM, which they argue are indispensable for the success of any such claims-making crusade. In their study of the events surrounding the revisions involved in each successive edition of DSM, Kirk and Kutchins identify four characteristics that have been common to each stage in the evolution of the APA's diagnostic system. First, "none of the revisions has been stimulated by clinical practitioners demanding a new classification system" (p. 214). Second, the process of decision making has become increasingly elaborate, with more and more input from "advisors, work groups, task forces, governance committees, and boards" (p. 214). Third,

> new diagnostic categories are [progressively] added and old ones are split into two or more. . . . Diagnostic criteria, both inclusion and exclusion criteria, are continually churned, resorted, and redefined. With each shuffle, the claim is made that the outcome is greater validity and more precision in the diagnostic

system. The unmistakable implication is that reliability will be improved through this painstaking process. (p. 214)

The final characteristic is the "selling" of each new revision:

> The process of revising each version of the DSM begins with the first official questioning of the scientific status of the current nosology, proceeds to tout the superior process being used for the version being developed, moves to proclaim that the brand-new version represents vast improvements over the old, encourages everyone to purchase the new publication with its paraphernalia (casebooks, tapes, instructional aids, etc.), and ends with a new task force questioning the scientific status of the latest version. The cycle of denigration, enthusiasm, and denigration is recognizable in many claims of scientific achievement, where breakthroughs make an old system appear antiquated and a new system necessary. (p. 214)

Above all else, each new clinical discovery must always be presented as "good news" (p. 197) to those affected, and particularly to those with influence or the ability to intervene. It must be seen to meet the internal scientific and ethical standards of the profession itself, and to be secure from the contaminating influence of special interests. The new class, condition, or commodity should be exhibited and written about in the neutral language of science, progress, and reform.

And however politicized and private (and even surreptitious) these propagation strategies might be, the events must at all times *appear* to be unfolding in full view and within the public domain. Open debates, inclusive consultations (there were more than 100 members on the DSM-III Task Force, and 152 task force and committee members for DSM-IV; APA, 1994, pp. ix–xii), interdisciplinary input, and governmental and agency participation are to be stressed in all the available documents and presentations. The problem-solving claims should cast as wide a net as possible across an array of clinical and social problems, and stress the common crises being faced by various constituencies and cohorts. And, as Kirk and Kutchins note, the clinical products being marketed have to "sell in Peoria":

> Good news must be simple. . . . Good news loses its impact if it is embedded in too technical jargon. Laypersons do not want a complicated lesson about nuclear physics; they want to hear about cold fusion and how it may solve the energy problem. They do not want biochemistry; they want announcements that cancers can be cured. They do not want a treatise on econometrics; they want to know that the economy is improving, inflation is under control, and their jobs are not in jeopardy. What psychiatrists wanted to hear about DSM-III, they heard over and over again, in brief, clear language: Diagnostic reliability was much better than before and so much better than expected. As far as they needed to be concerned, the problem was solved. (p. 197)

In addition to these various strategies, mandates, and trends noted by Kirk and Kutchins, one other disquieting tendency has been increasingly in evidence over recent years—one that I consider in more detail below. That is, the discovery and marketing of diagnostic categories is fast becoming an end in itself, and arguably the *exclusive* mission of many clinical experts and organizations. Just as we have witnessed a global shift from treatment to classification and from rehabilitation to management in therapeutic, forensic, and correctional contexts (Castel, 1991; Cohen, 1985; Foucault, 1977; Menzies, 1989; Menzies et al., 1995), so too has the generation of new terms, labels, typologies, nosologies, tests, actuarial instruments, and diagnostic systems become a central (and highly profitable) endeavor. As Cohen (1985) has suggested in his famous study of penal practices and discourses, the "helping professions" in general have been generating an overabundance of categories across all institutions of treatment and control, which continue to proliferate to the point at which they threaten to overwhelm practitioners' ability to cope. The result is a kind of conceptual entropy and anarchism—a state of affairs where everyone is an amateur, with the exception of those holding a proprietary claim to the latest hot idea; where everyone is frantically engaged in the dodgy business of categorical catch-up; and where more of a practitioner's time and effort is devoted to the questionable task of absorbing and debating the latest proposals, manuals, and digests than to delivering services or attending to the human needs of his or her patients, clients, and consumers.

THE DANGERS AND DILEMMAS OF MENTAL HEALTH CLASSIFICATION

A galaxy of new disturbances and disorders has been spinning out in recent years from the minds and laser printers of academic experts and mental health professionals. These cover a quite extraordinary range of human experience and behavior. And the exponential growth patterns over time are readily apparent. Kirk and Kutchins (1992) observe that DSM-II, published in 1968, contained 182 disorders occupying fewer than 40 pages of description, and cost $3.50. By 1980, DSM-III embodied 265 specific categories, and the number rose again to 292 when DSM-III-R was published in 1987 (Kirk & Kutchins, 1992, pp. 116–119).

In contrast, by my own calculation, when all diagnostic codes (including principal diagnoses, subtypes, and specifiers) are accounted for (APA, 1994, pp. 13–24), there are a total of 566 potential diagnoses in DSM-IV. (Paula J. Caplan [1995, p. 188], counting only the categories and subcategories, identifies a grand total of 374.) These are grouped into 16 main categories, plus six other classes of "other conditions that may be a focus of clinical attention" and Five "additional Codes" (including the paradoxical diagnosis of "no diagnosis" [V71.09]), along with the five-part multiaxial system modified from DSM-III (APA, 1994, pp. 25–31). All told, it is difficult to imagine a species of pathology that could conceivably escape inclusion. In addition to the traditional diagnostic classes that populated earlier editions (schizophrenia, mood disorders, anxiety disorders, personality disorders, and so on), DSM-IV extends a litany of esoteric offerings, including mathematics disorder (315.2), conduct disorder (312.8), oppositional defiant disorder (313.81), caffeine intoxication (305.90), 11 different variations of cocaine-Induced disorders (292), delusional disorder, erotomanic type (297.1), hypoactive sexual desire disorder (302.71), borderline personality disorder (301.83), partner relational problem (V61.1), noncompliance with treatment (V15.81), malingering (V65.2), and (the unrivaled favorite of the students in my undergraduate seminar on psychiatry and law) academic problem (V62.3). The diagnosis of premenstrual dysphoric disorder, whose earlier incarnation elicited such controversy in the making of DSM (Caplan, 1995; Russell, 1995; Ussher, 1991), is diplomatically relegated in DSM-IV to Appendix B, which covers "criteria sets and axes provided for further study" (see APA, 1994, pp. 715–718).

It is noteworthy too, given the subject matter of this book, that impulse-related categories make their appearance in several sections of DSM-IV, and indeed that some of them constitute an entire diagnostic genus in their own right ("impulse-control disorders not elsewhere classified"). This latter group includes intermittent explosive disorder (312.34), kleptomania (312.32), pyromania (312.33), pathological gambling (312.31), trichotillomania (the compulsion to tear out one's hair—312.39), and, presumably in the interests of ensuring full coverage, impulse-control disorder not otherwise specified (312.30).

Nor is this clinical construction exercise confined to the pages of DSM or the APA's policies. Phil Brown (1980), among others, suggests that in recent times we have been bearing witness to a "neo-Kraepelinian" era (p. 390; see also Blashfield, 1984), in which ever-widening circles of individual and collective cognition and behavior are being subjected to the impulse to pathologize (Conrad & Schneider, 1992; Ingleby, 1981).

Examples abound. The above-noted furor over the inclusion in Appendix A of DSM-III-R of premenstrual dysphoric disorder (then known as late luteal phase dysphoric disorder) and the similarly suspect self-defeating personality disorder failed to seriously dampen their influence on an androcentric mental health establishment (Busfield, 1986; Caplan, 1995; Russell, 1995; Ussher, 1991). Citing Hobbes's maxim that "ultimate power is the power to make definitions," Kaye-Lee Pantony and Paula J. Caplan proposed, in a 1991 *Canadian Psychology* paper and the forum that followed, a new classification for stereotypically hypermasculine males—delusional dominating personality disorder, the symptoms of which include "inability to establish and maintain meaningful interpersonal relations," "a pronounced tendency to use a gender-based double standard in interpreting or evaluating situations or behaviour," "a tendency to feel inordinately threatened by women who fail to disguise their intelligence," and "emotionally uncontrolled resistance to reform efforts that are oriented toward gender equity" (p. 121). Not incidentally, and rather ironically in view of this last point, Caplan's efforts to have delusional dominating personality disorder included in DSM-IV met much opposition within the APA and ultimately proved futile (Caplan, 1995).

Elsewhere, the category of hyperactivity, so dominant during the 1970s and 1980s (Schrag & Divoky, 1975), has since given way to a host of new labels that are now being ascribed to troublesome children—including attention-deficit/hyperactivity disorder, attachment disorder, and adaptive moral deficiency syndrome (Millar, n.d.), along with, among others, the above-mentioned DSM-IV diagnoses of conduct disorder and oppositional defiant disorder. The current wars over delayed adult recollections of child sexual abuse (Loftus & Ketcham, 1994) appear to represent an instance in which neither side can resist the inclination to couch its position in clinical discourse, in the defense, respectively, of "repressed-memory syndrome" or "false-memory syndrome."

On a more ironic note, Richard Bentall (1992) submits that even happiness (which he calls "major affective disorder, pleasant type") can be construed as a pathological defect, as "happy people are often carefree, *impulsive* and unpredictable in their actions" (p. 94, emphasis added). Bentall adds that happiness "is statistically abnormal, [potentially life threatening], consists of a discrete cluster of symptoms, . . . and . . . is associated with various cognitive abnormalities—in particular, a lack of contact with reality" (p. 97). Glenn Ellenbogen (1986) proposes that a similar case can be made for the vegetarian personality, "characterized by ruthless acts of an oral-sadistic nature directed against vegetables" (p. 89). Why not? This inventory of pathological classes, categories, and labels—serious and satiric, fictional and real—could be extended almost indefinitely. As Kirk and Kutchins maintain in one of the passages quoted earlier, there are "no limits" to this list "beyond public tolerance" and "the desire of the profession to avoid public ridicule" (1992, pp. 185–186).

Kirk and Kutchins are scarcely alone in their condemnation of these latest trends in the enterprise of mental health classification. Indeed, ever-increasing numbers of clinicians, sociolegal scholars, feminists, and psychiatric survivors have been calling into question the very foundations of this new generation of diagnoses, and express much concern about its potential to upset the fragile balance between the play of professional powers and the defense of social freedom and justice. Some of these critics believe that the application of these schemes represents a blatantly political exercise in the suppression of human diversity, and a highly successful (and profitable) effort to widen the net of state, professional, and legal regulation (Burstow & Weitz, 1988; Busfield, 1986; Cohen, 1990, 1994; Ingleby, 1981; Kovel, 1988; Sedgwick, 1982; Szasz, 1994; Ussher, 1991).

In other contexts, the scientific validity, reliability, objectivity, and neutrality of long-accepted DSM categories have been subjected to challenge on philosophical, political, conceptual, ethical, and methodological grounds (Bayer, 1981; Caplan, 1995; Cohen, 1990, 1994; Coleman, 1984; Conrad & Schneider, 1992; Kirk & Kutchins, 1994; Mirowsky, 1990; Zimmerman, 1988). The various new nosologies and diagnostic practices have been denounced as inherently biased along the lines of gender, race, ethnicity, class, age, and sexuality (Bayer, 1981; Breggin, 1991; Brown, 1990; Busfield, 1986; Pfohl, 1978; Scheff, 1975). Feminist critics have underscored the "double standard of health [that] exists for men and women" (Russell, 1995, p. 30) and the misogynist assumptions that are indelibly etched upon the concept of madness (Chesler, 1972; Ehrenreich & English, 1978; Showalter, 1987; Ussher, 1991). Survivors of psychiatric hospitalization and of such treatments as electroshock (Capponi, 1992; Chamberlin, 1978, 1994; Everett, 1994; Millett, 1990) have written eloquently about the failure of psychiatric schemes and diagnostic practitioners to account for the values and experiences of their human subjects, and about the potentially devastating implications for those who are so classified (including involuntary institutionalization; enforced treatment; loss of family, friends, and career; iatrogenic illnesses such as tardive dyskinesia; etc.). From all these vantage points, the impulse to extend one's institutional frontiers and to maximize capital and clientele—so characteristic of all large-scale industries—has in the final analysis spawned a cycle of overproduction in the mental health enterprise, leading to a radical devaluation of its stock and to an inevitable crisis of confidence among authorities, funders, practitioners, consumers, and public alike.

In his 1990 article "The Name Game: Toward a Sociology of Diagnosis," Brown conducts a compelling review of the social science research literature on the context, nature, and consequences of psychiatric diagnosis. Enlisting a variety of illustrations, Brown punctures many of the myths about DSM and related mental health diagnostic blueprints, convincingly showing how the constructed appearance of value-free science is belied by the grounded experience of social bias, practitioner discretion, and professional dominance (Freidson, 1986). As Brown argues, the clinical research typically harnessed to make the case for diagnostic science is rife with conceptual and methodological defects. Yet, despite these many failings and contradictions, the psychiatric discipline and its allies have continued to enjoy an era of seemingly limitless expansion. This growth has been propelled by both a "remedicalization" process (Brown, 1990, p. 389) associated with the reemergence of biomedical models of "mental illness," and a successful campaign on the part of APA and other professional organizations to demonstrate that psychiatry and allied disciplines are indeed sciences, thereby "solidify[ing] the psychiatric claim that it is a 'hard' medicine worthy of third-party reimbursement" (1990, p. 391). For Brown, the results are plainly in evidence, and the implications are ominous:

> Biopsychiatric neo-Kraepelinians lay claim to a project far grander than merely a comprehensive, objective diagnostic schema. Their goal is to lead the transformation of the mental health system. This is largely defined negatively—opposing the labeling/societal reaction perspective and the anti-institutionalist attitudes that have played such a large role. These new leaders seek to strip psychiatry of any context. They wish to place psychiatry in a technocratic framework rather than an interpretive, humanistic one. But even if the professional project goes beyond diagnosis, the diagnostic project is at the core of a larger goal. One reason for the centrality of diagnosis is that diagnosis plays a coordinating role in laying out the terms of medico-psychiatric diagnosis. Professional leaders have taken the diagnostic terminology of DSM and reified it into the essential statement and rationale of biopsychiatry. Another reason is that the significant social powers to whom organized psychiatry asks for support view the diagnostic schema as the proper codification of psychiatry. Third-party payers, both private and governmental, as well as state and federal bureaucrats who run mental health agencies, have established a diagnostic determinism. Quite literally, the mental health of a client only becomes "official" when the proper DSM code is affixed. (Brown, 1990, p. 404)

Finally, Caplan's 1995 book, *They Say You're Crazy: How the World's Most Powerful Psychiatrists Decide Who's Normal,* is a poignant and highly personalized account of the author's own encounters with the diagnostic enterprise throughout the development of DSM-III-R and DSM-IV. Caplan's involvement in, and eventual resignation from, the task forces on self-defeating personality disorder and late luteal phase dysphoric disorder provide an illuminating window through which the APA's inner politics of diagnosis can be observed. Moreover, her failed efforts to get delusional dominating personality disorder included in DSM-IV (see above) graphically reveal the APA establishment's resistance to pathologizing a form of male behavior plainly equivalent to certain women's "disorders," which they have unhesitatingly endorsed.

Following a devastating indictment of the DSM "gatekeeping process" (Larkin & Caplan, 1992), Caplan (1995) suggests that the construction and legitimation of diagnostic labels have, at their core, little to do with science. The impressive reliability statistics provided by the authors of DSM field trials and other experimental studies, she argues, are both disingenuous and false:

> The DSM authors diverge from responsible scientific practice . . . by designing and conducting studies in sloppy ways, by distorting their findings to make them look better than they are, and by revealing them too late to give non-DSM people time to respond before the next edition of the handbook is published. . . . A deeply disturbing consequence of the DSM's lack of science is that reasonably intelligent people assume that the labels in the handbook corre-

spond to disorders or problems that are known to exist. When categories are presented as though they are real, it is inevitable that some people will be classified as belonging to those categories and will be given various treatments aimed to cure their supposed mental disorders. For nonexistent disorders, this is a waste of time, energy, and money if the patient is lucky, and it is profoundly harmful if the patient is less fortunate. (1995, pp. 191, 195)

Declaring that "to assign a name is to act as though you are referring to something that exists, something real" (1995, p. 272), Caplan cautions that the ultimate outcome of this aggressive drive to pathologize human life—to classify all our ailments and failings, and to locate them within the defective hearts and minds of "mentally disordered" subjects—is the perpetuation of the manifold social problems that are left untouched by these systems of mental health diagnosis.

A major consequence of the DSM's medicalization of problems in living—recasting so much loneliness, mourning, disempowerment, insecurity, shame, anxiety, and anger as "diseases" or "disorders"—is that the real sources of many of those upsetting feelings are masked. . . . [I]t is clear that a great deal of pain is caused—or exacerbated—by social factors that could be changed if our society took more serious and sweeping steps toward eradicating poverty, prejudice, and violence. . . . DSM-backed assumptions that mental and emotional problems are caused by biochemical or brain defects mask the damage done by oppressive social arrangements. One way to describe the DSM process would be to say that a relatively small number of people take what they regard as deviant or different and then declare those things medical problems, mental disorders. (Caplan, 1995, pp. 278–279)

THE SCIENCE AND POLITICS OF IMPULSIVITY

All of this brings me full circle, back to the impulsivity construct itself.

Like the various other categories of psychiatric and psychological diagnosis that have been canvassed by the above-cited authors and addressed throughout this chapter, impulsivity has gained a considerable following in recent years (APA, 1994, pp. 609–621; Clarke Institute of Psychiatry, 1992; Doob, 1990; Hollander & Stein, 1995; Wishnie, 1977). The very fact of the present book's publication is clear evidence of the concept's healthy and growing reputation among clinicians, psychological researchers, and correctional authorities. Indeed, in their 1995 reader entitled *Impulsivity and Aggression,* Hollander and Stein cite literally dozens of studies on the subject that have appeared during the 1980s and 1990s; they also cite a multitude of tests, instrument schedules, questionnaires, and personality profiles for the detection of impulsivity, which date back nearly half a century to the 1949 Guilford–Zimmerman Temperament Survey (Hollander & Stein, 1995, p. 9). Impulsiveness was a core feature of Eysenck's personality theories, which have been prominent in behavioral psychology circles since the 1960s (Eysenck, 1977; Eysenck & Eysenck, 1978). It has accompanied the revival of psychopathy and is included as an item in the revised Psychopathy Checklist (Hare, 1991). Risk research (Monahan & Steadman, 1994) and violence prediction (Webster, Harris, Rice, Cormier, & Quinsey, 1994) have invoked impulsivity as a potential attribute of dangerous people. The American Psychological Association has embraced the idea in a recent publication (McCown et al., 1993). As noted earlier, it is conspicuously displayed in various forms throughout DSM-IV (APA, 1994). Clinical research programs (Clarke Institute of Psychiatry, 1992) and conferences (Webster, Jackson, & Brunanski, 1994) have been devoted to the study of impulsivity. Moreover, the topic makes an appearance in various textbooks and readers, particularly on the subjects of criminal, forensic, and correctional psychology (Andrews & Bonta, 1994; Blackburn, 1993; Hodgins, 1993).

Consistent with the patterns of category expansion described in earlier sections of this chapter, impulsivity has been tied and attributed to, or held responsible for, a quite extraordinary range of dysfunctional and pathological behavior. For example, in the first two pages alone of their paper entitled "The Nature of Impulsivity," Plutchik and van Praag (1995, pp. 7–8) claim a correspondence between impulsivity and (in order of their recitation) borderline personality disorder, antisocial personality disorder, hyperactive syndrome, alcoholism, substance abuse, brain damage, anorexia nervosa, bulimia, suicidal and violent behavior, neurological "soft signs," rage and aggression, homicide, sexual assault, risk taking, error-prone information processing, bipolar disorders, kleptomania, pyromania, addictions, perversions, some sexual disorders, and self-mutilating behavior.

It is also apparent that the majority of available research has focused not on the social, institutional, or cultural realm, but on the individual defects of "impulsive subjects" at the levels of biology, chemistry, neurology, and personality. Whereas Hollander and Stein (1995), for example, commendably concede that "sociological explanations suggest that poverty, lack of education, the breakdown of the nuclear family, substance abuse and alcohol abuse, lack of jobs and opportunity, racism, despair, and the widespread availability of guns and automatic weapons are *contributing factors*" (p. 1, emphasis added), they proceed to stress that "this book focuses on the phenomenology, neurobiology, and treatment of impulsivity and aggression" (1995, pp. 1–2).

The attractions of this clinical approach to impulsivity are abundantly clear. The idea that many of our collective crises and social problems might be attributable to psychologically or physiologically uncontrolled and undercontrolled people—those who, on account of internal defects, are unable or unwilling to reflect on their conduct or impose self-restraint—is both compelling and potentially empowering at a variety of levels. A "coordinating concept" (Webster, Jackson, & Brunanski, 1994, p. vii) of this kind could help us unify and make sense of the otherwise daunting array of human frailties and foibles that continue to plague our contemporary social world. Were it possible to marshal the impulsivity construct in a reliable and valid fashion, to map its biopsychological properties, to devise accurate assessment instruments, and to establish its connections to the various defects and dysfunctions catalogued above, perhaps a comprehensive program aimed at suppressing violence and promoting our social health and safety could result. As with the elusive clinical grails of dangerousness prediction and risk assessment mentioned above (Menzies, 1989; Menzies et al., 1995; Monahan & Steadman, 1994; Pfohl, 1978; Webster et al., 1994), the political, institutional, and professional benefits would be profound. But I, for one, harbor some serious misgivings on both scientific and political grounds.

First, the generally uncritical endorsement of the impulsivity construct within clinical circles may in itself be a cause for concern. By endeavoring to disperse the category across such a broad band of human disorder and malfeasance, its inventors have distended its meaning to the point of near-incomprehensibility. Both theoretically and practically, its sheer conceptual range renders impulsivity a rather protean and fragmented idea, with limited explanatory power in any given specific organizational or clinical context. Blackburn (1993) contends:

> The classification of impulse control disorders . . . does not identify specific psychological disorders having distinguishable referents. Rather are these classes explanatory fictions introduced when people are unable to attribute their repeated deviant acts to an "acceptable" or "rational" cause. Repetitive aggression, shoplifting, or arson can serve a variety of functions, which may sometimes be related to personal crises, conflicts, or dysfunctions in ways which the person does not fully comprehend. While there is a case for subdividing particular forms of repetitive deviant behaviour according to categories of motive (or reinforcer), a classification which effectively rests on arbitrary distinctions between "rational" and "irrational" has no scientific utility. (p. 74)

Second, it is difficult, if not impossible, to disentangle impulsivity from the galaxy of other attributes and traits that have been compiled over the years in the medical and psychological quest to identify troublesome people and to explain and predict their behavior. Most commentators recognize that behavior deemed impulsive is, in various combinations and degrees, associated with the timing and tempo of one's comportment, failure to reflect, impetuosity, lack of self-restraint, irrationality, explosiveness, unpredictability, nonutilitarianism, and other such qualities. Yet, on reflection, not only are these various descriptors inescapably mired in cultural expectations and social biases, but there is little evidence that they collapse into anything approaching a discrete cluster with systematic, stable, or measurable properties. Like dangerousness (Menzies & Webster, 1994; Menzies, Webster, & Hart, 1994), impulsivity has evolved into a kind of residual category, to be invoked to account for criminal, violent, or other vexatious conduct that cannot otherwise be explained. Once again, Blackburn (1993) makes roughly the same point:

> The validity of impulse control disorders as a distinct class is questionable on conceptual grounds. An "impulse" is a circular inference of cause from the behaviour it supposedly impels, and "failure to resist an impulse" is similarly inferred from the observation that an act has been performed. Moreover, these disorders are distinguished by the exclusion of acts having an immediately "obvious" motive. . . . Labels implying "compulsion" are . . . applied when neither the perpetrator nor an observer can account for the behaviour in terms of motives which are current, popular, or culturally sanctioned. (p. 74)

Third, although in these respects impulsivity has arguably become an overinclusive and overextended idea, in yet another sense—at the level of culture and political organization—it remains dolefully underdeveloped. In reviewing the literature, we find virtually no references to the systemic and institutionalized attributes of impulsivity, or to the many features of contemporary society that both precipitate impulsive conduct and reward its expression. Nor do we encounter analyses of the "culture of impulsivity" that characterizes modern life and to which we are all daily exposed, or of the social conditions under which impulsive conduct may be variously invited or abhorred, or the complex systems of reward and regulation that both spawn impulsive people and undertake their treatment and control. As one illustration, little attention has to date been paid to the extensive theory and research on masculinity that has surfaced in recent years (e.g., Brittan, 1989; Brod & Kaufman, 1994; Segal, 1990; Seidler, 1994). We inhabit a society where "hegemonic masculinity" reigns (Connell, 1987), and where the impulsivity (decisiveness? assertiveness? impetuosity? rashness?) of one's conduct is appraised through an intensely gendered filter. Men and women, boys and girls, are differentially credited and rebuked for showing impulsive inclinations; in this respect, impulsivity could well be an appropriate addition to Pantony and Caplan's (1991) differential diagnostic inventory for delusional dominating personality disorder (see above). We might therefore profit enormously from theory and research that consider the relationship between masculinity and impulsivity, and that recognize the role of male-dominated institutions, languages, and cultures in the genesis of impulsivity and other forms of violence and trouble.

Fourth, the messages conveyed earlier in this chapter, yielded from the various feminist and other critical analyses of diagnostic categories both within and without DSM, should not be forgotten. As Kirk and Kutchins (1992), Brown (1990), Caplan (1995), and others attest, the birth and dissemination of new clinical classifications (impulsivity included) are inherently about the ability of academics, clinicians, and other professionals to make and validate knowledge. Although the scientific qualities of this construction process may be open to debate, there is no contesting the political and ideological dimensions of ideas like impulsivity. To label an individual "impulsive" (or "personality-disordered," or "psychopathic," or "dangerous") is to effect a value judgment. Through the application of these culturally bound labels, professional clinicians and other officials wield immense power to change the lives of their human subjects, often with devastating consequences. And the purview of this professional authority is directly correlated with the number of such categories that are in circulation, with their psycholegal legitimacy and public acceptance, and with the capacity to present them as scientific truths instead of cultural products. For these reasons, the rise and diffusion of impulsivity are entirely fathomable from both a professional and an institutional standpoint. But for precisely the same reasons, the impulsivity construct, and those who would entrench it within mental health and correctional systems, must be held accountable and subjected to the most exacting scientific, legal, and ethical scrutiny.

SOME FINAL THOUGHTS

In reflecting on the future prospects and possibilities of the impulsivity construct, we need to be very mindful, I think, of the political context and consequences of this kind of categorical expansion, particularly in light of the various trends reviewed in this chapter. Our collective experience with other such ideas, both within and beyond the mental health apparatus, would suggest that impulsivity—not only as a state of mind and being and as a behavioral complex, but also as a "coordinating concept" (Webster, Jackson, & Brunanski, 1994, p. vii)—may turn out to be a risky notion indeed.

We clearly need to be posing a number of pointed questions about the costs and benefits that may be associated with the continuing, and even accelerated, infusion of this notion into the theories and practices of mental health and allied systems. For example, what are the clinical, social science, ethical, and ideological criteria by which we might go about assessing the benefits and risks of impulsivity? Do we have available any pure scientific indices of the idea, and can these conceivably be disentangled from the moral choices that operate in so many other spheres of private and public life? Can we demonstrate the construct's reliability and validity in any consistent fashion? And can we guarantee that impulsivity will enhance our power to identify and remedy social problems involving public health and safety, while simultaneously ensuring that justice is preserved and citizens are not subjected to arbitrary measures of treatment and control? On all these questions and more, I would suggest that the jury is still out, and that in the interim we have to be very circumspect in pushing such ideas onto the clinical and social agenda. In this general spirit of recommended restraint, I conclude with four final cautionary thoughts.

First, I would contend that the rise of impulsivity, like that of risk and other such constructs, is best understood as a cultural entity—specifically, a conceptual byproduct of the recent "splintering" of the dangerousness idea, which has been justifiably discredited (Pfohl, 1978; Menzies, 1989; Webster & Menzies, 1987), into a number of subconstructs, each of which comes to take on a clinical life of its own. The rise of the risk construct (Menzies et al., 1994; Monahan & Steadman, 1994) and the renaissance of psychopathy in the 1980s and 1990s (Hare, 1991) are two cases in point. Ironically, our work at METFORS (Metropolitan Toronto Forensic Service) over the years (Menzies, 1989; Webster & Menzies, 1987; Webster, Menzies, & Jackson, 1982) has no doubt reflected (and even contributed to) this categorical "big bang," through the invention of instruments like the Dangerous Behaviour Rating Scheme (Menzies, Webster, McMain, Staley, & Scaglione, 1994; Menzies, Webster, & Sepejak, 1985), which spits out such purportedly risk-related items as anger, hostility, rage, tolerance, manipulativeness, capacity for empathy, capacity for change, and so on. But our own research seems to show quite convincingly that, even when pooled, this kaleidoscope of constructs fails to add much meaning or predictive power to our diagnostic and forecasting projects. Nor is this an especially surprising outcome, given what we know about our inability to predict dangerousness or to assess risk.

Second, in order even to begin the process of evaluating impulsivity against a legitimate set of scientific, social, and ethical criteria, we need to open up the concept to critical scrutiny, and to locate it within a historical context. A number of related subjects have to be addressed, and continuing effort must be devoted to this—certainly more work than can possibly be mustered into a single edited book of this kind. There is much that remains to be learned. For example, what is the genealogy of the impulsivity construct; how and why has it been adopted, in varying forms, into selected clinical, social, and criminological theories; and what are its attributes and implications? Furthermore, is there anything really new or innovative about this most recent incarnation of impulsivity? And can it genuinely contribute to our understanding of psychosocial life, above and beyond the daunting arsenal of clinical descriptions and depictions that has been accumulating over the course of decades and centuries?

Third, it simply must be acknowledged that impulsivity is as much a cultural and moral ascription as it is a clinical commodity. That being the case, the onus should most decidedly rest on the side of those who would proclaim its scientific authenticity and applicability. Moreover, there is a need to explore the construct's political connotations. Surely, for example, the very behaviors that we might deplore as impulsive in some contexts can be highly adaptive, and even imperative, elsewhere. In the terrain of human conflict, our victors are recurrently lauded and lionized for their assertiveness, decisiveness, spontaneity, fast thinking, and quick action, whereas the defeated, deviant, and deficient are deplored for their impetuousness, rashness, recklessness, irrationality, nonutilitarianism, lack of control—in short, their impulsivity. We collectively reward and celebrate the capacity for aggressively unreflective conduct in many of our social circles (typically male-dominated), such as the military, policing, athletics, professional circles, financial institutions, and so on. Elsewhere, when similar activities under dissimilar conditions come under legal or clinical authority, diagnostic labels are speedily brought to bear. But is it really possible to discern, in any systematic or authoritative way, the psychometric distinctions between the adrenalized stockbroker careening around the commodities exchange floor and the homeless street kid spending his or her days and nights fixing, fighting, and fornicating? In either case, are the behaviors under scrutiny adaptive or maladaptive? Decisive or rash? Rational or pathological? Willful or impulsive? And who gets to decide? How are we to abstract the experts' judgments from the structural, cultural, linguistic, and just plain human circumstances within which these people are playing out their lives?

Fourth and finally, the postmodernists have been reminding us since the 1970s (Connor, 1991; Harvey, 1989; Lyotard, 1984; Nicholson, 1990) that, in order to confront and ultimately to transcend the destructive forces that have accompanied more than two centuries of "Enlightenment" thinking and practices (and the attendant domination by those who espouse the virtues of modernism, rationalism, positivism, science, and "progress"), we should be doing everything possible to deny and deconstruct the received categories that energize our institutions, forms of thought, languages, and social activities. The last thing we need, according to this view, is the invention of yet *more* linguistic instruments for the identification and segregation of those alleged to depart from some ambiguous (and often arbitrary) standard of normality and morality. To borrow from the title of a paper presented at the conference that spawned this book (Boyd, 1994), it may well behoove us to shift "from impulsivity to deliberateness" in our own academic and clinical work, when it comes to the pursuit of these categorical holy grails. This will require an active effort to engage with, to critique, and (when necessary) to decenter and even discard our own values, ideologies, and conceptual schemes. In short, it demands scientific humility. A genuine humanization of the "human sciences" and "helping professions" would constitute an outright abandonment of the rigid, centralized, expert-driven, top-down, instrumental (and, not incidentally, highly profitable) classificatory schemes of the institutional monopolies like the APA and the World Health Organization, in favor of localized, personalized, reciprocal, reflexive, and nonhierarchical models of the kind advocated in recent years, for example, by women working in feminist therapeutic contexts (Russell, 1995; Ussher, 1991).

Now, I for one doubt that such a utopian scenario is likely to unfold in the near or even distant future. The stakes are simply too high. There are far too many incentives to hang onto the old theoretical and linguistic structures, and to add new appendages whenever the appropriate conditions or perceived social and clinical problems arise. So we may, in the final analysis, predict a bright future for impulsivity, risk, attention-deficit/hyperactivity disorder, oppositional defiant disorder, borderline personality disorder, premenstrual dysphoric disorder, and the innumerable other members of this new generation of clinical categories. Whatever the contradictions and constraints this may entail, all the signs point in the direction of continuing diagnostic consolidation, elaboration, and extension. Kirk and Kutchins (1992, p. 238) reach much the same conclusion in their meticulous analysis of DSM: "An expanding list of mental disorders that contains everything . . . offers an ideology for understanding a potpourri of dysfunctional or devalued behaviors as medical disorders rather than as diverse forms of social deviance. . . . Diagnostic decisions made in mental health organizations for reimbursement purposes institutionalize this medicalization in a way that cannot be easily reversed."

REFERENCES

American Psychiatric Association (APA). (1994). *Diagnostic and statistical manual of mental disorders* (4th ed.). Washington, DC: Author.

Andrews, D. A., & Bonta, J. (1994). *The psychology of criminal conduct.* Cincinnati, OH: Anderson.

Bayer, R. (1981). *Homosexuality and American psychiatry: The politics of diagnosis.* New York: Basic Books.

Bentall, R. P. (1992). A proposal to classify happiness as a psychiatric disorder. *Journal of Medical Ethics, 18,* 94–98.

Blackburn, R. (1993). *The psychology of criminal conduct: Theory, research, and practice.* Chichester, England: Wiley.

Blashfield, R. K. (1984). *The classification of psychopathology: Neo-Kraepelinian and quantitative approaches.* New York: Plenum Press.

Boyd, N. (1994). Dependence on alcohol and other drugs: From impulsivity to deliberateness. In C. D. Webster, M. A. Jackson, & D. M. Brunanski (Eds.), *Impulsivity: New directions in research and clinical practice. Proceedings of a conference* (pp. 23–24). Vancouver, British Columbia: Simon Fraser University.

Breggin, P. R. (1991). *Toxic psychiatry: Why therapy, empathy and love must replace the drugs, electroshock and biochemical theories of the "new psychiatry."* New York: St. Martin's Press.

Brittan, A. (1989). *Masculinity and power.* Oxford: Blackwell.

Brod, H., & Kaufman, M. (Eds.). (1994). *Theorizing masculinities.* Thousand Oaks, CA: Sage.

Brown, P. (1990). The name game: Toward a sociology of diagnosis. *Journal of Mind and Behavior, 11,* 385–406.

Burstow, B., & Weitz, D. (Eds.). (1988). *Shrink resistant: The struggle against psychiatry in Canada.* Vancouver, British Columbia: New Star Books.

Busfield, J. (1986). *Managing madness: Changing ideas and practice.* London: Unwin Hyman.

Caplan, P. J. (1995). *They say you're crazy: How the world's most powerful psychiatrists decide who's normal.* Reading, MA: Addison-Wesley.

Capponi, P. (1992). *Upstairs in the crazy house: The life of a psychiatric survivor.* Toronto: Viking.

Castel, R. (1991). From dangerousness to risk. In G. Burchell, C. Gordon, & P. Miller (Eds.), *The Foucault effect: Studies in governmentality* (pp. 281–298). Chicago: University of Chicago Press.

Chamberlin, J. (1978). *On our own: Patient-controlled alternatives to the mental health system.* New York: Hawthorn.

Chamberlin, J. (1994). A psychiatric survivor speaks out. *Feminism and Psychology, 4,* 284–287.

Chesler, P. (1972). *Women and madness.* New York: Avon.

Chunn, D. E., & Menzies, R. (1990). Gender, madness and crime: The reproduction of patriarchal and class relations in a psychiatric court clinic. *Journal of Human Justice, 1,* 33–58.

Clarke Institute of Psychiatry. (1992). *Impulsivity programme annual report 1991–1992.* Toronto: Author.

Cohen, D. (Ed.). (1990). Challenging the therapeutic state: Critical perspectives on psychiatry and the mental health system [Special issues]. *Journal of Mind and Behavior, 11*(3–4).

Cohen, D. (Ed.). (1994). Challenging the therapeutic state, part two: Further disquisitions on the mental health system [Special issues]. *Journal of Mind and Behavior, 15*(1–2).

Cohen, S. (1985). *Visions of social control: Crime, punishment and classification.* Cambridge, England: Polity Press.

Coleman, L. (1984). *The reign of error: Psychiatry, authority, and law.* Boston: Beacon Press.

Connell, R. W. (1987). *Gender and power: Society, the person and sexual politics.* Cambridge, England: Polity Press.

Connor, S. (1991). *Postmodernist culture.* Oxford: Blackwell.

Conrad, P., & Schneider, J. W. (1992). *Deviance and medicalization: From badness to sickness.* Philadelphia: Temple University Press.

Doob, L. (1990). *Hesitation: Impulsivity and reflection.* New York: Greenwood Press.

Ehrenreich, B., & English, D. (1978). *For her own good: 150 years of the experts' advice to women.* Garden City, NY: Doubleday/Anchor.

Ellenbogen, G. C. (1986). Oral sadism and the vegetarian personality. In G. C. Ellenbogen (Ed.), *Oral sadism and the vegetarian personality: Readings from the Journal of Polymorphous Perversity* (pp. 87–94). New York: Ballantine Books.

Everett, B. (1994). Something is happening: The contemporary consumer and psychiatric survivor movement in historical context. *Journal of Mind and Behavior, 15,* 55–70.

Eysenck, H. J. (1977). *Crime and personality* (2nd ed.). London: Routledge & Kegan Paul.

Eysenck, S. B. G., & Eysenck, H. J. (1978). Impulsiveness and venturesomeness: Their position in a dimensional system of personality description. *Psychological Reports, 43,* 1247–1255.

Foucault, M. (1977). *Discipline and punish: The birth of the prison.* New York: Pantheon.

Freidson, E. (1986). *Professional powers: A study of the institutionalization of formal knowledge.* Chicago: University of Chicago Press.

Hare, R. D. (1991). *Manual for the Hare Psychopathy Checklist—revised.* Toronto: Multi-Health Systems.

Harvey, D. (1989). *The condition of postmodernity.* Oxford: Blackwell.

Hodgins, S. (Ed.). (1993). *Mental disorder and crime.* London: Sage.

Hollander, E. & Stein, D. J. (Eds.). (1995). *Impulsivity and aggression.* Chichester, England: Wiley.

Ingleby, D. (1981). *Critical psychiatry: The politics of mental health.* Harmondsworth, England: Penguin Books.

Kirk, S. A., & Kutchins, H. (1992). *The selling of DSM: The rhetoric of science in psychiatry.* New York: Aldine de Gruyter.

Kirk, S. A., & Kutchins, H. (1994). The myth of the reliability of DSM. *Journal of Mind and Behavior, 15,* 71–86.

Kovel, J. (1988). A critique of DSM-III. *Research in Law, Deviance, and Social Control, 9,* 127–146.

Larkin, J., & Caplan, P. J. (1992). The gatekeeping process of the DSM. *Canadian Journal of Community Mental Health, 11,* 17–28.

Loftus, E. F., & Ketcham, K. (1994). *The myth of repressed memory: False memories and allegations of sexual abuse.* New York: St. Martin's Press.

Lyotard, J.-F. (1984). *The postmodern condition: A report on knowledge.* Minneapolis: University of Minnesota Press.

McCown, W. G., Johnson, J. L., & Shure, M. B. (Eds.). (1993). *The impulsive client: Theory, research, and treatment.* Washington, DC: American Psychological Association.

Menzies, R. (1989). *Survival of the sanest: Order and disorder in a pretrial psychiatric clinic.* Toronto: University of Toronto Press.

Menzies, R., Chunn, D. E., & Webster, C. D. (1995). Risky business: The classification of dangerous people in the Canadian carceral enterprise. In N. Larsen (Ed.), *The Canadian criminal justice system: An issues approach to the administration of justice* (pp. 209–240). Toronto: Canadian Scholars' Press.

Menzies, R., & Webster, C. D. (1994). Faulty powers: The regulation of carceral and psychiatric subjects in the "post-therapeutic" community. In K. R. E. McCormick (Ed.), *Carceral contexts: Readings in control* (pp. 43–72). Toronto: Canadian Scholars' Press.

Menzies, R., Webster, C. D., & Hart, S. D. (1994). Observations on the rise of risk in psychology and law. In *Proceedings of the fifth symposium on Violence and Aggression* (pp. 91–106). Saskatoon, Saskatchewan: University of Saskatchewan Extension Press.

Menzies, R., Webster, C. D., McMain, S., Staley, S., & Scaglione, R. (1994). The dimensions of dangerousness revisited: Assessing forensic predictions about violence. *Law and Human Behavior, 18,* 1–28.

Menzies, R., Webster, C. D., & Sepejak, D. J. (1985). The dimensions of dangerousness: Evaluating the accuracy of psychometric predictions of violence among forensic patients. *Law and Human Behavior, 9,* 35–56.

Millar, T. P. (n.d.). *Adaptive moral deficiency syndrome.* Unpublished manuscript.

Millett, K. (1990). *The loony-bin trip.* New York: Simon & Schuster.

Mirowsky, J. (1990). Subjective boundaries and combinations in psychiatric diagnoses. *Journal of Mind and Behavior, 11,* 407–424.

Monahan, J., & Steadman, H. J. (Eds.). (1994). *Violence and mental disorder: Developments in risk assessment.* Chicago: University of Chicago Press.

Nicholson, L. (Ed.). (1990). *Feminism/postmodernism.* London: Routledge.

Pantony, K. L., & Caplan, P. J. (1991). Delusional dominating personality disorder: A modest proposal for identifying some consequences of rigid masculine socialization. *Canadian Psychology, 32,* 120–133.

Pfohl, S. J. (1978). *Predicting dangerousness: The social construction of psychiatric reality.* Lexington, MA: Lexington Books.

Plutchik, R., & van Praag, H. M. (1995). The nature of impulsivity: Definitions, ontology, genetics, and relations to aggression. In E. Hollander & D.J. Stein (Eds.), *Impulsivity and aggression* (pp. 7–24). Chichester, England: Wiley.

Prins, H. (1990). *Bizarre behaviours: Boundaries of psychiatric disorder.* London: Routledge.

Russell, D. (1995). *Women, madness and medicine.* Cambridge, England: Polity Press.

Scheff, T. J. (Ed.). (1975). *Labelling madness.* Englewood Cliffs, NJ: Prentice-Hall.

Schrag, P., & Divoky, D. (1975). *The myth of the hyperactive child.* New York: Pantheon.

Sedgwick, P. (1982). *Psycho politics.* New York: Harper & Row.

Segal, L. (1990). *Slow motion: Changing masculinities, changing men.* London: Virago.

Seidler, V. J. (1994*). Unreasonable men: Masculinity and social theory.* London: Routledge.

Showalter, E. (1987). *The female malady: Women, madness and English culture, 1830–1980.* London: Virago.

Szasz, T. S. (1994). *Cruel compassion: Psychiatric control of society's unwanted.* New York: Wiley.

Ussher, J. M. (1991). *Women's madness: Misogyny or mental illness?* Amherst: University of Massachusetts Press.

Webster, C. D., Harris, G. T., Rice, M. E., Cormier, C., & Quinsey, V. L. (1994). *The violence prediction scheme: Assessing dangerousness in high risk men.* Toronto: University of Toronto, Centre of Criminology.

Webster, C. D., Jackson, M. A., & Brunanski, D. M. (Eds.). (1994). *Impulsivity: New directions in research and clinical practice. Proceedings of a conference.* Vancouver, British Columbia: Simon Fraser University.

Webster, C. D., & Menzies, R. (1987). The clinical prediction of dangerousness. In D. N. Weisstub (Ed.), *Law and mental health: International perspectives* (Vol. 3, pp. 158–209). Elmsford, NY: Pergamon Press.

Webster, C. D., Menzies, R., & Jackson, M. A. (1982). *Clinical assessment before trial: Legal issues and mental disorder.* Toronto: Butterworths.

Wishnie, H. (1977). *The impulsive personality: Understanding people with destructive character disorders.* New York: Plenum Press.

Zimmerman, M. (1988). Why are we rushing to publish DSM-IV? *Archives of General Psychiatry, 45,* 1135–1138.

4

A Legal Perspective on the Concept of "Impulsivity"

JAMES R. P. OGLOFF

Strictly speaking, the words "impulse," "impulsive," and "impulsivity" do not have any specific meaning within the law. Indeed, the definition that *Black's Law Dictionary* (Black, 1979) offers for "impulse" does not differ much from the lay definition. *Black's* defines impulse as follows: "sudden urge or inclination; thrusting or impelling force within a person" (p. 682). Nonetheless, the law is replete with examples of how the concept of "impulsivity"—although it may not be termed as such—is used to develop legal principles, to carve out exceptions to legal rules, or even to increase the severity of punishment.

It would be impossible, within the confines of a single chapter, to provide a comprehensive overview of the use of the concept of impulsivity in the law. This task would be amply futile if one attempted to review the law across jurisdictions and countries. Therefore, two brief examples are first used here to highlight the variety of purposes impulsivity serves in the law. Then a review of the legal underpinnings of criminal responsibility is presented, as a foundation for the discussion of two criminal defenses that rely on impulsivity for their success: "irresistible impulse" and "automatism." Also, because the focus of the chapter is on the concept of impulsivity in the law, rather than on the state of the law in any given jurisdiction, examples are used from both Canadian and U.S. law, with some reference to British law.

TWO EXAMPLES OF IMPULSIVITY IN THE LAW

An example of how the law has relied upon impulsivity; in the case of impulsive statements, occurs in one of the traditional exceptions to the hearsay rule. Stated simply, "hearsay" occurs when witnesses testify about what another person has told them, rather than about what they have observed firsthand (Cleary, 1984; Delisle, 1993; Sopinka, Lederman, & Bryant, 1992). The rule exists because if a statement made by a third party is admitted into evidence at trial, there is no way to question the third party to determine the accuracy of the statement. As might be expected, though, many complicated exceptions to the hearsay rule exist. For our purposes, the one of interest is the traditional *"res gestae"* exception. Although more carefully refined now, the *res gestae* exception developed in common law to admit statements that might otherwise be hearsay if those statements were "spontaneous declarations" or "excited utterances" (Cleary, 1984). The rationale behind the *res gestae* exception is that statements made in haste, without time for careful thought and reflection, are probably truthful and therefore do not need to be subjected to scrutiny at trial. As we will see below, though, there are situations in the law when it is felt that a person whose behavior is impulsive presents a real danger to society and needs to be incarcerated.

Aside from evidentiary rules, the concept of impulsivity arises elsewhere in the legal system. In a rather bizarre and tragic case, *Regina v. Evans* (1991), a young man was convicted of brutally killing two women. The accused, Wesley Evans, was a young man who had suffered brain damage after being hit by a truck when he was 9 years old. When Evans was examined after having been charged, both a psychologist and a psychiatrist found that his IQ was in the borderline retarded range. Evans was not the suspect in the case initially. Instead, police suspected that his brother was responsible for the murders. The police arrested Evans on a marijuana charge, hoping that he would provide evidence against his brother. Although the police initially informed the accused of his right to counsel, Evans answered "no" when asked whether he understood his rights. Furthermore, when the police began to believe that Evans rather than his brother was responsible for the murders, they failed to advise him formally that he was being detained for murder; nor did they repeat that he had a right to counsel. During the long interrogation, Evans provided incriminating evidence, culminating in a confession to the murders. At trial, a jury found Evans guilty of two counts of first-degree murder. The primary evidence against him was the confession he gave to the police, admitting to having killed both women.

Evans appealed the guilty verdict, arguing that his right to liberty and counsel had been violated when the police did not formally inform him during his interrogation that they considered him a prime suspect in the case, and when they did not repeat the warning that he had the right to counsel. In upholding the conviction, the British Columbia Court of Appeal held that although there was a violation of Evans's rights, the evidence was compelling and suggested that Evans would harm others. Furthermore, the Court of Appeal believed that freeing Evans would bring the administration of justice into disrepute. In her decision, Madame Justice Southin (*Regina v. Evans*, 1988) wrote:

> Seventy-five years ago, Wesley Evans would have been hanged for these murders. Twenty-five years ago he would probably have had his death sentence commuted to life imprisonment. . . . (p. 564) Wesley Evans is a pathetic creature. . . . Society must be protected from those who are incapable of resisting the *impulse* to kill innocent strangers. (p. 568, emphasis added)

This example shows how concerned courts are with those people whose behaviors are uncontrollable or impulsive. Thus, in such situations, impulsivity may serve as an aggravating factor in guilt determinations and sentencing. It is interesting that in *Evans* the British Columbia Court of Appeal was apparently willing to "overlook" significant constitutional infractions in order to protect society from Evans's impulsive behavior.

To finish the story of the *Evans* case, it is important to note that the Supreme Court of Canada did not agree with the trial court or with the British Columbia Court of Appeal. In its decision, the Supreme Court quoted segments of the interrogation with the police, as well as a conversation Evans had with an undercover police officer who was placed in jail with him. The information shows that the police did not provide the necessary warnings, and that Evans apparently had no memory of the murders. When asked about the murders by the undercover police officer, Evans answered, "You know it's funny, I don't remember killing them. . . . Yeah. Usually I won't forget somein [*sic*] like that" (*Regina v. Evans*, 1991, p. 310). Furthermore, in a telephone conversation with his brother that the police tape-recorded, Evans again denied his guilt. Indeed, when asked by the undercover police officer why he confessed, Evans referred to the police pressure: He stated "they wouldn't give me a rest until I confessed. . . . So what else, what else was I gonna do . . . ?" (p. 310).

Taking all of the factors noted above into account, and writing for the majority of the Supreme Court, Madame Justice McLachlin noted:

> In all circumstances, the appellant's statements must be regarded as highly unreliable. It would be most unfair to convict him entirely on their strength. . . . In my view the violation of the accused's right to counsel in this case was highly serious. The police, despite knowledge of the appellant's deficient mental status and despite his statement to them that he did not understand his right to counsel, proceeded to subject him to a series of interviews and other investigative techniques. . . . Few things could be more calculated to bring the administration of justice into disrepute than to permit the imprisonment of a man without a fair trial. Nor, as a practical matter, can it be said that such

imprisonment would achieve the end sought by Southin J.A., namely, the prevention of further murders by the killer of Ms. Seto and Ms. Willems [the victims]. Only a conviction after a fair trial based on reliable evidence could give the public that assurance. . . . The conviction should be set aside and an acquittal entered. (pp. 310–312)

As this quotation suggests, contrary to the British Columbia Court of Appeal, the Supreme Court of Canada did not believe that Evans's "impulsive behavior" (if he did commit the murders) justified the liberties the police took with his constitutional rights during the course of the interrogation process.

As the examples above underscore, impulsivity arises under a number of circumstances in the legal system, and *res gestae* statements that are made impulsively are generally considered reliable. The British Columbia Court of Appeal decision in *Evans* shows that impulsive behavior is treated with considerable concern because it is felt that people cannot, by definition, control their impulses. What is interesting about these two examples, though, is that the law treats impulsivity quite consistently. The reason why impulsive statements are believed, and why impulsive behaviors are treated with great concern, is that the products of the impulsivity (i.e., the statements and behaviors) are believed to be somewhat beyond the control of the person.

Perhaps most interesting and best developed among the law's consideration of impulsivity, though, is the use of impulsivity as a criminal defense. Indeed, as the *Evans* case suggests, a defendant's being impulsive alone can increase a court's scrutiny of the defendant's behavior, rather than exculpating him or her. That is, courts are sensitive to the fact that a defendant who is impulsive will have difficulty controlling his or her behavior, and therefore is likely to pose a greater than ordinary risk to society. However, when impulsive behavior is coupled with mental illness, or when it is independent of an individual's conscious intent, impulsivity has been used as part of a criminal defense. I now present the underpinnings of criminal responsibility before turning to a discussion of those defenses that have incorporated impulsivity most directly: irresistible impulse and automatism.

THE FOUNDATION OF CRIMINAL RESPONSIBILITY

Much of the English-speaking world's legal system has been based on the principle of free will. The law assumes that people have control over their actions. As a result, if an individual commits an act that violates the law, the law holds the person responsible and punishes the person accordingly. Such sentiments can be found in the following passage, which was written in 1736 by the well-known English jurist Lord Hale:

> Man is naturally endowed with these two great faculties, understanding and liberty of will. . . . The consent of the will is that which renders human actions either commendable or culpable. . . . And because the liberty or choice of the will presupposeth an act of understanding to know the thing or action chosen by the will, it follows that, where there is a total defect of the understanding, there is not free act of the will. (Hale, 1736/1847, pp. 14–15)

Here, Lord Hale indicated that the concept of free will is linked to that of understanding or cognition. Indeed, as Hale wrote, the ability to exercise free will implies that one understands and intends what one is doing, and conversely, that, if one has a lack of understanding or intent, one's actions will not be caused by free will.

The logic expressed by Hale over 250 years ago was reflected in a decision by the Supreme Court of Canada in 1992. The Court in *Regina v. Parks* (1992) stated that "only those who act voluntarily with the requisite intent to commit an offense should be punished by criminal sanction" (p. 908). As this quotation implies, free will and intent are considered as inextricably entwined, rather than as separate concepts. Indeed, as the quote indicates, to hold an accused person responsible for his or her acts, the law now considers two fundamental elements. First, the law requires that the accused had the "*actus reus*" to commit the crime. To satisfy the *actus reus* requirement, the act that the accused committed must have been voluntary. Second, the law requires that the accused had the requisite "*mens rea*"—or criminal intent—to commit the act. The voluntariness requirement is known as the "volitional component" of criminal responsibility, and the criminal intent requirement is known as the "cognitive component." Therefore, before an accused person is convicted of an offense and punished, the prosecution must prove that the accused committed an illegal act voluntarily, and that he or she had intended to commit the act.

In regard to impulsive acts per se, it is clear that the law has never applied a blanket exoneration to acts that occurred impulsively. Rather, the law has concerned itself with the *cause* of the impulsivity. As we will see in the following brief review of the law, it is only when the criminal act occurs as a result of mental illness that the insanity defense will be successful. As the quote from the British Columbia Court of Appeal in the case of *Regina v. Evans* (1988) makes clear, rather than leading to an acquittal, impulsivity alone can serve to increase the severity of punishment. When used successfully as a defense, impulsivity must be combined with mental illness that either deprives an individual of the ability to understand the act (i.e., it affects the *mens rea*) or causes the individual to lose the ability to control his or her actions (i.e., it affects the *actus reus*). Indeed, the only two constants across specific insanity defense standards and jurisdictions are (1) that the person who committed that act was mentally ill at the time of the act, and (2) that the act occurred "impulsively." For the meaning of "impulsively" here, we can rely on the definition found in *Black's Law Dictionary* (1979). That is, the act must have occurred either as a result of a "sudden urge or inclination" or as a result of a "thrusting or impelling force within a person" (p. 682).

Figure 4.1 depicts the general way in which the law considers the relationship between determinism (or impulsive behavior) and mental disorder. Generally speaking, the more severe the mental disorder, the less likely it is that an individual will be found criminally responsible; it is assumed that the mental illness substantially incapacitates the accused's free will and produces deterministic or impulsive behavior (i.e., behavior that is unintentional or uncontrollable). As we will see later in the chapter, in the case of automatism (at least in Canada), a person need not even be mentally ill to be acquitted of an offense, as long as the offense occurred involuntarily.

Over the centuries, defenses have been developed in the law for acts committed without the requisite *actus reus* or *mens rea.* With respect to an individual's ability to form criminal intent, the defenses of "insanity" or "diminished capacity" have been developed. As we will see below, the insanity defense has traditionally focused on the cognitive component of criminal responsibility and is used when, as a result of mental illness, an individual either does not have the ability to understand the nature of his or her acts, or is not able to know or appreciate the difference between right and wrong. In addition, though, the "irresistible impulse" test was developed for the situation where, again as a result of mental illness, the defendant was unable to control his or her behavior.

The notion of "madness" can be traced far back in history; however, exculpating mentally ill people for their acts is a relatively recent phe-

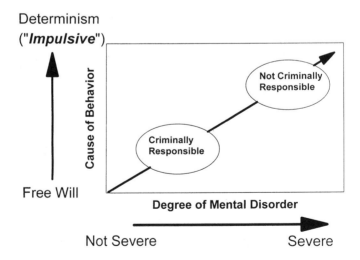

FIGURE 4.1. The law's view of the relationship between determinism (impulsive behavior) and mental disorder.

nomenon (Perlin, 1989; Walker, 1985). Although ancient Greeks and Romans recognized that some forms of mental illness may affect a person's behavior, Plato reported in 350 B.C. that the mentally ill and their families were held responsible for the actions of the mentally ill (Walker, 1985). Nonetheless, by the time the Digest of Justinian, a collection of the doctrines of Roman jurists, was compiled into volumes (about A.D. 230), it was held that "a madman [who] commit[s] homicide . . . is excused by the misfortune of his fate" (cited in Walker, 1985, p. 26). Apparently, it was believed that the mentally ill should be excused because they do not have the capacity to form the requisite *mens rea* for a criminal act and they are already punished by virtue of their mental condition (Walker, 1985). Thus, there appears to have been rather widespread belief that the mentally ill should not be generally held responsible for their actions.

The first recorded case of an individual's being acquitted by reason of insanity in English law occurred in 1505 (Walker, 1968). Simon and Aaronson (1988) note that by the end of the 16th century, "the doctrine of the lack of a guilty mind (or felonious intent)—and hence, lack of criminal responsibility—was well established" (p. 10).

By the 18th century, courts were developing "wild beast" standards for acquitting mentally ill offenders. For example, in 1724 an English jury was instructed that one acquitted for insanity must be "totally deprived of his understanding and memory, and doth not know what he is doing, no more than an infant, than a brute, or a wild beast" (*Rex v. Arnold*, 1724, pp. 764–765; see also Perlin, 1989; Walker, 1985).

Lord Hale (1736/1847), whose work has been cited above, was among the first legal commentators in modern times to focus rather extensively on the subject of the insanity defense (see also Low, Jeffries, & Bonnie, 1986). Regardless of the early attempts at determining whether insanity would be grounds for acquittal, and if so, what standard of insanity should be employed, no real progress was made towards developing a uniform standard of insanity until the nineteenth century. The modern "insanity test" approach to the insanity defense was established in the early part of the 19th century by the acquittals, by reason of insanity, of James Hadfield in 1800 (*Rex v. Hadfield*, 1820) and Daniel M'Naghten (*Regina v. M'Naghten*, 1843; see also Moran, 1985). Just as in the case of John W. Hinckley, Jr.'s attempted assassination of then-President Ronald Reagan in 1981 (*United States v. Hinckley*, 1981), the intended victims of Hadfield's and M'Naghten's assassination attempts were powerful government figures—King George IV and Prime Minister Sir Robert Peel of Great Britain, respectively. Also, like *Hinckley*, these cases have had a profound influence on the historical course of the insanity defense.

The elements that underlie the cognitive component of contemporary insanity defense statutes and cases are derived from perhaps the best-known case regarding the insanity defense—that of Daniel M'Naghten (*Regina v. M'Naghten*, 1843). Daniel M'Naghten attempted to kill Prime

Minister Sir Robert Peel, but mortally wounded Peel's private secretary instead, believing him to be Peel (Moran, 1981, 1985). Daniel M'Naghten's father was able to secure a well-financed defense, assembling "four of the most able barristers in London, nine prominent medical men, and eight lay witnesses from Glasgow, including four public officials" (Moran, 1985, pp. 37–38). With this backing, the jury acquitted Daniel M'Naghten because of his insanity. Just over 2 months after the decision in *M'Naghten* was made public, 15 common-law judges in Great Britain were summoned to the House of Lords to help determine the proper standard for criminal responsibility of the criminally insane. Fourteen of the judges agreed that essentially the same standard as that employed in *M'Naghten* was the correct legal standard (Moran, 1985). The opinion delivered included the *M'Naghten* rules, the essence of which is as follows:

> A person is presumed sane unless it can be clearly proven that, at the time of the committing of the act, the party accused was labouring under such a defect of reason, from disease of the mind, as not to know the nature and quality of the act he was doing; or, if he did know it, that he did not know he was doing what was wrong. (*Regina v. M'Naghten,* 1843, p. 203)

There are three main substantive elements of the *M'Naghten* standard. First, the decision maker must determine that the defendant was suffering from "a defect of reason, from disease of the mind." Today, these words are interpreted to mean that the defendant is suffering from a mental illness. Next, the decision maker must decide whether the evidence shows that the defendant did not "know the nature and quality of the act he was doing." Therefore, the defendant must not have understood exactly what he or she did. Finally, the *M'Naghten* standard also requires an inquiry to determine whether the defendant knew "he was doing what was wrong." Therefore, the defendant who understands his or her act, yet does not have the capability of knowing that the act was wrong, may also be acquitted under the *M'Naghten* test. In the context of the insanity defense, the word "wrong" in this element has been defined by different courts as meaning either "legally wrong" or "morally wrong." Because the final two elements require a subjective exploration of the defendant's thinking, the *M'Naghten* test is referred to as a "cognitive" test of insanity (e.g., Low et al., 1986). It is clear from a strict reading of the *M'Naghten* standard that there is no room for acquitting defendants whose *actions* are caused by a mental illness—even when those actions are impulses or uncontrollable urges—unless the individual also has the requisite cognitive deficits.

Almost immediately, the *M'Naghten* standard was employed in cases throughout Great Britain, its colonies, and the United States (Low et al., 1986). The substantive requirements of the *M'Naghten* rule are still being used by numerous jurisdictions around the world, almost half of the

United States, Canada, and of course Great Britain (Ogloff, 1993; Ogloff, Schweighofer, Turnbull, & Whittemore, 1992).

From the time it was introduced, however, the *M'Naghten* standard has been criticized (Hermann & Sor, 1983). Most criticisms have been launched against the purely cognitive focus of the *M'Naghten* standard (Hermann & Sor, 1983; Low et al., 1986; Melton, Petrila, Poythress, & Slobogin, 1987; Perlin, 1989; Schopp, 1989; Simon & Aaronson, 1988). Indeed, the concern has been that people whose mental illnesses impair their ability to control their behavior, but do not necessarily impair their cognitive processing, still will be found criminally responsible. From the standpoint of impulsivity, then, those people whose mental illnesses cause them to be impulsive and to engage in behavior beyond their control will not be acquitted for their criminal activities.

As a result of the criticisms and shortcomings of the *M'Naghten* standard, a number of alternative insanity standards have been developed over the years that provide for the acquittal of people whose mental illnesses prevent them from controlling their behavior (Simon & Aaronson, 1988). There is no room, or need, here to retrace the long history of the development of insanity defense standards. Rather, for our purposes it is sufficient to contrast the cognitive *M'Naghten* standard with the "volitional" standards, particularly the irresistible impulse test.

The most common standard currently in use in the United States[1]— apart from the *M'Naghten* standard—is the standard that was developed by the American Law Institute (ALI) and stated in its *Model Penal Code* (ALI, 1962). In drafting the "new" insanity defense standard, an ALI subcommittee attempted to redress the shortcomings of *M'Naghten* and other subsequent tests (Perlin, 1989). In so doing, the ALI subcommittee recognized that defendants could be found "not guilty by reason of insanity" (NGRI) for both cognitive and volitional reasons.[2] Thus, to some extent at least, the ALI rule incorporated some of the logic from the earlier insanity defense standards.

The ALI standard, as set out in Section 4.01 of the *Model Penal Code*, is as follows:

> (1) A person is not responsible for criminal conduct if at the time of such conduct as a result of mental disease or defect he lacks substantial capacity either to appreciate the criminality (wrongfulness) of his conduct or to conform his conduct to the requirements of law.
>
> (2) As used in this Article, the terms "mental disease or defect" do not include an abnormality manifested only by repeated criminal or otherwise anti-social conduct. (ALI, 1962, 4.01)

The ALI standard was the standard in force in the District of Columbia when John Hinckley, Jr., was tried.[3] So controversial was Hinckley's acquittal by reason of insanity that the U.S. Congress passed the Insanity

Defense Reform Act (IDRA) in 1984[4] (Committee of the Judiciary, U.S. Senate, 1982; Subcommittee on Criminal Justice, Committee of the Judiciary, House of Representatives, 1983, 1984; Subcommittee on Criminal Justice, Committee of the Judiciary, U.S. Senate, 1983). In essence, the IDRA had the effect of lopping off the volitional prong of the ALI rule—leaving it substantively like *M'Naghten,* with its focus on the defendant's cognitions for purposes of determining whether he or she should be found NGRI (Perlin, 1986, 1989). Now the substantive federal insanity test is whether the defendant "lacks capacity to appreciate the wrongfulness of his conduct." In addition, the mental disease or defect specified under the new standard must be "severe" (subcommittee on Criminal Justice, Committee of the Judiciary, U.S. Senate, 1984). Regardless of the specific standard, though, the ALI rule was specifically narrowed to eliminate the possibility of persons' being acquitted for a lack of ability to control their behavior. The implicit policy statement underlying the IDRA is that it is permissible to find a person NGRI if the person's mental illness causes cognitive deficits that produce bizarre behavior, but not if the mental illness produces bizarre behavior without significant concomitant cognitive deficits. As we will see next, the situation in Canada is quite different.

Canada's insanity defense standard, and that which is used by the majority of jurisdictions in the United States, is based on the traditional *M'Naghten* perspective (Ogloff, 1993; Ogloff, Schweighofer, Turnbull, & Whittemore, 1992). Section 16 of the *Criminal Code of Canada* provides for the "not criminally responsible on account of mental disorder" (NCRMD) defense (formerly the insanity defense, or NGRI). As revised most recently on February 4, 1992, it states that: "No person is criminally responsible for an act committed or an omission made while suffering from a mental disorder that rendered the person incapable of appreciating the nature and quality of the act or omission, or of knowing it was wrong" (Criminal Code, 1985). As it is written, this standard, like *M'Naghten,* is based on a purely cognitive inquiry—that is, whether the accused had the capacity to appreciate what he or she did, and whether it was wrong.

Having provided some basic information about the development of the insanity defense, and the various standards that exist, I turn to a specific discussion of impulsivity as a criminal defense. Indeed, the two defenses discussed—the irresistible impulse and automatism—both employ the concept of impulsivity.

IMPULSIVITY AS A CRIMINAL DEFENSE

The Irresistible Impulse Test

Although the insanity defense standards that have emerged in Canada, the United States, and Great Britain have largely focused on an analysis of the accused's cognitive capacities, this perspective has been criticized on and off for over 150 years. Critics have noted that the exclusive focus on the accused's cognitive abilities disregards the volitional components of behavior. As a result, courts have developed alternative tests that focus on the accused's (in)ability to resist impulses.

According to Tollefson and Starkman (1993), the concept that delusions could deprive a person of the ability to control his or her behavior was made popular by Dr. Isaac Ray in his book *A Treatise on the Medical Jurisprudence of Insanity* (1838). In fact, it was a competing notion to that ultimately adopted in the *M'Naghten* rule. The concept of irresistible impulse was argued by defense counsel in Great Britain in a number of cases in the 1840s. In the 1840 case of *Regina v. Oxford,* an English court held that "if some controlling disease was, in truth, the acting power within him which he could not resist, then he will not be responsible" (p. 950).

A little-mentioned fact is that the irresistible impulse test was even argued as part of the defense's case in the trial of *M'Naghten* (*The Queen against Daniel McNaughton,* 1843). Indeed, M'Naghten's lawyer argued that the test for insanity should be whether the accused was "incapable of judging between right and wrong, or of exercising that self-control and dominion, without which the knowledge of right and wrong would become vague and useless" (pp. 919, 922–923, as cited by Tollefson & Starkman, 1993, p. 38). The lack of success of the irresistible impulse argument was apparent in the *M'Naghten* case when Lord Chief Justice Tindal failed to provide any reference to "incapacity to control" as a test for insanity (see Tollefson & Starkman, 1993). Although a detailed account is beyond the scope of this chapter, the concept of irresistible impulse emerged occasionally in Great Britain from the time of *M'Naghten* to at least the 1950s (Tollefson & Starkman, 1993). Though the concept of irresistible impulse was not employed successfully as an independent insanity test, "it was treated by the English courts as highly relevant to the question of whether the accused was capable of knowing that his act was wrong" (Tollefson & Starkman, 1993, p. 39).

In the United States, the irresistible impulse test was given birth by the Alabama Supreme Court in *Parsons v. State* (1886), and later was adopted—but then rejected—in at least 18 U.S. jurisdictions (Perlin, 1989). In the general form, the irresistible impulse test provided for defendants' acquittal if their mental disorder caused them to experience an "irresistible and uncontrollable impulse to commit the offense, even if he remained able to understand the nature of the offense and its wrongfulness" (Dix, 1984, p. 7). According to Goldstein (1967), the irresistible impulse test is based on four assumptions:

> First, that there are mental diseases which impair volition or self-control, even while cognition remains relatively unimpaired; second, that the use of *M'Naghten* alone results in findings that persons suffering from such diseases are not insane; third, that the law should make the insanity defense available

to persons who are unable to control their actions, just as it does to those who fit *M'Naghten*; fourth, no matter how broadly *M'Naghten* is construed, there will remain areas of serious disorder which it will not reach. (p. 67)

Although the irresistible impulse test enjoyed relative success early on in the United States, it was eventually used to supplement cognitive insanity tests, and ultimately was rejected as a free-standing insanity defense standard. The failure of the defense occurred as a result of its impractical nature. Perlin (1989) has raised a number of questions about the irresistible impulse test. First, how is one ever to distinguish an "irresistible impulse" from an impulse that merely is not resisted? Second, the test raises niggling questions about human nature. That is, others have asked, should a person be relieved of responsibility for a lack of self-control even if his or her cognitive understanding is not impaired?

The irresistible impulse test has never been endorsed explicitly by Canadian courts. In fact, as early as 1908 it was explicitly rejected in Canada (*Rex v. Creighton*, 1908). More recently, though, courts have acknowledged that under some circumstances, volitional impairment caused by mental illness may satisfy the criteria of Section 16 of the *Criminal Code of Canada* (the NGRI/NCRMD provision). The Supreme Court of Canada's recognition of an "irresistible impulse" perhaps began with Mr. Justice Hall's dissenting opinion in *Regina v. Borg* (1969). In that dissent, Hall wrote that "if there is medical evidence of disease of the mind as there was here and yet the only symptoms of that disease of the mind are irresistible impulses, the jury may conclude that the accused is insane" (p. 570). The Supreme Court visited this matter again in *Regina v. Abbey* (1982), where Chief Justice Dickson wrote:

Both the majority and minority opinion in *Regina v. Borg* [1969] S.C.R. 551, deny the existence of a defense as such of irresistible impulse. Both the majority and minority opinions in *Borg*, however, recognize that irresistible impulse may be a symptom or manifestation of a disease of the mind which may give rise to a defense of insanity. (p. 561)

Thus, the concept of irresistible impulse may form part of the basis for an insanity defense in Canada only if the irresistible impulse is accompanied by cognitive impairment, as specified in the NCRMD defense.

As the overview of the irresistible impulse standard shows, the defense was most successful in the United States, but has had some influence on the interpretation of the insanity defense standards employed in Great Britain and Canada. In any case, the development of the concept of irresistible impulse shows clearly that the law has considered an inability to control one's behavior as a successful criminal defense—when the volitional incapacity or irresistible impulse is caused by a mental illness. Apart from irresistible impulses caused by mental illness, impulses that occur independently of an individual's conscious intent have also led to acquittals in Canada. The "automatism" defense, as it has been employed in Canada, is described below.

The Automatism Test

In the small hours of the morning of May 24, 1987, Kenneth James Parks, aged 23, got into his car and drove some 23 kilometers on highways around Toronto until he finally arrived at the home of his parents-in-law. There, he savagely beat his mother-in-law and father-in-law with a tire iron and stabbed them with a knife. Eventually, he was charged with the murder of his mother-in-law and with the attempted murder of his father-in-law. Although tragic, the facts of the case are not particularly noteworthy—except for the fact that Parks was asleep during the entire episode.

> Immediately after the incident, Parks got back into his car and drove to the nearby police station where he told the police: "I just killed someone with my bare hands; Oh my God, I just killed someone; I've just killed two people; My God, I've just killed two people with my hands; My God, I've just killed two people. My hands; I just killed two people. I killed them; I just killed two people; I've just killed my mother- and father-in-law. I stabbed and beat them to death. It's all my fault." (*Regina v. Parks*, 1992, p. 879)

At trial, Parks raised the defense of automatism. All of the defense's medical experts at trial agreed that Parks was asleep during the entire episode. The experts also agreed that Parks did not have a mental disorder and that he would not repeat his dangerous acts again in his sleep, since there was no known case of repeated violence by the same sleepwalker. A jury acquitted Parks of the charges, and his acquittal was upheld by both the Ontario Court of Appeal and the Supreme Court of Canada. The courts accepted that sleepwalking is genuine automatism and is not caused by a mental disorder.

As noted above, the concept of irresistible impulse has had variable success in Canada as either a free-standing or a supplementary insanity defense standard. However, a different and rather distinctive concept developed in Canada to handle cases in which it was believed that an individual did not act voluntarily when committing a criminal act (Jang & Coles, 1995). Whereas the insanity defense is thought to address the *mens rea* element, automatism is used to challenge or rebut the *actus reus* requirement. Unlike irresistible impulse, in Canada automatism may be considered a free-standing defense that is separate from insanity or NCRMD. The Supreme Court of Canada in *Regina v. Rabey* (1980) endorsed a definition of automatism:

> Automatism is a term used to describe unconscious, involuntary behaviour, the state of a person who, though capable of action, is not conscious of what

he is doing. It means an unconscious, involuntary act, where the mind does
not go with what is being done. (p. 518)

From the Court's definition of automatism, it is clear that automatism
involves impulsivity. Unlike the irresistible impulse test, though, in which
mental illness must lead to uncontrollable behavior, automatism does not
require that a person be mentally ill. Instead, the person must be "unconscious" or have no awareness of the act. With both the irresistible impulse
and automatism, the act occurs as a result of an uncontrollable impulse.

As just noted, automatism does not require that a person be mentally
ill.[5] A further distinction has been made, however, between insane and
noninsane automatism. Indeed, this was an important concern in the *Parks*
case, reviewed above. In *Parks*, the defense argued that sleepwalking is
not caused by a mental disease, and that the behavior accompanied by
sleepwalking, in fact, is both unconscious and automatic. By contrast, the
Crown (the prosecution) attempted to prove that sleepwalking stems
from a disease of the mind, and as a result that the only proper defense
for sleepwalking is really the insanity defense. Thus, insane automatism
is considered to be automatism that is brought on by a disease of the mind
(or internal causes unique to the individual in question). By contrast,
noninsane automatism is unconscious and involuntary behavior that is
not brought on by a disease of the mind (but may be caused by external
factor that, if experienced by other individuals, may produce similar
behavioral sequelae).

Although the distinction between insane and noninsane automatism
may seem picayune and academic, it is in fact very important with respect
to the consequences of the outcome of the defense. Indeed, if, as in the
Parks case, the automatism is considered to be of the noninsane variety,
then the accused may be acquitted outright. That is, the accused is
absolutely free, beyond the control of the state. By contrast, if the unconscious, involuntary behavior is considered to be insane automatism, then
the accused may be found NCRMD; the question of his or her disposition
then comes under the control of the state, as provided for in the *Criminal
Code of Canada*.

CONCLUSIONS

As this chapter indicates, the concept of impulsivity has received considerable attention in the law, and the results have often varied. Impulsive
behavior alone may almost serve as an aggravating factor in guilt determinations and sentencing. However, impulsive or uncontrollable behavior has also developed as a challenge or defense to a criminal act. If, on
the one hand, the behavior was caused by a disease of the mind, and the
cognitive requirements of the insanity defense are satisfied, an accused

person may be found NGRI/NCRMD, regardless of whether the act, strictly speaking, is considered to be an irresistible impulse, or insane automatism, depending on the jurisdiction. By contrast, if the accused's behavior was unconscious and involuntary (truly impulsive), then the defense of noninsane automatism may be raised; if this is successful, the accused may be acquitted outright.

It is beyond the scope of this chapter to address the multitude of psychological questions that arise from this complicated situation. (For example, how do we distinguish "involuntary" behavior from that which is "unintended"? Even if we assume that an individual cannot consciously control his or her behavior, does that in any way adequately explain the behavior that occurs?) However, it seems appropriate to briefly discuss one of the questions that is more centrally related to the volitional insanity standards and the irresistible impulse test. The British and Canadian cases, as well as some of the commentary concerning the irresistible impulse standard employed in the United States, raise an interesting question: Can "irresistible impulses" exist without some considerable degree of cognitive impairment, and, if so, to what extent? As it was employed in the United States, the irresistible impulse test was quite separate from the cognitive *M'Naghten* standard. In fact, some jurisdictions adopted both the irresistible impulse test and the *M'Naghten* test. This suggests that the law considered impulses or volitional impairment as separate, at least in some circumstances, from cognitive factors or impairment. By contrast, courts in Canada have generally refused to adopt the irresistible impulse test as an independent defense. To this day, the insanity defense in force in Canada does not include a statutory provision for volitional impairment. Nonetheless, courts have interpreted the *M'Naghten*-based standards liberally enough to include volitional impairment (e.g., *Regina v. Abbey*, 1982). Thus, it would appear that courts in Canada have considered volitional and cognitive impairments as difficult to separate, at the very least.

The apparent confusion on the part of the courts and legislatures, insofar as they consider the nexus between volitional and cognitive impairment, has received relatively little attention from mental health professionals. This is surprising, because this matter lies at the heart of one of the key distinctions between law and psychology. Indeed, Carson (1995) writes that

> lawyers believe that people have "free will" whether to commit a criminal act, and . . . psychologists believe that people are "determined" into behaving in particular ways, including criminal behaviour, whether through social background, learned responses or heredity. If a person's behaviour is not "voluntary" then, the law agrees the actor commits no crime. But what is the nature of this "voluntariness," is it a denial of the *mens rea*, the *actus reus*, causation, or does its absence constitute a defense? (p. 279)

Following from Carson's description above, it is clear that we are far from being able to address the difficult questions that arise from the law in this area. However, Rogers (1987) has noted that, from a psychological perspective, there is always a cognitive component to an impulse. A similar conclusion appears to have been drawn by the bar and by psychiatry. Indeed, the American Bar Association and the American Psychiatric Association have written that it is impossible to determine whether an act was an irresistible impulse (the same could be said for automatism) (Schopp, 1989). As a result of this position, both associations have supported *M'Naghten*-like insanity standards that place the emphasis of the inquiry on whether the accused suffered cognitive impairment to the extent necessary to prevent the person from appreciating the wrongfulness of his or her act.[6] It would be useful for researchers to focus more attention on this important matter.

As the discussion in this chapter (and some of the more bizarre cases that have occurred) shows, it is important that the law, in its effort to distinguish forms of behavior and cognition, does not veer too far from the path of what is known or even plausible psychologically. Much of the discussion of irresistible impulses and insane or noninsane automatism really boils down to how broadly one construes the legal question of what is a mental disorder. This explains the fact that a person in Canada can be acquitted for acts committed when sleepwalking (*Regina v. Parks*, 1992), while in Britain the same person may be found "legally insane" (*Regina v. Burgess*, 1991). Such arbitrary distinctions are ill founded intellectually and, given the difference in disposition, have serious implications both for accused persons and for the societies in which they live. By further exploring "impulsive behavior" and its causes and effects, perhaps we can come to develop a more consistent and valid method of determining the extent to which people are responsible for their criminal behavior.

ACKNOWLEDGMENTS

This chapter was completed during a sabbatical spent in the Department of Mental Health Law and Policy at the Florida Mental Health Institute at the University of South Florida. I am grateful to Professor John Petrila and the faculty and staff there for their support and assistance with the preparation of the chapter.

NOTES

1. It should be noted that in the United States each state has its own criminal code and insanity defense standard, whereas in Canada and England there is one standard that is employed nationwide.

2. In formulating the ALI insanity test, members of the ALI relied on language similar to that proposed by the British Royal Commission on Capital Punishment (Goldstein, 1967).

3. D.C. Code Ann. 24-301 (1981). As discussed above, the D.C. Code has since been revised.

4. 18 U.S.C. 20 (1986 Supp.).

5. It is interesting to note briefly that in England and Wales—in contrast to the *Parks* case in Canada—acts committed during sleepwalking, while in a diabetic coma, or during epileptic seizures have been considered "insane automatism" (see *Regina v. Burgess*, 1991; *Regina v. Hennessey*, 1989; and *Regina v. Sullivan*, 1984, respectively). In these cases, which employed the insanity standard based on *M'Naghten*, the accused were considered to have a "disease of the mind."

6. It is worth noting here that this rather academic discussion may have little effect on what occurs in practice. In fact, both field and analogue studies suggest that jurors have considerable difficulty comprehending insanity defense standards, and that changes in the standards do not produce changes in verdicts (see Ogloff, 1991; Ogloff et al., 1992); they also indicate that changes in insanity standards in jurisdictions do not generally produce significant changes in insanity acquittal rates (Ogloff et al., 1992).

REFERENCES

American Law Institute (ALI). (1962). *Model penal code: Proposed official draft.* Philadelphia: Author.

Black, H. C. (1979). *Black's law dictionary.* St. Paul, MN: West.

Carson, D. (1995). Criminal responsibility. In R. Bull & D. Carson (Eds.), *Handbook of psychology in legal contexts* (pp. 277–314). Chichester, England: Wiley.

Cleary, E. W. (Ed.). (1984). *McCormick on evidence* (3rd ed.). St. Paul, MN: West.

Committee on the Judiciary, U.S. Senate. (1982). *The insanity defense* (Serial No. J-97-126). Washington, DC: U.S. Government Printing Office.

Criminal Code. (1985). *Revised Statutes of Canada,* ch. C-46.

Delisle, R. J. (1993). *Evidence: Principles and problems* (3rd ed.). Toronto: Carswell.

Dix, G. (1984). Criminal responsibility and mental impairment in American criminal law: Response to the Hinckley acquittal in historical perspective. In D. Weisstub (Ed.), *Law and mental health: International perspectives* (Vol. 1, pp. 1–44). Elmsford, NY: Pergamon Press.

Goldstein, A. (1967). *The insanity defense.* New Haven, CT: Yale University Press.

Hale, M. (1847). *The history of pleas of the Crown.* Philadelphia: R. H. Small. (Original work published 1736)

Hermann, D. H. J., & Sor, Y. S. (1983). Convicting or confining? Alternative directions in insanity defense reform: Guilty but mentally ill versus new rules for release of insanity acquittees. *Brigham Young University Law Review, 1983,* 499–638.

Jang, D., & Coles, E. M. (1995). The evolution and definition of the concept of "automatism" in Canadian case law. *International Journal of Medicine and Law, 14,* 221–238.

Low, P. W., Jeffries, J. C., & Bonnie, R. J. (1986). *The trial of John W. Hinckley, Jr.: A case study in the insanity defense.* Mineola, NY: Foundation Press.

Melton, G. B., Petrila, J., Poythress, N. G., & Slobogin, C. (1987). *Psychological evaluations for the courts: A handbook for mental health professionals and lawyers.* New York: Guilford Press.

Moran, R. (1981). *Knowing right from wrong: The insanity defense of Daniel McNaughton.* New York: Macmillan/Free Press.

Moran, R. (1985). The modern foundation for the insanity defense: The cases of James Hadfield (1800) and Daniel McNaughtan (1843). *Annals of the American Academy of Political and Social Science, 477,* 31–42.

Ogloff, J. R. P. (1991). A comparison of insanity defense standards on juror decision-making. *Law and Human Behavior, 15,* 509–531.

Ogloff, J. R. P. (1993). Juror decision making and the insanity defense. In N. J. Castellan (Ed.), *Individual and group decision making: Current issues* (pp. 167–201). Hillsdale, NJ: Erlbaum.

Ogloff, J. R. P., Schweighofer, A., Turnbull, S., & Whittemore, K. (1992). Empirical research and the insanity defense: How much do we really know? In J. R. P. Ogloff (Ed.), *Psychology and law: The broadening of the discipline* (pp. 171–210). Durham, NC: Carolina Academic Press.

Parsons v. State, 81 Ala. 577, 2 So. 854 (1886).

Perlin, M. L. (1986). The things we do for love: John Hinckley's trial and the future of the insanity defense in the federal courts. *New York Law School Law Review, 30,* 857–875.

Perlin, M. L. (1989). *Mental disability law: Civil and criminal.* Charlottesville, VA: Mitchie.

Ray, I. (1838). *A treatise on the medical jurisprudence of insanity.* Boston: Little, Brown.

Regina v. Abbey, [1982] 2 S.C.R. 24.

Regina v. Borg, [1969] S.C.R. 551.

Regina v. Burgess, [1991] 2 Q.B. 92.

Regina v. Evans (1988), 45 C.C.C. (3d) 523 (B.C.C.A.).

Regina v. Evans (1991), 63 C.C.C. (3d) 289 (S.C.C.).

Regina v. Hennessey, [1989] 2 All E.R. 9.

Regina v. M'Naghten, 10 Cl. and F. 200, 8 Eng. Rep. 718 (1843).

Regina v. Oxford, 173 Eng. Rep. 941 (1840).

Regina v. Parks, [1992] 2 S.C.R. 871.

Regina v. Sullivan, [1984] A.C. 156.

Regina v. Rabey, [1980] 2 S.C.R. 513.

Rex v. Arnold, 16 How. St. Tr. 694 (1724).

Rex v. Creighton (1908), 14 C.C.C 349.

Rex v. Hadfield, 27 St. Tr. 1281, 1312–1315 (1820).

Rogers, R. (1987). The APA position on the insanity defense: Empiricism vs. emotionalism. *American Psychologist, 42,* 840–848.

Schopp, R. (1989). Depression, the insanity defense, and civil commitment: Foundations in autonomy and responsibility. *International Journal of Law and Psychiatry, 12,* 81–98.

Simon, R. J., & Aaronson, D. E. (1988). *The insanity defense: A critical assessment of law and policy in the post-Hinckley era.* New York: Praeger.

Sopinka, J., Lederman, S., & Bryant, A. (1992). *The law of evidence in Canada.* Toronto: Butterworths.

Subcommittee on Criminal Justice, Committee of the Judiciary, U.S. House of Representatives. (1983). *Insanity defense in federal courts* (Serial No. 134). Washington, DC: U.S. Government Printing Office.

Subcommittee on Criminal Justice, Committee of the Judiciary, U.S. House of Representatives. (1984). *Reform of the federal insanity defense* (Serial No. 21). Washington, DC: U.S. Government Printing Office.

Subcommittee on Criminal Law, Committee of the Judiciary, U.S. Senate. (1983). *Limiting the insanity defense* (Serial No. J-97-122). Washington, DC: U.S. Government Printing Office.

The Queen against Daniel McNaughton, (1843). 4 St. Tr. (N.S.) 847.

Tollefson, E. A., & Starkman, B. (1993). *Mental disorder in criminal proceedings.* Toronto: Carswell.

United States v. Hinckley, 525 F. Suppl. 1342 (D.D.C. 1981).

Walker, N. (1968). *Crime and insanity in England: Vol. 1. The historical perspective.* Edinburgh: Edinburgh University Press.

Walker, N. (1985). The insanity defense before 1800. *Annals of the American Academy of Political and Social Science, 477,* 25–30.

5

A Cybernautical Perspective on Impulsivity and Addiction

J. MAXWELL CLARK

The present chapter departs somewhat from the traditional format for scholarly papers, in that it is a largely speculative piece on an emerging social phenomenon that may prove to be a vehicle for emancipation or enslavement. The computer interface, "cyberspace," and now "virtual reality" (VR) are part of the vanguard of innovative technologies that are rapidly revolutionizing the structure of human social organization. The emancipatory potential of this new technology is considerable and is a subject of fervent global discourse. Of course, much of the discussion is distinctly utopian in vision, and is thus largely responsible for inciting the engines of innovation. In this chapter, however, I would like to address the latter potential. It is a notion that, for the most part, has received little attention in cybernetic circles, but has become a recurring theme for a new genre of dystopian science fiction. In a general sense, it is the old notion of the (intelligence) machine's becoming master of its creators. However, herein I do not wish to proffer speculation in such a hypothetical domain, which assumes artificial intelligences and technology well beyond our current understanding; rather, I would like to consider this notion in contemporary terms—that is, without anthropomorphisms, and in light of current technological capabilities and forecasts.

Like any other novel, seemingly emancipatory vehicle, cyberspace has the potential for misuse, overreliance, and so forth. Certainly, its unique attributes are such that we must expect such abuses; however, the potential also exists for more extreme behaviors, notably impulsivity and addiction. Cursory consideration of this potential reveals at least the following. At present, these are frontier technologies (i.e., largely unexplored and ripe for exploitation). And, perhaps, like the homesteaders of the recent past, many of today's "cybernauts" (i.e., operators) are wont to leave their mark or make their claim in this frontier with a kind of "anything goes" abandon. As I have said, cyberspace is uniquely configured for just such possibilities. When immersed in these environments, operators are afforded anonymity, a sense of depersonalization (stronger in the case of VR), and largely uninhibited capabilities for accessing and manipulating information. As decades of research on conformity and group dynamics can attest, all of these are among the classic preconditions for nonconforming and impulsive behavior. These technologies stand to give rise to a new breed of nonconformity—one that is distinctly anonymous, indirect, and seductive. In fact, avenues of nonconformity already abound in these environments, as evidenced in the cases of hacking, "compuporn," and organized "hate" networks, among others. One has only to name one's brand of social deviance, and chances are that it either is out there already or soon will be.

To appreciate the potential verity of this proposition, let us consider an example from the emergent industry of VR. Rather than speaking broadly of impulsivity and addiction in VR *sui generis,* this chapter concentrates chiefly on an aspect of VR that is currently a hotbed of discussion and a most likely candidate for the behaviors described above. The particular aspect is "virtual sex." However, in order to come to terms with the manifold factors that may give rise to such behaviors and the production of such technology, it would be wise to begin this meditation with a consideration of the effects of the development of technology upon both the individual and humanity as a whole.

SOME PRELIMINARY REMARKS ON TECHNOLOGY AND VIRTUAL REALITY

For about the last 10,000 years, the human species has been undergoing a transformational phase in its evolutionary history. With the emergence of symbolic communication (i.e., language), strictly biological evolution has been superseded by an evolution in understanding, knowledge, or information more generally. The noted physicist Stephen W. Hawking (1993) has referred to this last 10,000 years of human history as the "external transmission" phase of human evolution; although DNA has changed little in this time, human experiential knowledge has progressed considerably. The last 300 years, in particular, have been witness to a near-exponential acceleration in the rate of information acquisition. Whereas biological evolution has proceeded within a time span of hundreds of thousands of years, the "information evolution" has arguably been reduced to a margin of approximately 50 years or less. (This figure is intended to reflect, in the present century, the appearance of revolutionary technological innovations.) The significance of the preceding statement is neatly exemplified by the following observation. As Hawking has noted, it has been suggested that approximately 100 million bits of information are contained in the human genes (1 bit being equivalent, in this example, to the answer of a yes–no question), while the Cambridge University library alone contains approximately 10 quadrillion bits of information. The near-incomprehensibility of this figure is compounded by the recognition that it is neither fixed nor limited to Cambridge University. Rather, information is being accumulated and shared at a tremendous rate at points around the globe each day.

If the present state of human evolution, technological or otherwise, would seem not to be wholly indicative of a species in its formative stages of development, then perhaps it is fair to say that humanity has reached its adolescence. This particular ontogenetic phase is marked by quite rapid and profound cognitive and biological changes, among others. It is also marked by an additional distinctive characteristic. The psychologist Erik Erikson (1982) observed that adolescence is a critical period for identity formation. During this time, individuals come to consolidate a working identity for themselves—one that integrates private and public definitions, as well as social and physiological demands. The psychological and physiological rigors of this period, however, make the process of identity achievement difficult. Consequently, individuals are prone to experience "identity diffusion" or an "identity crisis" (i.e., a failure to achieve an integrated sense of identity). Although Erikson considered adolescence a critical period for identity formation, he did not mean to say that it is fixed at this period alone; rather, in his view, identity achievement is a process that is continually revised throughout the course of the lifespan. By extension, identity diffusion and identity crisis may be (re)experienced at different points throughout life, depending on an individual's unique biopsychosocial status. Sometimes an identity crisis may be waylaid, however, with the adoption of what Erikson called a "negative identity." This is essentially an identity that does not meet personal and social prescriptions for health, productivity, commitment, or the like. Delinquency and addictions are typical negative identities. The various roles offered individuals in these antiestablishment subcultures often provide a ready-made sense of identity.

An additional point may serve to lend further credence to the "adolescence" analogy and the accompanying discussion of identity formation. As noted above, I think that this analogy and the discussion of identity formation may be suitably applied to our present state of development as a species. Numerous scholars have observed that humanity is currently traversing the gap between what I call a subjective world view and the purely objective world view of science. Auguste Comte, writing in the 19th century, made this observation in terms of metaphysical belief systems' yielding to a positivist (i.e., scientific) belief system; similarly, in the present day, technology aficionados, having fully embraced the scientific ethos, are now speaking of a transition from the "digital age" to the "virtual age" or "cyber-age" (i.e., from interface to cyberspace). In the present case, the vanguard ushering in this (re)evolutionary transition is technology. At present, the theoretical potential of this new technology is "virtually" unbounded; whatever its potential applications, it will require us to reconceptualize our most fundamental definitions of what it means to be human (just how is discussed shortly). The point to be made here is that technology is progressing at such a rate that it is almost requiring individuals to revise and reintegrate themselves with each new development. A difficulty or failure to do so may thus result in an identity crisis and the adoption of a negative identity.

In scientific circles, VR technology is being spoken of in somewhat Nietzschean terms as providing "the bridge over the abyss"—that is, as providing the material means by which humanity will become superhuman, or at least take its next evolutionary leap. And what does this leap entail, but a merging or direct interaction with pure information? This aspect of VR technology and its implications for human development are discussed briefly in what follows.

If the preceding statement regarding direct interaction between humans and information sounds vaguely Platonic to the reader, then he or she may not be far from the truth. One writer, Michael Heim (1993), has suggested that VR or cyberspace is the embodiment of Platonism. Consider Plato's metaphor of the cave, for example. In this story, Plato described the fate of people caught in the prison of corporeality. With their attention fixed upon the flickering shadows cast by a physical fire, the prisoners take these images (i.e., sensory objects) to be the highest and most interesting reality. Only when they are able to break free of their corporeal bonds, and thus leave the cave, do they come to perceive the real forms of things—things palpable not to the physical eye but to the mind's eye. In Plato's terms, this is the universal, intelligible world; it is a realm of active thought. In this realm truth is laid bare, stripped of the imprecise and distorted raiment given by the physical senses. As Plato also wrote, the way to this higher truth is not open to all. Formal training, education, is needed to redirect one's gaze beyond the superficial sensory realm; once one is trained, love (Eros) will guide the mind to the forms of the intellect. In VR the user, or cybernaut, is very much lost to the trappings of the phenomenal world and is instead immersed in a world of digitized forms—a landscape of pure information.

It should be noted that cyberspace is to be considered Platonic not in a literal sense, but in a distinctly modern and empirical sense. In cyberspace, information does not exist as pure concepts or formulas, but as proceeding from such and represented as well-formed cyberspatial entities. In essence, what VR does is take information and translate it into empirical referents that otherwise seem to possess the ideality of Plato's forms. As Heim (1993) writes, "the mathematical machine [the computer] uses a digital mold to reconstitute the mass of empirical material so that human consciousness can enjoy an integrity in the empirical data that would never have been possible before computers" (p. 89). Nowhere but in VR is one quite literally treated to landscapes of pure information. Besides constituting an ontological shift, VR also carries implications for knowledge production and for our relationship with our bodies in particular.

In the Western scientific tradition, the pursuit and acquisition of knowledge have typically been the provinces of the intellect, quite apart from the body. Knowledge has generally been gained through a passive cognitive process of taking in new information and making associations with old, but now VR promises to change all that. Its promise lies in its ability to objectify concepts and empirical data so that they are more readily tangible to the physical senses. For example, in synthesizing new medicines, chemists are now able to analyze the consequences of various molecular combinations through VR simulations. They are thus able to *feel* whether certain molecules are attractive or repellent to one another. Similarly, many physicians are developing bold new surgical techniques via experimental "virtual surgery" simulations. Moreover, in some cases, VR technology is able to place a physician inside the body of a patient at the site of a potential difficulty. The medium of VR would thus seem to hold profound implications for the representation of knowledge in terms of strictly abstracted symbols. In fact, one of the most pressing questions surrounding the advent of VR technology is that it threatens to do away with this practice altogether. Computers are already being assigned the task of processing hard data, leaving individuals free to explore the results for patterns, differences, and so forth. VR takes this one step further by allowing individuals to interact directly with the information. Thus, "knowing" may no longer be the exclusive province of cognition; feeling may come to play an equally integral role in the production of knowledge. In this way, mind and body truly become synchronous. That is to say, they become synchronous in their ability to interact with the digital environment. However, our own experience of our actions (i.e., self-reference) is likely to be challenged, if not rendered superfluous. Self–object distinctions may not be so clear-cut in cyberspace, because of the sheer computing challenge of creating convincing personal representations. In the absence of such boundaries, what may we suppose will become of personal identity, and what ramifications will this have for behavior?

Having a physical body makes each of us distinct from others. It is the most immediately tangible referent of our identity and individuality. In cyberspace, however, the issue of identity is somewhat vague and undefined. Consequently, the quality of human interaction may also become moot. In the virtual environment, we can exist in either a disembodied or a cyberspatial form. Whatever the case, as Heim (1993) has noted, we need reveal "only as much of ourselves as we mentally wish to reveal. Bodily contact becomes optional; [one] need never stand face-to-face with other members of the virtual community. [One] can live [one's] own separate existence without ever physically meeting another person" (p. 100). The sheath of anonymity and impersonality afforded to individuals in VR may present serious moral and ethical implications. The veritable freedom of the virtual environment, for example, could foster in individuals a kind of contempt for corporeality, for fleshly existence. Consequently, such simple human virtues as respect, warmth, and compassion for others may conceivably languish in cyberspace; so too may responsibility for one's actions. This theme is certainly echoed in William Gibson's (1984) novel *Neuromancer,* the seminal science fiction work on the future of VR. In the story, the protagonist, a VR addict, despairs at the prospects of not being able to enter cyberspace: "For Case, who'd lived for the bodiless exultation of cyberspace, it was the Fall. In the bars he'd frequented as a [cyberspace] hotshot, the elite stance involved a certain relaxed contempt for the flesh. The body was meat. Case fell into the prison of his own flesh" (1984, p. 6). Besides the intimations of depersonalization and/or dehumanization, this passage suggests an additional, equally tenable side of cyberspace: addiction.

In the preceding remarks, I have attempted to show that rapid gains in knowledge (i.e, information) and thus technology, as well as the very prospects of VR itself, are contributing to a kind of global psychosocial dislocation. As the rate of technological innovations in particular quickens, individuals may experience greater difficulty than heretofore in achieving and maintaining a consistent sense of identity. Following Erikson's (1982) theory, such difficulties may precipitate the adoption of a negative identity. Although possibly contributing to this sense of dislocation, cyberspace and VR also offer individuals a potential escape from social expectations—and reality in general—in the lattices of the computer matrix. Provided that an individual can acquire the suitable technology, the fix afforded to the individual in VR will be quick, easy, inexpensive, and "virtually unbounded." In the following, I plan to limit my discussion to what may arguably be one of the most controversial if not potentially addicting applications of VR. The prospect is "virtual sex," and it is a subject that was being discussed in VR circles even before the technology became a reality.

THE PROSPECTS OF VIRTUAL ADDICTION: VIRTUAL SEX

For Gibson, cyberspace is much more than a computer-simulated alternative reality; it is an ultimately liberating "potentiality" bounded only by the imagination. In this sense, it also has a deeply erotic allure to it; it is a place where one's dreams and desires may find satisfaction. In *Neuro-*

mancer, we see the effect that cyberspace has upon Case, a cybernaut whose desire for cyberspace has grown to addictive proportions:

> A year [in Japan] and he still dreamed of cyberspace, hope fading nightly. . . . Still he'd see the matrix in his sleep, bright lattices of logic unfolding across that colorless void. . . . He was no [longer] console man, no cyberspace cowboy. . . . But the dreams came on in the Japanese night like livewire voodoo, and he'd cry for it, cry in his sleep, and wake alone in the dark, curled in his capsule in some coffin hotel, his hands clawed into the bedslab, . . . trying to reach the console that wasn't there. (1984, p. 4)

A particularly salacious extension to the possibility of VR addiction is this notion of virtual sex, or "teledildonics," as it has been euphemistically termed. According to technology critic Howard Rheingold (1991), the term "teledildonics" was originally coined to describe a device capable of converting sound into tactile sensations. The "dildonic" aspect of this device depended on which part of the anatomy a user decided to interface with the machine's tactile stimulators. The potential of VR makes the technology of this device look crude in comparison. Perhaps the most suitable analogy that can be drawn in today's world with the prospect of a teledildonics network is the growing popularity of telephone sex networks. Like the promise of virtual sex, telesex offers consumers disembodied sexual experiences; unlike virtual sex, however, it relies largely on the imaginative and fantasy abilities of the user. In a way, virtual sex will leave nothing to the imagination. Cybercoitus promises a fully interactive, three-dimensional, multisensory experience. For practical purposes, users will probably not interact with human computer simulations (human simulation technology is still only possible in the worlds of *Star Trek* or *Red Dwarf*), but with other users—by means of somewhat crude representations—on the same network of the information superhighway. Conceivably, in order to achieve full consummation in virtual sex, the amorous cybernaut will need to don, in addition to the seemingly requisite head-mounted three-dimensional display unit, a form-fitting electronic body prosthesis—in other words, a bodysuit, containing arrays of sensors and tactile stimulators. Thus equipped, the cybernaut will be ready for cyberspace and the titillating adventures that await. When plugged into the network, individuals will probably see computerized representations of themselves, along with representations of other network users. From there on, the possibilities are better left to the imagination. All that need be said is that the experience(s) will be multisensory; moreover, a teledildonics network, like the telesex networks, will also offer prospective users anonymity, innumerable partners, and freedom from sexually transmitted diseases and unwanted pregnancies. Furthermore, if one is displeased with one's encounter, one can terminate the experience with the flick of a switch.

Although it all sounds so promising, the reality is that virtual sex is not quite "just around the corner." Rheingold (1991) has noted a number of factors that first must be overcome before an on-line global teledildonics network can become a reality. First, in order to accommodate the amount of information that will be required for a tactile VR system, extensive fiber-optic networks will have to be created, interlinking not only individual network users but countries; second, the sheer computing power required to process the calculations necessary for tactile stimulation is so far unavailable; third, perhaps the most formidable obstruction to a global, real-time, shared cyberspace is the physical size of the planet. Basically, the larger the cyberspace network, geographically speaking, the larger the "system lag time"—until, perhaps, the speed-of-light barrier is broken. The tactile bodysuit mentioned earlier has also yet to become a reality; however, research teams on three continents are currently hard at work on this project, and already a number of prototypes are being developed.

CONCLUSIONS

If the prospect of virtual sex would not seem to be next year's technological triumph, its eventual reality seems inevitable. One thing is certain: When virtual sex becomes possible in cyberspace, it promises to change the face of human intimacy forever. It will challenge our most fundamental personal and social definitions for what constitutes erotica; it will also force us into a radical reconsideration of conventional moral codes. In addition, Rheingold (1991) has raised a perplexing implication for identity: "With our information machines and our bodily sensations so deeply 'intermingled', . . . will our communication devices be regarded as 'its' or will they be part of 'us'?" (p. 353). Indeed, as the pace of technological innovations quickens, we will become more reliant on our machines personally to augment and restructure our physical deficits in processing the ballooning quantities of data that we must contend with in this information age. This information (re)evolution, then, might give us reason seriously to contemplate Rheingold's seemingly outrageous science-fiction-like proposition. Are we destined to be subsumed by the "machine," or are we to become hybrids or "cyborgs"—part human, part machine, possessing qualities of both, but never fully being one or the other? This question, however strange it may seem, nevertheless fixes our gaze upon mechanisms that may be central to any understanding of impulsive and addictive behaviors in cyberspace.

VR has been dubbed "the plug-in drug" of the next century, but I have previously noted that the ingredients for such behaviors are already "built into" our cyberspace network. These ingredients include the following:

Power in accessing, manipulating, and otherwise controlling data in such a vast information space.

Erotic allure, in its original or Platonic sense—love stemming from a narcissistic fascination with the products of one's labors and from the expression and enrichment of one's intellect.

Mystery and opportunity, in exploring and exploiting an as yet un-mapped frontier.

Freedom of access and expression.

Anonymity and depersonalization—freedom to reveal only as much of oneself as one desires, and, in addition, freedom to fabricate a myriad of pseudoidentities.

Limited accountability and responsibility, which are consequences of the preceding characteristics, but particularly the latter.

Community and belonging—opportunities to communicate with denizens of the globe who share similar beliefs and convictions, or who at least share a vested interest in a particular issue.

And, of course, the medium itself—an alternative "interactive" reality capable of enhancing or restricting one's life, or simply of providing a means by which one can escape from one's daily routines.

Taken collectively, these ingredients already constitute a recipe for impulsivity and addiction. Given the preceding remarks, it is not at all surprising that such behaviors are becoming more readily apparent on the internet. But rather than directing our efforts solely toward under-standing the individuals who exhibit such tendencies, and/or the prod-ucts of our labors themselves (i.e., the services or technologies that may foster such proclivities), we might do well to direct our attention to the preconditions that may be giving rise to such behaviors and technolo-gies in the first place. As I have intimated throughout this chapter, I believe that these have less to do with the technologies themselves than with a struggle to adjust to a new stage of evolutionary development. This is a struggle to exact meaning and identity from a medium that is bereft of such human qualities. This dystopic aspect of cyberspace, VR, and information technology in general is suggestive of a kind of crisis of identity.

Technological revolutions are dramatically changing the face of the workplace; they are also exerting a no less dramatic, but considerably more subtle, influence over our personal and social identities. As our relationship to information and information technologies becomes in-creasingly challenging, perhaps because of the pace of progress itself, we might expect to witness an increase in behaviors that constitute impul-sivity and/or addiction. Understanding such a phenomenon will require a careful examination of our relationship with information—that is to say, the psychology of information and information technologies.

REFERENCES

Erikson, E. (1982). *The life cycle completed.* New York: Norton.

Gibson, W. (1984). *Neuromancer.* New York: Ace Books.

Hawking, S. W. (1993, June). *Speculations on the possibility of life in the universe.* Lecture, Vancouver, British Columbia.

Heim, M. (1993). *The metaphysics of virtual reality.* New York: Oxford University Press.

Rheingold, H. (1991). *Virtual reality.* New York: Touchstone.

II

FOUNDATIONS

It came in a biology class. Biehl explained about Darwinism—the survival of the fittest. It still applies, he said, even in our society, but it is mitigated because we alleviate its consequences.

After he had said that, there was a pause. It was a rich moment.

He had not looked at anyone in particular. He never addressed himself, as it were, to individuals. Still, maybe I was the one, at the moment, who understood him best. Those who were on the inside, the majority, that is, found it hard to get his point, mostly they were just pleased that they were on the inside, that they were the fittest. For those on the outside, the fear and abandonment amount to almost everything, everybody knows that.

Understanding is something one does best when one is on the borderline.

—PETER HOEG, *Borderlines* (1995, pp. 36–37)

Moreover, the patients in the second hospital defied the tidy classification so beloved by psychiatrists. None of them were clear-cut cases of schizophrenia, yet they would exhibit schizophrenia-like symptoms. Others were depressed, but they sometimes added outbursts of rage to their depression. I could not understand what one pleasant elderly lady, who bore herself well and talked rationally, was doing on the ward—until she disappeared to a closed ward after a suicide attempt.

—STUART SUTHERLAND, *Breakdown: A Personal Crisis and a Medical Disease*, revised edition (1987, p. 83)

6

The Biopsychology
of Impulsivity:
Focus on Brain Serotonin

DONALD V. COSCINA

In order to discuss the "biopsychology" of "impulsivity," I must first define my perspectives on the meaning of both terms.

Over the past few decades, the term "biopsychology" has been used to describe a variety of fields whose common focus is on identifying and describing the mechanisms of any number of biological processes that influence behavior. This encompasses broad areas of research in such traditionally separate disciplines as anatomy, biochemistry, pharmacology, physiology, and nutrition. For the purposes of this chapter, the primary focus is on neurochemistry—a division of biochemistry that specializes in studying the chemical processes occurring in nervous tissue. The reason for this choice is that the vast majority of recent biopsychological research has been grounded in this field, with input from all the other disciplines mentioned providing additional information that can be seen to converge on this domain.

As for definitions of "impulsivity," it is evident from reading the rest of this book as well as others on this topic (e.g., McCown, Johnson, & Shure, 1993; Zuckerman, 1991) that this construct can be defined in many ways. However, one feature that all definitions seem to have in common is that of acting (i.e., behaving) without much forethought of the outcome or consequences of those actions. This fact accords well with a general dictionary definition, which includes the following features:

im.pulse (im′puls), **n.** [L. *impulsus*, pp. of *impellere*; see IMPEL], **1.** *a*) an impelling, or driving forward with sudden force. *b*) an impelling force; sudden, driving force; push; thrust; impetus. *c*) the motion or effect caused by such a force. **2.** *a*) incitement to action arising from a state of mind or some external stimulus. *b*) a sudden inclination to act, without conscious thought. *c*) a motive or tendency coming from within. **3.** in *mechanics,* the change in momentum effected by a force, measured by multiplying the average value of the force by the time during which it acts. **4.** in *physiology,* a stimulus transmitted in a muscle or nerve, which causes or inhibits activity in the body. (*Webster's New World Dictionary, College Edition,* 1956)

A particularly important distinction has been made recently in the many forms that impulsivity can take—that is, a distinction between "functional" and "dysfunctional" subtypes (Dickman, 1990). The former variant consists of tendencies toward spontaneous, thoughtless actions when such a style is optimal in certain situations and/or produces beneficial results. One example of this might be found in an individual whose job it is to buy and sell commodities on a stock exchange. A person who does so in an inordinately quick fashion but just at the right time, and is successful in making money doing so, can be thought of as being "functionally impulsive." The latter variant consists of similar tendencies toward thoughtless, spontaneous action; however, in this case the consequences are deleterious to the person acting and/or to others with whom he or she interacts. Although these two tendencies are not correlated with each other, it is interesting that most common usages of the term "impulsivity" in daily life seem to refer to the dysfunctional subtype. This fact is most clearly apparent in contemporary accounts of various crimes as recounted in the popular media. Commercial, sensationalistic motivations of such reporting aside, this is not surprising if one considers that any undesirable outcomes of human actions are legitimate societal concerns— particularly if those actions affect the lives of innocent or incompetent people adversely. Perhaps for this reason, most human research designed to elucidate biological factors that seem to cause or sustain impulsive states has focused on behaviors viewed as deleterious either to the impulsive persons or to those with whom they interact. That fact is also reflected in this chapter, although I return to the distinction between the functional and dysfunctional subtypes at the chapter's conclusion.

AROUSAL AND IMPULSIVITY

It is axiomatic in all fields of behavioral science that in order for an organism to act (i.e., move or behave), it must be endowed with built-in biological mechanisms that (1) permit the occurrence of actions and (2) motivate the organism to act. Aside from specific mechanical bodily systems (e.g., muscle, bone, connective tissue, and peripheral sensory networks) that enable animals and humans to move physically through space, there are other specialized biological tissues capable of integrating the necessary external and/or internal information (i.e., stimuli) that give rise to coordinated, appropriate actions to those stimuli (i.e., responses). In more highly evolved organisms like vertebrates, which are capable of relatively broad ranges of motoric acts compared to invertebrates, the central nervous system (CNS—i.e., the brain and spinal cord) is widely studied in order to understand how these critically important functions are monitored, coordinated, and executed. Interacting with these CNS subsystems are others that, in an allied fashion, integrate motivational controls with motoric capabilities. It is therefore quite reasonable that investigations into the causes or sustaining factors of impulsivity have focused to a great degree on the CNS in general and the brain in particular.

In the late 1940s, a very important quality of the brain was discovered—that is, its capacity for "arousal" (see Carlson, 1991). Experiments in animals showed that small amounts of electrical stimulation to a portion of the brainstem called the "reticular formation" produced a more alert, behaviorally active organism. Indeed, because of the functional outcome of such stimulation, this brain region has also become known as the "reticular activating system." This fundamental observation was very important in setting the stage for subsequent work into CNS controls over impulsive actions, since, by their very nature, such behaviors represent overactivated and/or highly directed motoric or motivational states. Consequently, much of the subsequent research into the biopsychological processes affecting impulsivity has focused directly or indirectly on various brain mechanisms that in some way mediate enhanced arousability.

GENERAL OVERVIEW
OF CENTRAL NERVOUS SYSTEM NEUROCHEMISTRY

A cardinal feature of research in any field is its attempt to isolate definable factors that are capable of explaining discrete phenomena. Since the primary goal of research in biopsychology is to understand the biological bases of behavior, and the CNS is of paramount importance for integrating and controlling behavior, it is not surprising that this field has important historical as well as contemporary linkages with neurochemistry. For this fundamental reason, research efforts to understand CNS controls over behavior took an enormous leap forward in the early 1960s, when a new neurochemical technique was developed in Sweden that ultimately permitted the direct visualization of certain discrete chemical systems within the brain and spinal cord believed to subserve information transfer between neurons. Although it had been known for some time that nervous tissue throughout the periphery (i.e., the rest of the body) as well as the CNS contained these so-called "neurotransmitter" substances, it was not possible before then actually to visualize them in structurally intact tissue, and hence to trace their pathways and interconnections. This procedure, known as "histochemical fluorescence" (Falck, Hillarp, Thieme, & Torp, 1962), took advantage of the fact that certain small neurotransmitter molecules known as "monoamines" (so called because they possessed one amino or NH_2 moiety), when exposed to dry formaldehyde vapors under very specific conditions, developed a characteristic fluorescent color under particular wavelengths of light. CNS tissue processed in this way could then be examined with the appropriate microscopic equipment and could reveal, in sequential serial tissue sections, the pathways that these distinct chemical-containing neurons followed within the brain and spinal cord.

Two classes of particular neurotransmitters to which this technique was applied were ones implicated a decade earlier as potentially subserving important functions related to mood, affect, and behavior in humans (Brodie & Shore, 1957). They were the two catecholamines norepinephrine (NE) and dopamine (DA), and the single indoleamine serotonin (5-HT, which stands for its chemical name, 5-hydroxytryptamine). All three compounds are fairly small molecules synthesized in nervous tissues from simple amino acids, the building blocks of proteins. In the case of NE and DA, which both contain catechol groupings (i.e., a six-member carbon chain with hydrogen moieties that interconnect to form a closed ring), the starting material or "precursor" is the "essential" (i.e., required in our diets, since it cannot be synthesized in the body) amino acid tyrosine. This substance is taken up by a specific transport system into NE- and DA-producing neurons, in which the presence of a specific enzyme, tyrosine hydroxylase, adds a hydroxyl or -OH group to the amino acid, creating the intermediate compound commonly called L-DOPA (L-dihydroxyphenylacetic acid). Then this compound is quickly decarboxylated (i.e., a -COOH group is removed and an -H is added) by a ubiquitous enzyme, L-aromatic amino acid decarboxylase, to form DA. In the case of NE neurons, DA is further converted to this neurotransmitter by the presence of an additional enzyme, dopamine-β-hydroxylase, which adds another hydroxyl group to the DA molecule. In the case of 5-HT, the synthetic process is fundamentally similar; however, in this instance the starting material is another essential amino acid, tryptophan. This precursor substance is taken up by 5-HT neurons, again by a selective transporter system, and first hydroxylated (this time by the enzyme tryptophan hydroxylase) and then decarboxylated (also by L-aromatic amino acid decarboxylase) to form the end product 5-HT. A particularly interesting feature of 5-HT synthesis is the fact that it can, in part, be altered by modifying the amount of tryptophan consumed in our diets.

This is because the initial enzyme in the synthetic pathway has the capacity to hydroxylate much more tryptophan than is usually available. This fact has been utilized in certain research studies to improve our understanding of how 5-HT contributes to behavior in general and impulsivity in particular.

In the case of all three monoamines just described, once these neurotransmitters have been made, they are largely stored in "vesicles" located at the ends of neurons (which are called "axon terminals") until appropriate electrical stimulation of the neurons produces their release into extracellular spaces—most importantly at "synapses," which are junctions between individual neural elements where the transfer of such chemical information occurs. Released monoamines interact with different "receptor" subsystems on pre- and/or postsynaptic sites in order to exert their biological functions. Portions of monoamines released into extracellular spaces are metabolized by various enzymes, which inactivate them, after which they are taken up by microcirculatory systems for return to the bloodstream and eventual elimination from the body. Larger proportions of these monoamines are reabsorbed into the presynaptic elements from which they were released. The majority of these molecules are reused again for neurotransmission, while other subsets are inactivated by various intracellular enzymes for eventual removal and disposal by the bloodstream, much as described after extracellular inactivation.

Another CNS neurotransmitter system that has figured prominently in our understanding of arousal mechanisms is the acetylcholine (ACh) system. The first neurotransmitter substance to be identified earlier in this century, it was initially isolated in the periphery but later shown through biochemical extraction techniques to exist in the brain as well. Subsequent research, which allowed the mapping of the enzyme that inactivates it, permitted tracing of ACh neurons throughout the brain. Like the monoamines already described, ACh is a fairly small molecule. It is synthesized in neurons that contain an uptake mechanism for choline, a moiety derived from the breakdown of lipids. Once inside these specialized neurons, choline has an acetate ion attached to it under the influence of another enzyme, choline acetyltransferase. Like the monoamines, ACh is stored in vesicles until appropriate neural impulses release it to permit its actions on specific receptor subtypes; it is recyclable through reuptake systems; and it is inactivated by specific enzymes in the general manner described above.

NEUROCHEMICAL SPECIFICITY OF AROUSAL

There are a great many other neurotransmitter substances in the CNS (current estimates number well over 100), many of which play roles in arousal processes. However, the four mentioned above have been studied the most thus far, in large part because we have known about them the longest and have developed ways and means of studying their actions most effectively. Research into the different ways each compound appears to influence arousal has resulted in various theories. One particularly interesting hypothesis (Robbins, Everitt, Muir, & Harrison, 1992) holds that specific regions of the brain that utilize NE, DA, ACh, and 5-HT modulate the processes of distraction, basal latency to respond, accuracy, and impulsive responding, respectively. The linkage of brain 5-HT systems with impulsivity in this model does not derive only from data generated by Robbins's group; it can also be traced back to a major influential review that preceded it. Soubrie (1986) espoused a critical role for this monoamine not only in the control of behavioral arousal, but more importantly in the abilities to withhold responding before acting and to tolerate delays, in both animals and humans. Given the limited space available in this chapter, the remainder of my discussion focuses primarily on the role of CNS 5-HT functioning and impulsivity. This choice does not derive only from the implications of the models put forth by Soubrie (1986) and Robbins et al. (1992). It also reflects the fact that the majority of research over the past 10 years, which I examined in order to write this chapter, identified 5-HT as a cardinal focus of investigation (i.e., 76 out of 150 studies). In addition, it is also the case that most current attempts to treat impulsivity-related disorders pharmacologically have employed drugs whose biological actions are partially or wholly aimed at altering 5-HT metabolism. However, as we shall see, there are instances where the putative involvement of altered 5-HT neurotransmission in impulsivity can best be thought of as an interaction process with other transmitter systems, most notably DA systems.

FUNDAMENTAL QUALITIES OF SEROTONIN SYSTEMS

Before summarizing key contemporary literature that links aberrations of 5-HT metabolism to problems with impulsive control, I comment on some intrinsic properties of this neurochemical axis that lend themselves to playing such a role.

Phylogenetic Considerations

5-HT neural systems are phylogenetically old. They exist in fairly simple invertebrate organisms, suggesting that they have regulated important basal functions from a very early point in the evolution of the animal kingdom. Perhaps the most widely studied of such creatures in a behavioral context is *Aplysia californica,* a sea mollusk lacking any shell. Kandel and Schwartz (1982) reported that the gill withdrawal response of such animals, which is clearly a motoric process, is mediated by 5-HT release. This type of fundamental behavioral role for 5-HT can be viewed as a primordial link to other action-related mechanisms, which relate in more highly evolved organisms to movements we can think of in the context of impulsivity.

Anatomical Considerations

One of the most remarkable qualities of the brain's 5-HT system in mammals is its widespread nature (Azmitia & Whitaker-Azmitia, 1991). Emanating largely from two diffuse groupings of cell bodies in the midline of the upper brainstem (called the "raphe"), subdivisions of these two groupings send axonal projections to almost every level of the forebrain, as well as significant areas of the lower brainstem. Of further interest is the fact that such axonal projections send multiple branches out from single cell bodies. This structural feature permits neuronal activity in single cells to influence multiple terminal sites. In addition, 5-HT projections connect or "innervate" structural elements other than neurons—things like blood vessels and "astroglia," a form of tissue that surrounds neurons and other brain structures and provides nutrient and other supportive processes to neuronal functioning. These brief comments should make it clear that by their anatomical nature alone, 5-HT brain systems are well designed to influence a variety of CNS functions, including the diverse neurobiological processes that underlie arousal and impulsivity.

Ontogenetic Considerations

It has already been mentioned that once molecules of 5-HT are released from neurons at synaptic sites, they interact with various receptors to exert some of their biological actions. Another interesting feature of the brain 5-HT system, which it shares with other neurotransmitter systems, is the fact that it is not fully developed at birth (Whitaker-Azmitia, 1991). Rather, it shows significant postnatal expansion that mirrors the appearance of a number of behavioral states. In addition, the different receptor sites at which 5-HT molecules act in the adult show different levels of sensitivity to this transmitter at birth versus during adulthood. This receptor expression changes during ontogeny, but in varying ways, depending on the location and type of receptors involved. Specific 5-HT receptor subtypes appear to be involved in influencing a number of developmental processes, including cell growth and differentiation. Seen in this way, it is clear that the brain 5-HT system has important organizational roles to play, and that these vary according to the point in the lifespan at which the dynamics of this system are operating. Since all behaviors are ultimately shaped by biological and/or environmental factors during development, these ontogenetic characteristics of the brain 5-HT system point to one more quality that makes it an important player in the establishment and/or maintenance of impulsive actions.

Biochemical Considerations

Recall that 5-HT is synthesized from the amino acid tryptophan, which must be consumed in our diet, since we are unable to produce it ourselves from other nutrients. Recall also that trytophan hydroxylase, which converts tryptophan to the intermediate moiety known as 5-HTP, is normally unsaturated with this substrate. This means that within certain limits, more 5-HT can be made in the brain (and to a lesser extent in the body), if more tryptophan is consumed. This relatively unique quality of brain 5-HT systems among neurotransmitters implies that the functional states it subserves can be influenced in part by the amount of amino acid precursor made available for 5-HT production. Since proteins are made up of different amino acids that are liberated during digestion, the amounts and types of proteins we eat can in part contribute to the capacity of the 5-HT system to function. Of additional interest is the fact that when insulin levels are elevated in mammals, there is a preferential increase in blood tryptophan compared to the other amino acids, with which it normally competes for uptake into the brain (Colmenares, Wurtman, & Fernstrom, 1975). Since one releaser of insulin in normal humans is the consumption of sugars, the amounts and types of carbohydrates we consume can also influence the availability of 5-HT in the brain. Based on these types of information, recent work by Wurtman (1993) has postulated that affect and mood are controlled in part by the foods we consume via their effects on brain 5-HT function. Since low levels of brain 5-HT have traditionally been linked to depression, it has been suggested that consuming sweets is one means by which people may try to normalize otherwise deficient 5-HT systems. Other researchers interested in 5-HT's linkage to impulsivity have also considered the role of tryptophan availability as a factor in explaining this state. Some of that literature is discussed below.

SEROTONIN AND AGGRESSION

Of the many behavioral forms that impulsivity can take, aggression toward the self (suicide, self-mutilation) or toward others (murder or other violent acts) seems to be the one most highly studied. This is not surprising, since aggressive actions are clearly threats to survival. Some of the earliest evidence suggesting that impairments of normal brain 5-HT functioning are linked to increased aggression came from animal research. Studies employing rats showed that experimentally induced damage to the 5-HT-synthesizing cell bodies in the midbrain's dorsal and median raphe nuclei (Grant, Coscina, Grossman, & Freedman, 1973), or pharmacological treatment that impeded the synthesis of 5-HT neurotransmission (Valzelli, Bernasconi, & Dalessandro, 1981), increased the incidence of mouse-killing behavior or "muricide." More recent work with male rhesus monkeys living in a totally natural habitat has confirmed this linkage between 5-HT and aggression. Based on quantitative behavioral observations during social interactions, Mehlman et al. (1994) have reported that a small ($n = 26$) aggressive subset of a large ($n = 4,500$) free-ranging population had abnormally low levels of 5-HT's major metabolite, 5-hydroxyindoleacetic acid (5-HIAA), in their cerebrospinal fluid (CSF). Low levels of 5-HIAA are traditionally viewed as reflecting poor synthesis and/or release of 5-HT. Of additional interest was the fact that these low levels of 5-HIAA were inversely correlated with "escalated aggression" (i.e., a higher ratio of chasing and assaulting other monkeys, relative to all aggressive acts displayed), as well as with risk-taking behavior (i.e., long leaps from tree tops), which can be viewed as a form of "impulsivity" and associated with "sensation seeking" (Zuckerman, 1984).

The most widely cited study that seems to have first powerfully linked violent aggression/impulsivity with aberrations of 5-HT metabolism in humans is that of Asberg, Traskman, and Thoren (1976). They observed a bimodal distribution of 5-HIAA in the CSF of patients with major unipolar depression, wherein patients with the lowest levels of this metabolite were the most likely to have attempted or succeeded in committing suicide in a violent manner. The essence of this study has been replicated many (but not all) times and extended to include individuals with a predisposition toward mild hypoglycemia, early-onset alcohol and drug abuse, familial trends toward alcoholism, and altered circadian (day–night) activity patterns (see review by Linnoila & Virkkunen, 1992). Similarly, other work by Linnoila, DeJong, and Virkkunen (1989) has pointed to subnormal functioning of brain 5-HT metabolism as a factor contributing to the impulsivity of arsonists or violent offenders who were also suicidal. Of particular interest is a more recent study by Nielsen et al. (1994). It showed that in a cohort of extremely impulsive, alcoholic, violent offenders from Finland, there was a significant relationship between variations in the gene responsible for producing tryptophan hydroxylase and low levels of 5-HIAA in their CSF. This same genetic variation was also linked with a history of suicide attempts in a larger subgrouping of violent offenders, regardless of their tendencies toward impulsiveness.

Independent investigations by Coccaro and colleagues also support the general notion that deficient 5-HT neurotransmission is a contributory factor in impulsive aggression. Rather than directly measuring an index of 5-HT metabolism such as 5-HIAA, they measured levels of the hormone prolactin in the blood of personality-disordered patients after administering different drugs that directly stimulate 5-HT receptors known to control the release of 5-HT from the pituitary gland. In one study (Coccaro, Gabriel, & Siever, 1990), infusions of buspirone—a compound that stimulates brain 5-HT_{1A} receptors—produced differential prolactin release in 10 such patients, which correlated inversely ($r = -.76$) with their self-assessed "irritability." A later paper that summarized a variety of related results (Coccaro, 1992) stated that infusions of a more general 5-HT receptor stimulant, m-chlorophenylpiperazine, again produced a negative correlation ($r = -.66$, $n = 10$) between blood prolactin levels and an index of impulsivity (the Buss–Durkee "assault + irritability" dimensions). Since the latter findings were independent of patients' mood states, and CSF levels of 5-HIAA did not correlate with prolactin measures, this type of research suggests that certain forms of impulsive aggression are related to a diminished sensitivity to 5-HT at postsynaptic sites that might otherwise respond normally to 5-HT stimulation. In keeping with these findings in humans is a more recent study by Botchin, Kaplan, Manuck, and Mann (1993) in adult male cynomolgus monkeys (*Macaca fascicularis*). They reported that low-prolactin responders to the drug fenfluramine, which mimics 5-HT actions in the brain, displayed higher indices of "overt aggression" (e.g., fighting episodes with conspecifics involving physical contact; chasing and lunging forms of aggression) than did high-prolactin responders. This was so despite similar dominance status between the groups. In addition, low responders were more socially withdrawn and showed less body contact with other animals. So, even in nonhuman primates, deficiencies in 5-HT-stimulated prolactin release seem associated with higher levels of certain forms of aggression, as well as lower levels of positive social interactions.

The findings cited above can be seen as compatible with other research by Mann, McBride, Anderson, and Mieczkowski (1992). They found that levels of 5-HT in the blood platelets from a subset of 29 depressed patients with comorbid personality disorder correlated positively ($r = .44$, $n = 22$) with a measure of hostility (Brief Psychiatric Rating Scale), as well as with a measure of long-term aggression (Brown–Goodwin Aggression History Scale; $r = .41$, $n = 21$). Since platelet levels of 5-HT are viewed as a model of how much 5-HT in the brain might bind to receptors there, it is conceivable that tonic low levels of circulating brain 5-HT occur in such individuals because there is an abnormally high level of transmitter binding to receptors. Such chronic receptor stimulation could lead to compensatory desensitization of such receptors, expressing itself in this case as a blunted prolactin response to acute stimulation by 5-HT-like drugs.

Other lines of evidence exist that link abnormally low brain 5-HT functioning with aggressive acts. In a review article by Young, Pihl, and Ervin (1988), which summarized a variety of the authors' work, normal males who were given an amino acid drink devoid of tryptophan (de-signed to lower 5-HT levels) reported an acute depression of their mood, but no effects on tests of aggression. However, a separate study of vervet monkeys, who were apparently quite highly aroused under test condi-tions, showed that a comparable amino acid load did indeed enhance aggressive acts. Young et al. point out that since the firing of 5-HT neurons (an index of this transmitter's release) is high during arousal but low in depressed states, the inability to detect aggressive effects in humans might simply reflect the inability of the tryptophan-deficient drink to lower 5-HT functioning in the human subjects' relatively unaroused state. Other research by Kent et al. (1988) supports a role for low 5-HT in patients with a history of periodic losses of self-control and outbursts of violent acts against property, animals, or people. The uptake of 5-HT into blood platelets of 15 such individuals was 18% lower than in 15 matched controls, and was negatively correlated with the BIS-10 form of the Barratt Impulsiveness Scale ($r = -.62$).

Additional evidence suggests that deficient brain 5-HT metabolism is related to other forms of human aggressiveness. One form of such aggression that captures particular attention in the mass media consists of sexual transgressions against others. Studies by Kafka (1991a, 1991b) and Kafka and Prentky (1992) have shown that both paraphilic and nonparaphilic "sexual addictions" can be treated with the now commonly prescribed antidepressant fluoxetine, which enhances brain 5-HT func-tioning. Of course, the fact that an enhancer of 5-HT functioning is effective in treating a particular disorder does not necessarily mean that a deficiency in the 5-HT system is the cause of the disorder. However, there is a scientific rationale for such treatment. It follows in part from earlier work (Brown et al., 1982), which showed that levels of CSF 5-HIAA were inversely correlated to the Psychopathic Deviate scale of the Minne-sota Multiphasic Personality Inventory in a small sample of patients with borderline personality disorder. More recent work by Faustman et al. (1991) has confirmed a similar finding in a group of unmedicated de-pressed patients. In addition, other work by O'Keane et al. (1992) has revealed that male murderers diagnosed as having antisocial personality disorder showed blunted prolactin responses to oral fenfluramine during quiescent, nonviolent periods. This type of evidence again supports the notion that individuals who act out against others may normally possess low levels of brain 5-HT neurotransmission and/or a general subsensitiv-ity of 5-HT receptive mechanisms within the CNS.

Subnormal functioning of the 5-HT system has been linked not only to acts of aggression against others, but also to forms of aggression against the self. I have already mentioned the classic study by Asberg et al. (1976), which showed that low levels of CSF 5-HIAA were linked to violent suicide. Another form of "autoaggression" is self-mutilation. Simeon et al. (1992) showed that in a group of self-mutilating personality-disordered patients (n = 12), an index of maximal 5-HT binding to blood platelets correlated inversely with the magnitude of their self-mutilation (r = −.57), impulsivity (r = −.61), and aggression (r = −.37), compared to a control group (n = 14) of nonmutilating personality-disordered patients. Of interest, though, is the fact that there were no differences between the groups in CSF 5-HIAA levels, even though the mutilators were rated as more depressed on the Hamilton Rating Scale for Depression (but not the Beck Depression Inventory). Still another form of behavior that can be viewed as "self-harming" is hair-pulling, or trichotillomania. A variety of past research has linked this disorder with movement disorders such as Gilles de la Tourette's syndrome, as well as with obsessive–compulsive disorder (OCD), all of which have been linked to functionally high levels of DA neurotransmission in the brain. Since it has long been known that one of the roles of brain 5-HT release is to inhibit DA neurotransmission, some investigators have had success in treating hair pulling with drugs that mimic this process. One study (Stein & Hollander, 1992) confirming this has shown that treating such patients with 5-HT reuptake blockers does indeed mitigate such symptomatology. However, in cases where the effect was mild or not long-lasting, additional treatment with the broad DA receptor blocking agent pimozide effected greater diminution and more sustained cessation of hair pulling. This finding points out an important issue that is discussed further below: That is, the CNS mechanisms by which aberrations in brain 5-HT metabolism may affect impulsivity (i.e., through interacting with brain DA systems).

This relatively small sample of studies points out that there is strong *prima facie* evidence across species, including humans, to support the notion that important linkages exist between various indices of abnormally low 5-HT functioning in the CNS and different states of aggression that have been linked to impulsivity.

SEROTONIN AND OTHER FORMS OF IMPULSIVITY

Lest readers get the impression that abnormally low brain levels of 5-HT have been *specifically* linked to heightened states of aggression, I hasten to point out that a great deal of additional research more broadly implicates 5-HT deficiencies in a myriad of other impulse-related disorders. Space limitations preclude extensive discussion of these conditions here. However, they include the eating disorders anorexia nervosa and bulimia nervosa (Sohlberg, Norring, Holmgren, & Rosmark, 1989), overeating and obesity (Mustajoki, 1987), inability to delay gratification in preschoolers (Mischel, Shoda, & Rodriguez, 1989), substance abuse (Fishbein, Lozovsky, & Jaffe, 1989; Moeller et al., 1994), and pathological gambling (Moreno, Saiz-Ruiz, & Lopez-Ibor, 1991). In some individuals, more than one of these impulsive disorders can coexist; for example, eating disorders can coexist with alcoholism, autoaggression, suicidality, shoplifting, and drug abuse (Fichter, Quadflieg, & Rief, 1994; Higuchi, Suzuki, Yamada, Parrish, & Kono, 1993). Separate research has linked abnormally low functioning of the 5-HT system to all of these problems in a variety of indirect ways. This raises an important point. The fact that dysfunction of the brain 5-HT system can be linked to so many disorders that can be thought of broadly as problems of impulsivity raises at least two general issues that need to be addressed: (1) the specificity of the construct "impulsivity," and (2) the specificity of the chemical abnormality putatively involved (in this case, low functioning of the 5-HT system). The first issue is one to which many other chapters in this volume have been devoted, so I do not discuss it here. With regard to the second, I touch briefly on the types of problems associated with this concern; I reflect on the types of studies described above that employed different measures of the 5-HT system to imply abnormalities of its operation.

SPECIFICITY OF SUBNORMAL MEASURES
OF BRAIN SEROTONIN FUNCTIONING

5-Hydroxyindoleacetic Acid

Attempts to define subnormal 5-HT functioning by measuring CSF levels of 5-HT are fraught with problems of validity. The description earlier in this chapter of the massive distribution of the 5-HT system throughout all levels of the upper and lower CNS, including the spinal cord, should make something immediately apparent. Taking samples of CSF at the base of the spinal cord in the low back (the site where such samples are routinely obtained) runs the risk of ultimately assessing an index of 5-HT functioning that disproportionately represents a region of nervous tissue unrelated to the upper CNS structures normally thought of as controlling the types of complex behaviors associated with impulsivity. At best, CSF levels of 5-HIAA can only reflect an incredibly diverse mix of this metabolite derived from any number of CNS structures. At worst, it can largely reflect only a subset of them—those that lie near the cerebrospinal spaces, which course through only a portion of this long and varied matrix of tissue. Second, although they are not outlined here for purposes of brevity, a number of other minor metabolites of 5-HT are normally formed in the process of its natural degradation. Under behavioral conditions viewed as abnormal, it is possible that more of these substances are made than under normal conditions, thus leading to lesser amounts of 5-HIAA being generated. A failure to obtain additional measures of these substances runs the risk of underestimating the true metabolic profile of 5-HT, and hence of deriving false positives implying that its metabolism is indeed faulty. Third, we have seen from some studies above that other indices of low 5-HT functioning were found in "impulsive" persons, but that simultaneous measures of CSF 5-HIAA in such persons failed to reveal deficiencies. At best, then, this implies that measures of 5-HIAA cannot serve as a robust indicator of subnormal 5-HT neurotransmission.

Prolactin

Researchers who desire to measure a more functional postsynaptic consequence of low 5-HT functioning in brain have often opted to examine the release of prolactin after administering 5-HT-stimulating compounds. Although measurement of prolactin is conceptually closer to a meaningful "output" index than measurement of 5-HIAA, quantifying levels of this hormone can again be misleading. For one thing, neuroactive substances other than 5-HT can trigger prolactin release. Conceivably, aberrations of 5-HT neurotransmission—even if they exist—may not be the sole reason why subnormal prolactin levels are found in targeted patient populations. In addition, the brain site where 5-HT is acknowledged to act in releasing prolactin is quite circumscribed (i.e., the hypothalamus). Among the vast human and animal literature that has implicated sites in the brain where impulsive actions may be mediated, the hypothalamus is rarely mentioned. Therefore, abnormal 5-HT receptive mechanisms in this part of the CNS may not necessarily mirror abnormalities in other parts of the brain (e.g., portions of the neocortex, limbic system, and/or extrapyramidal system) where aspects of impulsivity are thought to be mediated. Related to this is the fact that there are many published studies showing that receptor binding mechanisms in the hypothalamus can differ radically from those in other parts of the brain, including those just mentioned. Therefore, even if hypothalamic 5-HT mechanisms controlling prolactin release are faulty in impulsive individuals, this does not have to mean that they are faulty elsewhere in the brain. Another factor to consider is that the myriad of 5-HT receptor subtypes already identified (see Dourish, 1995) bind 5-HT to different degrees. Hence, the capacity of a particular receptor stimulant to effect prolactin release is unlikely to mirror accurately the capacity of 5-HT to alter in the same manner the particular receptor subtypes involved in mediating impulsive acts.

Blood Platelet Binding of Serotonin

The fact that 5-HT or some drug used to mimic its binding properties (usually the antidepressant imipramine) shows abnormal adherence to blood platelets when measured in a test tube cannot be viewed as a perfect model of what happens in the brain. Although much research has attempted to validate this peripheral model for the purpose intended, it is hard to imagine that whatever platelet binding changes can be documented can serve as a powerful correlate of 5-HT receptor binding in specific parts of the CNS associated with impulsivity. The reasons for this have already been noted in the section above on prolactin (i.e., 5-HT binding to receptors is not uniform across different brain regions; different receptor subtypes may be involved in mediating impulsive acts that are not wholly represented by the binding to platelets of 5-HT or drugs that serve as indices of 5-HT action).

For a more complete discussion of issues relevant to the chemical specificity of 5-HT measurements as they relate to aggression, suicide, and other aspects of impulsivity, readers are referred to a recent review by Golden et al. (1991).

INTEGRATION OF FINDINGS

Despite the cautionary notes expressed above, the sheer volume and diversity of the literature that has linked subnormal 5-HT metabolism to impulsivity makes it highly likely that this brain neurochemical system is indeed functionally important to certain expressions of this personality/behavioral construct. If we accept that this is the case, the next logical question to ask is this: In what general domains might aberrant 5-HT metabolism account for this involvement?

Several investigators have postulated ways in which decrements in brain 5-HT metabolism might be linked to impulsivity. For many years, van Praag has questioned the linkage of such 5-HT deficiencies to specific disease states (e.g., van Praag et al., 1988). More recent work from his group (Plutchik & van Praag, 1993) supports this contention by pointing out a number of interconnections between trait anxiety on the one hand and impulsivity, suicide, violent behavior, and deficient 5-HT metabolism on the other. Cloninger (1986) has also focused on anxiety as an overarching construct, but has gone somewhat further by hypothesizing that interactions among 5-HT, NE, and DA account for certain inherited personality traits, among which impulsivity is represented. Of interest here is Cloninger's suggestion that increased activity in brain 5-HT systems is linked to high harm avoidance, decreased activity in NE systems to reward dependence, and low activity in DA systems to novelty seeking. Such a combined neurochemical profile is seen as characteristic of obsessional individuals who, because of faulty integration of environmental sensory information, misperceive environmental cues and are thus in states of chronic anxiety. Although such an attempt at formulating a unified biopsychosocial theory to explain many personality dimensions is likely to be oversimplified, it is nonetheless laudable for its neurochemically and behaviorally multifaceted nature. Since it is also specific about the directions in which these altered neurochemical events are hypothesized to operate, it provides a heuristic model for future investigations to probe. Indeed, some recent research (Benjamin et al., 1996; Ebstein et al.,

1996) has found that human genes responsible for the DA receptor subtype D4 are abnormal in individuals with high novelty-seeking scores, and thus provides some support for part of Cloninger's (1986) theory.

If we accept for the moment that many impulsivity-related disorders are linked with anxiety and depressive conditions, there is one additional model that should be discussed in the context of 5-HT abnormalities. Jacobs (1994) has recently published a fascinating overview of some research he began over two decades ago, in which he sought to understand the relationship of neuronal firing in the midbrain raphe nuclei (measured electrophysiologically) and its relationship to feline behaviors. Jacobs has assembled compelling evidence that as cats become aroused, there is an increased frequency of electrical discharge in the raphe complex. Indeed, in some studies, he and his colleagues were able to demonstrate that such neuronal firing could increase linearly as the rate or strength of four-legged movements took place on a treadmill. Similar firing patterns were observed in conjunction with other repetitive motor actions (e.g., chewing food). As mentioned earlier, the firing rate of 5-HT neurons is generally felt to be a covariant of how much of the neurotransmitter is released at synaptic regions throughout the broad neural axis to which it projects. Therefore, these and related findings have led Jacobs (1994) to suggest that a major function of the brain's 5-HT system is to prime and facilitate gross motor movements when they occur chronically and/or repetitively. Since low levels of 5-HT release are believed to contribute to depressive mood states, Jacobs has further suggested that voluntarily enhancing motor movements (e.g., exercising) may increase 5-HT release and help ameliorate depression. This notion is consistent with the facts that many depressed people show psychomotor retardation, and that most effective antidepressant medications enhance 5-HT neurotransmission and increase movement. Recent data from studies in rats trained to exercise provide support for this proposed relationship among 5-HT release, exercise, and antidepressant efficacy (Dey, 1994). Such a theory is also compatible with evidence cited above suggesting that some of 5-HT's control over impulsivity is linked to obsessional tendencies, since Jacobs has hypothesized that the repetitive actions of individuals with OCD may represent attempts at "self-medication" (i.e., their increased movements produce increased release of endogenous 5-HT). The particulars of how this theory might apply to specific aberrations of impulse control remain to be determined.

At face value, there appears to be a disparity between Jacobs's (1994) proposal that OCD may be a result of low endogenous levels of 5-HT and Cloninger's (1986) assessment that "obsessional personalities" are highly anxious in part because of high harm avoidance stemming from *elevated* 5-HT levels. This difference is more apparent than real. A careful reading of Cloninger's hypothesis reveals his acknowledgment that low 5-HT states exist in highly anxious, aggressive/violent people; this admission is based on essentially the same types of literature discussed above with regard to these conditions. As I see it, Cloninger's theory may appear to deviate from Jacobs's proposal in its attempt to include low DA activity as a prime mediator of high novelty seeking. In many ways, Cloninger's fundamental focus on reward and related processes requires such a construct, and conceptualizing low DA as a motivator mediating this role fits well with a large separate literature on this topic (e.g., Wise & Rompre, 1989). However, since 5-HT and DA functioning are often found to be inversely related, it follows that 5-HT would have to be conceptualized by Cloninger as functioning highly in obsessionals. Most other researchers view OCD much as Jacobs does; that is, 5-HT neurotransmission is considered to be dysfunctional in OCD. Indeed, Katz (1991) has gone so far as to propose that deficient 5-HT neurotransmission may be the biological substrate of Freudian repression in persons so affected.

CONCLUDING REMARKS

I have attempted in this broad overview to provide a general context within which readers of this book can obtain some sense of the interesting but complex relationships that exist in current thinking about the neuro-chemical substrates of impulsivity. The particular focus here has been on brain 5-HT because of the preponderance of knowledge accumulated on this subject. However, it should now be apparent that any comprehensive understanding of this transmitter's role in mediating impulsive actions requires additional knowledge of the other chemical systems with which this indoleamine interacts. A major challenge for biopsychologists is to derive valid multivariate biological studies in order to pursue this matter further. In that sense, we would do well to emulate the work of our colleagues who attempt to plumb the depths of complex personalities by employing multifactorial approaches in their studies. This task is made difficult by the methodological limitations often imposed on biopsycholo-gists in the measurement domains of basic biological properties. It is hoped that as technological advances continue to occur (at a sometimes dizzying rate), we may soon find ourselves better able to apply more sophisticated, multiple-measurement methods to this important question. Certainly, one dimension of the biological basis of impulsivity that appar-ently has not been probed yet is the neurochemical distinction that may exist between functional and dysfunctional variants (see Dickman, 1990). Are we to expect that there are different biochemical profiles for individu-als who possess differing forms of such hastiness to act? If so, such fine biological differences may be exceedingly difficult to discern. Even if such a possibility were realized, it would not address a more fundamental aspect of impulsivity as a construct—that is, the value judgments placed upon it within different societal or cultural contexts. As pointed out recently by Stein (1994), the biological study of impulsive aggression—which has been the major focus of this chapter—can inadvertently carry with it a negative stigmatization of individuals so identified, because of misperceptions that such people are inherently flawed. In other words, their "natural" or "genetic" makeups may be viewed as somehow constitutionally abnormal. Such a conclusion may be greatly in error, and, as such, may do a great disservice to those individuals and to our societal structure because of the implicit suggestion that these people are irreparably damaged. Ultimately, the role of biopsychologists and allied biological researchers is to define the physiological mechanisms that mediate such processes as "arousal," "motivation/willingness to act," "reward," and the like. How these basic processes are woven together to create the final fabric that constitutes each individual is invariably shaped by the person's environment and by the social/moral values assigned to behaviors within the environment. To conclude with an extension of this analogy, the biopsychologist merely tries to identify the characteristics of the various strands that contribute to the finished cloth we call "personality." It is the task of society to act as the loom upon which the fiber strands are woven to create the persona. And it is the more difficult role of other psychologists to describe the factors that turn this material into the diverse "wardrobe" that ultimately makes up a particular society.

ACKNOWLEDGMENTS

The research for and initial sections of this chapter were written when I was head of the Section of Biopsychology Research at the Clarke Institute of Psychiatry in Toronto. However, shortly after this project was initiated, I took up my current position as professor and chair of the Department of Psychology at Wayne State University. The majority of this chapter was written there. As a result, I must acknowledge the support of both institutions for the various resources made available to me in order to complete this work. I also acknowledge the financial support of the Natural Sciences and Engineering Research Council of Canada, which provided my lab with financial support for 9 years before my departure from Canada. The work conducted with their resources—though not specifically discussed here—permitted a variety of research to be performed that indirectly stimulated my interest in this topic and in the general area of impulsivity.

REFERENCES

Asberg, M., Traskman, L., & Thoren, P. (1976). 5-HIAA in the cerebrospinal fluid: A biochemical suicide predictor? *Archives of General Psychiatry, 38*, 1193–1197.

Azmitia, E. C., & Whitaker-Azmitia, P. M. (1991). Awakening the sleeping giant: Anatomy and plasticity of the brain serotonergic system. *Journal of Clinical Psychiatry, 52*(12, Suppl.), 4–16.

Benjamin, J., Li, L., Patterson, C., Greenberg, B. D., Murphy, D. L., & Hamer, D. H. (1996). Population and familial association between the D4 receptor gene and measures of novelty seeking. *Nature Genetics, 12*, 81–84.

Botchin, M. B., Kaplan, J. R., Manuck, S. B., &, Mann, J. J. (1993). Low versus high prolactin responders to fenfluramine challenge: Marker of behavioral differences in adult male cynomolgus macaques. *Neuropsychopharmacology, 9*(2), 93–99.

Brodie, B. B., & Shore, P. (1957). A concept for a role of serotonin and norepinephrine as chemical mediators in the brain. *Annals of the New York Academy of Sciences, 66,* 631–642.

Brown, G. L., Ebert, M. H., Goyer, P. F., Jimerson, D. C., Klein, W. J., Bunney, W. E., & Goodwin, F. K. (1982). Aggression, suicide, and serotonin: Relationship to CSF amine metabolites. *American Journal of Psychiatry, 139,* 741–746.

Carlson, N. R. (1991). *Physiology of behavior* (4th ed.). Boston: Allyn & Bacon.

Cloninger, C. R. (1986). A unified biosocial theory of personality and its role in the development of anxiety states. *Psychiatric Developments, 3,* 167–226.

Coccaro, E. F. (1992). Impulsive aggression and central serotonergic system function in humans: An example of a dimensional brain–behavior relationship. *International Clinical Psychopharmacology, 7,* 3–12.

Coccaro, E. F., Gabriel, S., & Siever, L. J. (1990). Buspirone challenge: Preliminary evidence for a role for central 5-HT_{1A} receptor function in impulsive aggressive behavior in humans. *Psychopharmacology Bulletin, 26,* 393–405.

Colmenares, J. L., Wurtman, R. J., & Fernstrom, J. D. (1975). Effects of ingestion of a carbohydrate–fat meal on the levels and synthesis of 5-hydroxyindoles in various regions of the rat central nervous system. *Journal of Neurochemistry, 25,* 825–829.

Dey, S. (1994). Physical exercise as a novel antidepressant agent: Possible role of serotonin receptor subtypes. *Physiology and Behavior, 55*(2), 323–329.

Dickman, S. J. (1990). Functional and dysfunctional impulsivity: Personality and cognitive correlates. *Journal of Personality and Social Psychology, 58*(1), 95–102.

Dourish, C. T. (1995). Multiple serotonin receptors: Opportunities for new treatments for obesity? *Obesity Research, 3*(Suppl. 4), 449S–462S.

Ebstein, R. P., Novick, O., Umansky, R., Priel, B., Osher, Y., Blaine, D., Bennett, E. R., Nemanov, L., Katz, M., & Belmaker, R. H. (1996). Dopamine D4 receptor (DrDR) exon III polymorphism associated with the human personality trait of novelty seeking. *Nature Genetics, 12,* 78–80.

Falck, B., Hillarp, N.-A., Thieme, G., & Torp, A. (1962). Fluorescence of catecholamines and related compounds condensed with formaldehyde. *Journal of Histochemistry and Cytochemistry, 10,* 348–354.

Faustman, W. O., King, R. J., Faull, K. F., Moses, J. A., Jr., Benson, K. L., Zarcone, V. P., & Csernansky, J. G. (1991). MMPI measures of impulsivity and depression correlate with CSF 5-HIAA and HVA in depression but not schizophrenia. *Journal of Affective Disorders, 22,* 235–239.

Fichter, M. M., Quadflieg, N., & Rief, W. (1994). Course of multi-impulsive bulimia. *Psychological Medicine, 24,* 591–604.

Fishbein, D. H., Lozovsky, D., & Jaffe, J. H. (1989). Impulsivity, aggression, and neuroendocrine responses to serotonergic stimulation in substance abusers. *Biological Psychiatry, 25,* 1049–1066.

Golden, R. N., Gilmore, J. H., Corrigan, M. H. N., Ekstrom, R. D., Knight, B. T., & Garbutt, J. C. (1991). Serotonin, suicide, and aggression: Clinical studies. *Journal of Clinical Psychiatry, 52*(12, Suppl.), 61–69.

Grant, L. D., Coscina, D. V., Grossman, S. P., & Freedman, D. X. (1973). Muricide after serotonin depleting lesions of the midbrain raphe nuclei. *Pharmacology, Biochemistry and Behavior, 1,* 77–80.

Higuchi, S., Suzuki, K., Yamada, K., Parrish, K., & Kono, H. (1993). Alcoholics with eating disorders: Prevalence and clinical course. A study from Japan. *British Journal of Psychiatry, 162,* 403–406.

Jacobs, B. L. (1994). Serotonin, motor activity and depression-related disorders. *American Scientist, 82,* 456–463.

Kafka, M. P. (1991a). Successful treatment of paraphilic coercive disorder (a rapist) with fluoxetine hydrochloride. *British Journal of Psychiatry, 158,* 844–847.

Kafka, M. P. (1991b). Successful antidepressant treatment of nonparaphilic sexual addictions and paraphilias in men. *Journal of Clinical Psychiatry, 52,* 60–65.

Kafka, M. P., & Prentky, R. (1992). Fluoxetine treatment of nonparaphilic sexual addictions and paraphilias in men. *Journal of Clinical Psychiatry, 53,* 351–358.

Kandel, E. R., & Schwartz, J. H. (1982). Molecular biology of learning: Modulation of transmitter release. *Science, 218,* 433–443.

Katz, R. J. (1991). Neurobiology of obsessive–compulsive disorder—a serotonergic basis of Freudian repression. *Neuroscience and Biobehavioral Reviews, 15*(3), 375–381.

Kent, T. A., Brown, C. S., Bryant, S. G., Barratt, E. S., Felthous, A. R., & Rose, M. (1988). Blood platelet uptake of serotonin in episodic aggression: Correlation with red blood cell proton T_1 and impulsivity. *Psychopharmacology Bulletin, 24*(3), 454–457.

Linnoila, M. I., DeJong, J., & Virkkunen, M. (1989). Psychobiological concomitants of history of suicide attempts among violent offenders and impulsive fire setters. *Archives of General Psychiatry, 46,* 604–606.

Linnoila, M. I., & Virkkunen, M. (1992). Aggression, suicidality, and serotonin. *Journal of Clinical Psychiatry, 53*(10, Suppl.), 46–51.

Mann, J. J., McBride, A., Anderson, G. M., & Mieczkowski, T. A. (1992). Platelet and whole blood serotonin content in depressed inpatients: Correlations with acute and life-time psychopathology. *Biological Psychiatry, 32,* 243–257.

McCown, W. G., Johnson, J. L., & Shure, M. B. (Eds.). (1993). *The impulsive client: Theory, research, and treatment.* Washington, DC: American Psychological Association.

Mehlman, P. T., Higley, J. D., Faucher, I., Lilly, A. A., Taub, D. M., Vickers, J., Suomi, S. J., & Linnoila, M. (1994). Low CSF 5-HIAA concentrations and severe aggression and impaired impulse control in nonhuman primates. *American Journal of Psychiatry, 151,* 1485–1491.

Mischel, W., Shoda, Y., & Rodriguez, M. L. (1989). Delay of gratification in children. *Science, 244,* 933–938.

Moeller, F. G., Steinberg, J. L., Petty, F., Fulton, M., Cherek, D. R., Kramer, G., & Garver, D. L. (1994). Serotonin and impulsive/aggressive behavior in cocaine dependent subjects. *Progress in Neuro-Psychopharmacology and Biological Psychiatry, 18,* 1027–1035.

Moreno, I., Saiz-Ruiz, J., & Lopez-Ibor, J. J. (1991). Serotonin and gambling dependence. *Human Psychopharmacology, 6,* S9–S12.

Mustajoki, P. (1987). Psychosocial factors in obesity. *Annals of Clinical Research, 19,* 143–146.

Nielsen, D. A., Goldman, D., Virkkunen, M., Tokola, R., Rawlings, R., & Linnoila, M. (1994). Suicidality and 5-hydroxyindoleacetic acid concentration associated with a tryptophan hydroxylase polymorphism. *Archives of General Psychiatry, 51,* 34–38.

O'Keane, V., Moloney, E., O'Neill, H., O'Connor, A., Smith, C., & Dinan, T. G. (1992). Blunted prolactin responses to *d*-fenfluramine in sociopathy: Evidence for subsensitivity of central serotonergic function. *British Journal of Psychiatry, 160,* 643–646.

Plutchik, A. A., & van Praag, H. M. (1993). Anxiety, impulsivity and depressed mood in relation to suicidal and violent behavior. *Acta Psychiatrica Scandinavica, 87,* 1–5.

Robbins, T. W., Everitt, B. J., Muir, J. L., & Harrison, A. (1992). Understanding the behavioural functions of neurochemically defined arousal systems. *International Brain Research Organization News, 20*(3), 7.

Simeon, D., Stanley, B., Frances, A., Mann, J. J., Winchel, R., & Stanley, M. (1992). Self-mutilation in personality disorders: Psychological and biological correlates. *American Journal of Psychiatry, 149*(2), 221–226.

Sohlberg, S., Norring, C., Holmgren, S., & Rosmark, B. (1989). Impulsivity and long-term prognosis of psychiatric patients with anorexia nervosa/bulimia nervosa. *Journal of Nervous and Mental Disease, 177*(5), 249–258.

Soubrie, P. (1986). Reconciling the role of central serotonin neurons in human and animal behavior. *Behavioral and Brain Sciences, 9,* 319–364.

Stein, D. J. (1994). Is impulsive aggression a disorder of the individual or a social ill?: A matter of metaphor. *Biological Psychiatry, 36,* 353–355.

Stein, D. J., & Hollander, E. (1992). Low-dose pimozide augmentation of serotonin reuptake blockers in the treatment of trichotillomania. *Journal of Clinical Psychiatry, 53*(4), 123–126.

Valzelli, L., Bernasconi, S., & Dalessandro, M. (1981). Effect of tryptophan administration on spontaneous and p-CPA-induced muricidal aggression in laboratory rats. *Pharmacological Research Communications, 13,* 891–897.

van Praag, H. M., Kahn, R. S., Asnis, G. M., Wetzler, S., Brown, S. L., Bleich, A., & Korn, M. L. (1988). Beyond nosology in biological psychiatry: 5-HT disturbances in mood, aggression and anxiety disorders. In M. Briley & G. Fillion (Eds.), *New concepts in depression* (pp. 96–119). New York: Macmillan.

Webster's new world dictionary, college edition. (1956). New York: World.

Whitaker-Azmitia, P. M. (1991). Role of serotonin and other neurotransmitter receptors in brain development: Basis for developmental pharmacology. *Pharmacological Reviews, 43*(4), 553–561.

Wise, R. A., & Rompre, P.-P. (1989). Brain dopamine and reward. *Annual Review of Psychology, 40,* 191–225.

Wurtman, J. J. (1993). Depression and weight gain: The serotonin connection. *Journal of Affective Disorders, 29,* 183–192.

Young, S. N., Pihl, R. O. & Ervin, F. R. (1988). The effect of altered tryptophan levels on mood and behavior in normal human males. *Clinical Neuropharmacology, 11*(Suppl. 1), S207–S215.

Zuckerman, M. (1984). Sensation seeking: A comparative approach to a human trait. *Behavioral and Brain Sciences, 7,* 413–471.

Zuckerman, M. (1991). *Psychobiology of personality.* New York: Cambridge University Press.

7

Brain Impairment in Impulsive Violence

MARILYN L. BOWMAN

People suffer brain damage under many different circumstances, including accidents, electrocutions, acute or chronic poisonings, strokes, tumors, and progressive dementias. Some proportion of these people will show aggression or violence that appears to be a result of brain changes associated with the damage. This chapter considers the extent to which violence may be attributed to damaged cerebral mechanisms.

Aggression and violence are viewed here as aspects of impulsivity, varying in terms of the severity of the behavior. "Impulsivity" is used as a broader term that refers to problems in regulating, and especially in inhibiting, emotions, thoughts, and behavior. Dysfunctions arising out of cerebral impairment may affect any of these functions and in turn may be associated with forms of aggression ranging from chronic irritability to episodes of violence.

Problems in emotional regulation related to aggression can include chronic irritability, emotional lability, and excessive temper. Cognitive problems associated with aggression include regulatory dysfunctions, such as ill-judged responses to new stimuli, inappropriate perseverations or obsessions, memory inefficiencies that lead to confusion and frustration, problems in identifying errors, and lack of insight and perspective. Problems in regulating overt behavior may be seen in aggressive and violent acts even when cognition appears to be intact after an insult to the brain.

Problems with aggression or violence can be found in association with cerebral impairment arising out of all the most common sources of brain damage, including acute or cumulative brain injury, progressive dementias, and stroke. This chapter focuses mainly (but not exclusively) on aggression associated with traumatic brain injury (TBI) from sudden or cumulative harmful stimuli, such as accidents, electrocution, or noxious fumes. Males are subjects of TBI twice as frequently as females, so masculine pronouns are used in this chapter.

NATURAL HISTORY OF AGGRESSION ARISING FROM BRAIN INJURY

There is a natural history of the aggressive behavioral changes that are seen in the acute and chronic (long-term) stages after brain injury.

Acute Effects

During the immediate period following a head injury with altered consciousness, the patient is often agitated as he emerges from a state of confusion. This agitation is shown in disinhibited behavior, which may include aggressive attacks on catheters, tubes, and people; sexually explicit language; verbally abusive behavior; and other overreactions to minimal stimulation, including uncontrollable laughter. These behaviors occur during a stage when the brain is undergoing acute changes as a result of the injury. With successful medical care, this tumultuous display is reduced.

In one study, the acute and aggressively agitated syndrome appeared to affect about 11% of TBI patients when criteria were applied systematically in a consecutive sample of hospital admissions for head injury in the early weeks following admission (Brooke, Questad, Patterson, & Bashak, 1992). The behavior is not associated with preinjury personality or psychiatric disorders, but is directly associated with the brain injury. The aggression is not well focused and is not psychologically meaningful. Among the most disturbed cases during early recovery, there seems to be no correlation between the occurrence of violent agitation requiring restraints or of sexually explicit behavior, with duration of coma or eventual outcome (Levin & Grossman, 1978). Thus, these behaviors have no necessary relationship with either coma status or long-term problems.

When aggression continues long after the period of acute injury, the question arises as to whether it represents residual organic effects of the original injury or whether additional factors are contributing to the behavior.

Long-Term Effects

The long-term prevalence rates for aggression and violence after recovery from the acute state of a brain injury have not been well established, because doing so requires a longitudinal prospective study from initial hospitalization onward, and such studies are expensive and rare. Although studies have looked at specific outcome groups to estimate prevalence rates of problem behaviors, these groups represent many different kinds of outcome status ranging from chronic inpatient status to discharge and return to normal home and work life; each kind of postinjury group shows different incidence rates for aggression and other kinds of problem behavior.

The best evidence to date suggests that aggression and violence are weakly related to injury factors (e.g., severity) across the long-term period of recovery and disability. (In terms of injury severity, Miller and Jones, 1985, found that approximately 95% of head injuries in a sample of 1,919 were mild [84%] or moderate [11%].)

Once patients have recovered from the acute trauma, a minority show continuing general emotional lability, including temper problems with aggression. The prevalence of this heightened emotionality is hard to determine; although it appears to increase across time in some patients after hospital discharge, the apparent increase may in part reflect changes in the focus of family observations, which are initially directed to patient survival and only later shift to interpersonal behavior. One survey of the relatives of patients who had suffered a severe head injury 5 years earlier and had been discharged to home life found that the prevalence of personality change had increased across time, with 74% of the patients described as showing personality change (Brooks, Campsie, Symington, Beatty, & McKinlay, 1986). Threats or gestures of violence were uttered by 54%, and there had been actual assault in 20% of cases. A similar figure was reported in a study of U.S. Vietnam veterans with penetrating head injury (Schwab, Grafman, Salazar, & Kraft, 1993). Twenty percent of the sample of 520 (out of the larger population of 1,112) showed problems with violent behavior; violence was ranked 8th out of a list of 15 impairments in order of frequency within the sample.

A different kind of aggression occurs in a small percentage of brain injury patients whose accident precipitates a major mental disorder. These cases are rare enough that they are usually reported as individual case studies in the psychiatric literature. Levin and Peters (1976), for example, described an affective psychosis with hypomanic dyscontrol and hypersexuality that was precipitated by the injury. In a series of 800 consecutive brain-injured patients studied by Levin and Grossman (1978), only 10 cases of such major decompensation were identified.

Problems with impulse control, including aggression, are also associated with deterioration of the brain from causes other than TBI. For example, approximately one-third of psychogeriatric inpatients show impulsive aggressive behavior, and aggression in this population is seen as the primary patient management problem in long-term care facilities

(Bolger & Dougherty, 1993). Poststroke patients show heightened lability at a rate of about 10%; it seems to be associated with subcortical damage, in that the patients have insight and are often embarrassed by their own poorly controlled behavior (House, Dennis, & Molyneux, 1989).

Although violence is found in association with brain damage, it is not an invariable result or even the most typical long-term outcome of brain damage when the population consists of ambulatory individuals who have returned to their homes. In my professional experience with home-dwelling TBI survivors of work accidents, even the minority of patients who show increased aggressiveness rarely commit acts of violence. More typically, they swear, yell, use crude language, and sometimes throw or break things around the house. A minority from this group utter threats to do personal harm; fewer than 5% of the more than 200 I have examined acted upon these threats.

The problems of impulsive aggression seen in TBI patients are often related in a meaningful way to their cognitive inefficiencies. These may be seen in prototypical situations among patients who have returned home and in whom temper remains a problem. The most typical aggression narratives that head-injured patients and their spouses tell concern episodes in which a patient displaces his rage when his memory problems lead to significant inefficiencies in performing long-held skills. His frustration at being unable to do things as accurately and quickly as before builds up into a high level of unhappiness with himself, which is easily displaced into rage against another when triggered by some other minor event. Both head-injured men and their spouses or partners tell independently of situations in which a patient is trying to do something useful (e.g., drywall a basement room) because he has free time and is restless staying at home. In the course of the job, he perpetually loses his tools through misplacing them; he measures expensive materials incorrectly despite several attempts to cross-check things and has to buy additional supplies; he generally finds that his work is full of expensive errors, delays, and frustrations. Once he is in this mood of disappointment, it takes only very minor household problems to trigger the outburst of anger.

Another prototypical situation in which impulsive aggression arises out of cognitive inefficiencies concerns the patient who is being expected to behave in a normal way in the life of the family, but cannot do so because his memory is unreliable and he has become confused. He may have been told a number of times about an upcoming family social event; yet when the day and hour arrive, he does not remember any of the previous conversations. He concludes that no one tells him anything, becomes furious that he has been excluded from the family's plans, and angrily refuses to take part in something about which he believes he has been allowed to have no choice or comment. In other situations, the patient responds to his confusion by denying the memory problem that led to the confusion, and attributing it instead externally—to inadequacies in the behavior of his wife/partner or children. This externalizing of responsibility then justifies an angry outburst at them for their uncaringness or ineptitude.

From these prototypical examples, it is possible to see that the temper outburst is not solely an organic effect of a damaged brain's directly producing aggressive behavior. Instead, anger and aggression result from a combination of many individual and contextual factors. In the cases of cerebral impairment from head injury, toxic poisoning, or electrocution that I have seen, outright violence is relatively infrequent, but about one-quarter of patients' families report that the patients now have a bad temper and that this has become a serious problem for the families. In the relatively small group within which violence occurs, a pattern of violent acting out had existed prior to the head injury and alcohol was always a triggering factor, usually on the part of both a patient and his spouse/partner. There has not been a single case in which violence occurred without some powerful personal contextual factors, including premorbid problems. These data suggest that among TBI patients who have been discharged to normal living situations, problematical long-standing individual traits, disturbed relationships, and long-standing conflicts contribute powerfully to the expression of anger as actual violence.

Effects on the Family

Among those cases of brain-injured patients who do show persistent aggression in daily life, the consequences of the behavior are frequently devastating to their families. Eruptions of aggression against children lead to disturbed behavior in the children and to marital disputes. Aggression against spouses/partners contributes further to marital strains and to the destruction of family life. There are important interaction effects involving cerebral impairment, premorbid family patterns, and personality that must be included in attempting to understand the origins of impulsive violence within such a family. One study of 31 male patients who had been referred for evaluation of marital violence found that 61% had histories of severe head injury, and 48% had histories of alcohol abuse (Rosenbaum & Hoge, 1989). In logistic regressions in a later controlled study of discordant marriages, head injury functioned as a good predictor of partner-battering (Rosenbaum et al., 1994). In such studies, it is also important to determine what proportion of cases had alcohol use and violence as factors contributing to the original head injury, before any physiological interpretations relating the head injury to the family problems as if it were causal are attempted.

THE BRAIN AND AGGRESSION

In a 1995 conference on the genetics of violence, held in London, researchers reviewed evidence concerning the possibility of genetic predispositions to violence. There Sir Michael Rutter, a distinguished researcher in developmental psychiatry, stressed that although there is no such thing as a "crime gene," genetic factors do appear to have a significant link to adult criminal behaviors (Stevenson, 1995). Much has yet to be done concerning this hypothesis and the neural mechanisms through which as yet unidentified genetic factors might operate. The mechanisms that have been studied independently of a genetic model are reviewed in the following sections.

Although there are no anatomical "aggression centers" in the brain that singly determine violent behavior in humans, there are functional brain systems that include specific areas as part of networks in which damage to some components of the network may have more significant effects on aggression than damage to other parts. Dysfunctions involving brain chemicals have also been associated with impulsive aggression, but again there are no specific "aggression chemicals" in the brain that will solely trigger violence.

Neuroanatomy

The Frontal Lobes

The frontal lobes are considered to be important in the overall management of cognitions that organize, plan, and evaluate behavior. If there is sufficient damage to the frontal cortex to weaken these "executive" cognitive functions, an affected patient may use poor judgment and show disinhibited behavior that includes violence. The frontal lobes are the most common site of brain injury (Spreen, 1981).

There appear to be two main patterns to the altered regulation of inhibition associated with frontal lobe damage (Miller, 1990). In one pattern a patient demonstrates marked apathy and indifference, whereas in the other a patient exhibits impulsive outbursts of aggressiveness. The latter syndrome was described as "organic personality syndrome, explosive type" in the *Diagnostic and Statistical Manual of Mental Disorders,* third edition, revised (DSM-III-R; American Psychiatric Association, 1987); this was changed to "personality change due to a general medical condition, aggressive, labile, or disinhibited type" (depending on the most prominent symptom) in DSM-IV (American Psychiatric Association, 1994). The two frontal patterns are associated with damage to different regions of the frontal lobes; the syndrome of impulsive aggression has been associated with damage to the orbital–frontal cortex. A recent case, for example, reported the onset of antisocial personality disorder following surgery for a pituitary tumor that affected only the left orbital–frontal region; a 33-year-old man showed no cognitive changes, yet his interpersonal behavior changed markedly (Meyers & Berman, 1992). Despite such interesting case reports, in the more typical "frontal lobe syndrome" there is a bland and casual unconcern about important life problems, rather than impulsive aggression.

The Temporal Lobes and Limbic System

The limbic system is another brain network that has been implicated in violence. It is an old functional midbrain unit underlying the temporal lobes. Within the limbic system, the hippocampus and amygdala have been extensively studied in experimental animal research concerning fear and rage responses. With stimulation of the amygdala in humans, heightened emotionality with fear and rage emerges after an initial orienting response (Joseph, 1990).

In humans, research on the amygdala–aggression relationship has been derived from experience with individual cases involving surgery (Mark & Ervin, 1970), from computed tomography (CT) scan data (Martinius, 1982), and from autopsy studies. Case reports have described damaged limbic structures in humans showing episodic violence. Most of the surgery has concerned cases of intermittent explosive disorder, and there is now a literature of case studies in which previously uncontrolled episodic bursts of violence were significantly reduced following surgical removal of tumors affecting the amygdala (e.g., Sachdev & Smith, 1992). In a recent example, temporal lobe damage resulting from herpes simplex viral encephalitis in a 14-year-old boy resulted in a new syndrome of aggression (Greer & Lyons-Crews, 1989). Charles Whitman, the notorious University of Texas sharpshooting killer of 14, was found upon autopsy to be suffering from a tumor pressing on the amygdala (Joseph, 1990). In the weeks leading up to Whitman's rampage, he had kept notes revealing how troubled he was with feelings of violence, which overwhelmed his daily life and which he experienced as being very much out of character. Because his violent acts were planned, however, they do not represent a true dyscontrol rage comparable to that seen in animals with specific brain lesions.

In addition to episodic violence, temporal and limbic system damage is often related to abnormal electrophysiological activity, which may include seizures. One review found that epilepsy associated with lesions in the temporal lobe was associated with aggression in 37% of cases prior to surgery, of which about half showed improvement following surgery (Strauss & Wada, 1991).

Despite evidence from individual cases, and although electrophysiological and neuroanatomical data show an association between limbic functioning and aggression, it is important to note that there can be limbic system pathology without aggressive behavior, and aggressive behavior without limbic pathology (Eichelman, 1983). Damage to the amygdala, for example, does not invariably contribute to violence; it has also been associated with nonviolent problem behaviors, including sexual preoccupations, hyperreligiosity, and pseudomystical ideas (Schiff, Sabin, Geller, Alexander, & Mark, 1982).

Diffuse Damage with Acceleration–Deceleration

In contrast to these descriptions of brain damage associated with highly localized brain areas affected by lesions, many patients with cerebral impairment from brain injuries have suffered acceleration–deceleration trauma, which is generally understood to cause diffuse microscopic damage (Jennett, 1986). These widespread lesions "consist of varying neuronal damage throughout the brain, together with shearing lesions of nerve fibers in the subcortical region and brain stem, and contusions and lacerations of the cerebral cortex" (Jennett, 1986, p. 5212). It appears that a majority of the damage usually occurs above the level of the brainstem, and this damage is less obvious in neurological examination than the highly visible signs of loss of consciousness associated with brainstem injury.

Acceleration–deceleration injuries to the brain can occur in accidents where there has been no direct hit to the head, but instead an abrupt and forceful movement and stopping of the entire body. Diffuse brain injuries can also occur in blunt head trauma, where there may be a combination of focal and diffuse injuries. Brooks (1988) concluded that in blunt head injury the diffuse damage that is sustained actually overrides the effect of focal lesions, even though focal lesions are more readily observed on neural imaging procedures and in terms of narrowly defined functional deficits.

The functional effects of diffuse brain damage on behavior are far less well established, although there is some agreement that diffuse effects within the frontal lobes will be manifested as general failures in the overall regulation of behavior, as described above. In cases where the brain injury cannot be seen and localized by means of CT or other neural imaging techniques, yet there is good evidence of an acceleration–deceleration accident followed by disturbed behavior including aggression, diffuse injuries may be contributing to an attenuated version of the "frontal lobe syndrome."

Neural Electrochemistry

Violent behavior has been related to disturbances in endogenous brain chemistry involving sex hormones and neurotransmitters, as well as to epileptic seizure activity. Testosterone, the naturally occurring male hormone, appears to play some role in violence and aggression (Gladue, 1991; Susman & Inoff-Germain, 1987), and there have been chemical attempts to reduce general or specifically sexual aggression through the use of antiandrogens and estrogens (Arnold, 1993; Horn, 1987). There are receptors for both estrogen and androgens in the amygdala. In animals, most aggression that is not for self-defense or food predation is related to reproduction, so hormones play a role in aggression (Carlson, 1988). Despite this, the evidence of a strong causal connection is "unconvincing" (Leger, 1992), and correlational studies cannot be used as evidence of the direction of the connection because increased aggression may cause increased testosterone levels. In animal studies, for example, experienced dominant males will continue to fight to maintain dominance even after removal of the testes, and subordinate males with histories of failed fights will fail to fight even after testosterone is increased. Furthermore, in humans, personality variables such as "Type A" characteristics have been observed to moderate testosterone–aggression relations in experimental studies (Berman & Gladue, 1993), and elevations of testosterone arising from general elation and happiness can be seen. Experimental studies by McCaul, Gladue, and Joppa (1992) found that testosterone levels rose in human males after dominance experiences. Individual life experience may thus be more powerful than the hormonal effects of androgens, both in animals and in humans.

Neurotransmitters have been studied for their roles in aggression, and low serotonin levels have been implicated (Coccaro & Kavoussi, 1992; Linnoila & Virkkunen, 1992; Virkkunen & Linnoila, 1993; see Coscina, Chapter 6, this volume). Normalization of serotonin levels as a means of reducing aggression has been carried out through the use of serotonin-enhancing drugs such as lithium (Haas & Cope, 1985). Excesses of excitatory neurotransmitters such as norepinephrine and acetylcholine also appear to be associated with increased activity and mania. Excessive levels of acetylcholine in the hypothalamus, for example, have been associated with increases in predatory aggression in animal studies, and increased manic activity in humans can be successfully reduced with lithium.

The complexity of the neurotransmitters and hormones implicated in aggression, and their diverse roles in brain activity and behavior, further reinforce the problems noted earlier concerning the neuroanatomy of aggression. There is no neurotransmitter or hormone that has functions solely related to violence, and all are essential neurochemicals for functioning outside the domain of aggression.

Exogenous Chemicals and Aggression: Alcohol and Other Drugs

Just as endogenous brain chemicals play a role in the relations between brain function and violent behavior, so too do some exogenous chemicals. Among normal subjects, experimental studies have shown that subjects will act with more and faster aggressive behavior following alcohol, cocaine, or morphine ingestion (Berman, Taylor, & Marged, 1993; Licata, Taylor, Berman, & Cranston, 1993; Weisman & Taylor, 1994). These substances interact with disposition and environmental cues, however, and the aggression is not entirely drug-related (Taylor & Chermack, 1993).

Among individuals with sudden-onset brain damage, intoxicants such as alcohol appear to be experienced as aversive. The majority of such patients reduce or avoid alcohol use, and this is true even for patients who had been heavy users premorbidly (Kreutzer, Wehman, Harris, Burns, & Young, 1991). Alcohol exacerbates problems with headache, dizziness, balance, speech slurring, and confusion, leading the majority of brain-injured patients to avoid these unpleasant neurological symptoms by reducing their intake of the drug or avoiding it altogether.

Is There Specificity in Brain–Violence Relationships?

Studies of the neuroanatomy and neurochemistry associated with violence show the kind of complexity in brain–behavior correlations that is found in studies of other human behavior that has evolutionary implications, such as sexual behavior, eating behavior, and other kinds of dominance. It is difficult to localize brain regions or to identify endogenous neurochemicals that are specifically or solely responsible for violent behavior in humans. The correlations between a specific brain region or neurochemical and violence are weak and are affected by confounding factors, including premorbid personality, life experience, and current environmental conditions (e.g., family and work life). For example, although male sex hormones may be implicated in some male violence, research as long ago as the classic work reported by Ford and Beach (1951) has shown that within higher species sexual behavior is significantly affected by past learning and experience, and that sexual aggression can be seen in males of many species even long after the loss of sex hormones through castration in adulthood.

Second, the brain regions or naturally occurring biochemicals that play a role in violence have multiple purposes within the brain other than the management of aggression. The amygdala, for example, is an important part of the limbic system and plays a key role in orientation and sustained attention, thus affecting learning and memory. Finally, in studies where altered biochemical concentrations are found in the brains of narrowly defined subjects (such as incarcerated violent criminals), some of the changes found may well be results of subject bias and confounding variables (such as isolation and incarceration stresses), rather than having been precipitating causes of the original violence (DeFeudis & Schauss, 1987). Biased subject samples pose an especially high risk in research looking for causal relationships when a correlational research method is used.

It is only in a minority of brain impairment cases that a specific focal brain region or specific neurochemical problem is known to be the cause of violent behavior. Attempts to localize brain areas or to identify brain chemicals responsible for violent behavior in humans who have suffered brain damage are speculative rather than definitive. Neural imaging techniques studying glucose uptake to identify active areas in the functioning brain may in the future yield insights into the brain functioning of violent individuals; however, there is insufficient evidence yet for any way of identifying a living brain that might be expected to initiate violent rather than depressed or demented behavior. The Brain Imaging Council of the Society of Nuclear Medicine is trying to create guidelines for interpreting brain scans to prevent misuse of the techniques for such premature ventures (Tikovsky, Alavi, Devous, & van Heertum, 1994).

Brain Damage and Criminal Violence

Because violent behavior is criminal, researchers have considered the question of whether criminals have a high prevalence of brain damage. The question is also of practical interest, in that brain injury is increasingly being used in criminal court cases as an explanation of the origins of violent criminal behavior, and as a defense against charges of violence (Restak, 1992). In 1985, the U.S. Supreme Court ruled (*Ake v. Oklahoma*, 1985) that a defendant is entitled to psychiatric assistance when the jury is considering the death penalty on the basis of the prosecution's argument that the defendant will continue to be dangerous. Since that ruling, it appears probable that evidence relating to organic brain disorder, including neuropsychological testing to assess the presence of organic impairment, will become increasingly common in defenses against criminal charges in the United States.

Results of studies of the prevalence of cerebral impairment in incarcerated prisoners have been variable. Brain damage—either localized damage or disturbed neurochemical functioning—has been identified as an important feature associated with violent behavior in some studies (e.g., Martell, 1992; Volavka, Martell, & Convit, 1992). Other studies have reported impaired performance by psychopaths on neuropsychological tests, suggesting neurocognitive impairments (e.g., Gorenstein, 1982; Nachshon, 1988). Nevertheless, the evidence is far from clear on the causal hypothesis. Alcohol use is an important premorbid factor and confound in studies of cerebral impairment in psychopaths. The cognitive and behavioral sequelae of head injury are so difficult to distinguish from those of chronic alcohol use that Levin and others typically exclude alcoholics from studies of cognitive outcomes after brain injury (Levin, Benton, & Grossman, 1982).

In studies that incorporate controlled comparisons of violent and nonviolent subjects, significant differences in neuropathology have not been clearly established. Langevin and Ben-Aron (1987) did not find differences, whereas Rosenbaum et al. (1994), using an unbiased assessment of medical history and behavioral and quantified measures of aggression, found that histories of head injury were significantly more frequent in partner-abusive men than in two comparison groups. A careful study by Hart, Forth, and Hare (1990), using clear criteria for psychopathy and controls for age, education, general psychopathology, and substance abuse in a large sample, found that the prevalence of clear signs of mild or worse brain impairment among criminal psychopaths was relatively low and around 7%. The authors concluded: "The results provide no support for traditional brain-damage explanations of psychopathy" (p. 374). Restak (1992) has argued that "the neurological defense" attributing violent criminal behavior to a damaged brain has little scientific support outside a small number of cases with damage specifically to the limbic system.

It appears that brain damage is rarely a significant cause of intermittent violence in otherwise normal people. Investigations concerning criminal violence will be of increasing interest as neural diagnostic procedures improve. With these improvements and better control of confounds, eventually the base rates of brain damage within violent criminal populations and the base rates of violence within noncriminal brain-damaged populations will become clearer.

MODELS OF THE BRAIN–AGGRESSION RELATIONSHIP

Research has tried to account for the core psychological mechanisms explaining the apparent relationship between brain damage and violence. One way of construing the connection is to see it as a failure of cognition. However, if cognition is viewed specifically as IQ or problem-focused reasoning ability, the cognitive failure model fails to account for the brain–aggression relationship, because IQ may be unchanged following brain damage and even following significant removal of brain tissue (e.g., Hebb, 1942, and sources cited in Luria, 1980).

In assessments of current neuropsychological functioning, global cognitive skills are often broken down to discriminate right- and left-hemisphere functions, and also caudally to discriminate the anterior "higher" cortical functions from the more posterior sensory–motor functions. Concerning the hemispheric lateralization hypothesis, early research by David Wechsler showed that "sociopaths" had consistently lower scores on the Verbal IQ portion of the Wechsler intelligence tests (Kaufman, 1990); this was interpreted as showing some relatively inferior left-hemisphere function or reduced left-hemisphere lateralization. Research continues to show that those found guilty of criminal acts as adolescents or adults show a cognitive skill pattern in which visual–spatial reasoning is significantly better than verbal reasoning, even when many relevant confounds are controlled for (e.g., test motivation, race, socioeconomic status, academic achievement, and impulsivity; Lynam, 1993). However, the interpretation of these cognitive results as if they truly represented hemispheric differences probably goes beyond the evidence; few cognitive skills are tightly lateralized in people with intact brains, and thus it would be going well beyond the data to conclude that criminal acts are associated with a more active or effective right hemisphere. Moffitt (1988) looked at the anterior–posterior comparison in antisocial 13-year-olds and concluded that frontal lobe functions were not impaired, whereas functions such as memory and language (associated with somewhat more posterior cortical areas) showed deficits.

If cognition is studied in terms of general social knowledge, there is some evidence that this hypothesis is also insufficient as an explanation for a cognition–aggression relationship. In one case study of the social knowledge hypothesis, conceptual flexibility and comprehension of behavioral consequences were tested to see whether problems in these cognitive skills were the hallmarks of "frontal" antisocial behavior. The case was a prototypical ventromedial–frontal patient with "acquired sociopathy" arising out of this damage (Saver & Damasio, 1991). The patient was studied to see whether his abilities to generate behavioral options when faced with choices concerning social behavior, and to predict probable consequences of different kinds of behavioral responses, were deficient in comparison to those of five male controls. Across a range of measures focused on social knowledge of this sort, the patient performed at levels equal to or better than those of his controls, despite actual social behavior that was unacceptably antisocial—suggesting that his core defect was not a lack of knowledge of social behavior.

In another model, brain-related cognitive inefficiencies may contribute to a change in threshold for behavioral acts such as aggression, which are normally subjected to judgment before being enacted. Miller (1990) has thus argued that cognitive skills may be the key to the postinjury change in impulsive aggression. He argues that individuals who were previously marginal in terms of antisocial behavior and cognitive competence become outright disinhibited following a head injury, as a direct outcome of diminished cognitive and coping skills. According to Miller, when these higher cognitive skills are impaired, the behavior that remains is impulsive, aggressive, and childish without compensatory thinking skills or judgment. Another approach has been to consider the interpersonal behavior problems related to brain injury as a kind of regression. Santoro and Spiers (1993), for example, compared the behavior of TBI patients with that of children on a social cognition task requiring taking another person's point of view. Children normally develop this recursive thinking capacity between the ages of 7 and 9; the researchers found that TBI patients performed significantly more poorly on this task than controls matched for general cognitive competence on a test of vocabulary level.

In general, it has been difficult to identify specific cognitive deficits that might be at the heart of the behavioral dyscontrol seen in cases with cerebral damage, whether the data come from individual cases with well-identified lesion areas (Meyers & Berman, 1992), from uncontrolled groups (Kaye & Grigsby, 1990), or from small controlled group studies (Damasio & Tranel, 1990).

Other models have gone beyond the cerebral and cognitive factors to look at contextual variables as part of the mechanisms of aggression in cerebral impairment. Kandel and Freed (1989) have put forward a speculative and interactional diathesis-stress model, in which behavior affected by minimal frontal brain dysfunction (inferred from neuropsychological test data) is then seen as being excessively affected by noxious social conditions, resulting in antisocial behavior.

The most interesting research has considered deeper dimensions of higher cognitive functions, such as the general regulation of inhibition. Caplan and Shechter (1990) wanted to see whether impulsivity (rapid physical response) might be the core variable in the brain–aggression relationship, and they tested to see whether it was differentially associated with lateralized lesions. In a controlled study, they tested the speed of response to a visual matching task in elderly samples. Although they found hints of greater impulsivity with right-hemisphere lesions and in both lesioned groups in comparison with normals, Caplan and Shechter retreated from any general thesis of impulsivity, noting that the right-hemisphere-lesioned groups also suffered from incomplete visual scanning, which may have contributed to their quicker responses. In contrast, Bolger and Dougherty (1993) more recently concluded from their study of 84 psychogeriatric patients that aggression is a generalized personality problem in inhibiting behavior, rather than being related more narrowly to impairment of higher cognitive functions.

Using a more somatic model of affective regulation, Damasio and Tranel (1990) studied the reactivity of brain-damaged individuals who had sociopathic behavior, to see whether differences in emotional responsivity would be characteristic of patients with frontal lobe damage. They found support for their hypothesis: Patients with frontal lesions showed defective electrodermal skin conductance responses to socially significant stimuli, compared to brain-damaged patients with lesions elsewhere, even though the patients with frontal damage nonetheless showed normal autonomic responsivity to unconditioned stimuli.

The evidence thus suggests that violence may be understood as an expression of general disinhibition associated with generalized impairments in regulatory functions commonly associated with the frontal cortex, rather than as a factor arising from specific cognitive impairments. To understand why regulation may be the core problem, rather than some more specific cognitive skill, the prevalence of aggression in relation to other disturbed behaviors among brain-damaged populations needs to be revisited.

Although problems with temper control are seen in perhaps 30% of brain-damaged patients if consecutive cases are studied, cerebral damage is much more frequently associated with a lethargic syndrome. The typical long-term results of a brain injury are general apathy, loss of initiative, and social withdrawal, rather than violent outbursts (Fordyce, Roueche, & Prigitano, 1983). This lethargy is seen especially in more severely damaged patients, who often show a bland demeanor and vague cordiality, with little insight or concern about their cognitive losses. One study followed 70 brain-injured patients after the initial period of recovery from acute trauma, and found that the most prominent symptoms differentiating patients, in terms of both severity of injury and long-term effects, were withdrawal and motor retardation rather than excitement and disinhibition (Levin & Grossman, 1978). In another study of 80 consecutive cases within 6 months of hospital discharge, three of the five most commonly reported symptoms were related to social withdrawal (social isolation, 56%; decreased community involvement, 43%; and major depression, 37%), in addition to problems associated with changes in family and economic arrangements (Swartzman & Teasell, 1993). Similarly, a study of chronically brain-impaired adults found that the most frequent psychological disorder was depression, with its associated psychomotor retardation and general withdrawal; disorders included TBI, multiple sclerosis, Huntington's disease, Parkinson's disease, and dementia of the Alzheimer's type (Drudge & Rosen, 1986). Although this apathetic syndrome appears to be very different from an impulsive violence syndrome, it may be most useful to consider this behavior as reflecting the other end of a single continuum of impaired regulation of initiative.

The great Russian neuropsychologist Luria (1980) long ago argued that regulation of emotions and thinking is one of the core problems when lesions affect higher cortical functioning. Damage to the deep parts of the temporal lobes may be manifested both in lethargy or stupor and in anxious agitation and even rage, when the regulation of emotion is the core difficulty. Damage associated with the frontal cortex may be manifested as a defect in inhibiting inappropriate or irrelevant behavior. The patient does not compare his own performance with his original plan and therefore fails to correct a wrong approach. This general error in regulation of behavior will be seen even if the patient's performance on formal tests of reasoning and knowledge is in the relatively normal range.

Within this framework, although impulsive violence seems to be the opposite of apathetic and lethargic behavior, both problems can exist within the same individual because the regulatory mechanisms are those that are impaired. With lack of effective regulation, there can be problems of both excessive and deficient responsivity in the same person. The same man who refuses to go outside for a walk or visit family members, and who prefers instead to sit isolated in front of the TV set on for days on end, may suddenly erupt in an abusive attack on a close family member over some trivial matter. Defective regulation of thinking is revealed in sudden and impulsive actions based on poor judgment, such as excessive purchases, sudden trips, and sudden marital or work changes. These general problems in regulating behavior can thus be associated both with social withdrawal and with its behavioral opposite, intermittent aggression. The impulsive behavior (including violence) that may be seen in patients with cerebral impairment may be most usefully understood as part of a more general syndrome—one that also includes the inappropriate inhibition of behavior at other times. In this sense, the impulsive aggression associated with cerebral impairment does not have the features of callous and calculating self-interest that can be seen in the aggression of individuals with personality disorders but without cerebral impairment.

ASSESSING AND PREDICTING VIOLENCE

Among the most commonly used standardized tests of clinical psychodiagnostic assessment, there is no particular psychological test that has high validity in the prediction of violence, although some of the commonly used clinical tests include scales with items sensitive to aggression and hostility. On the Minnesota Multiphasic Personality Inventory, for example, some of the basic clinical scales (e.g., Paranoia, Schizophrenia, and Hypomania), and some special scales (e.g., Overcontrolled Hostility), include item content concerning aggressive behavior. Other objective and projective techniques similarly include some consideration of hostility, callousness, and energy levels, which are key psychological features of violent behavior. In general, however, the record of validity for standard clinical psychological tests in predicting dangerousness is quite poor.

In line with Luria's (1980) regulatory model, Bolger and Dougherty (1993) made a recent attempt to construct an assessment instrument specific to the problem of aggression, focusing on behavioral inhibition as the core construct. They compared aggressive and nonaggressive psychogeriatric inpatients to assess the value of several tests of behavioral inhibition, as compared to measures of higher cognitive functions. Results suggested that one particular behavioral checklist concerning capacity for inhibition provided the best identification, with an average correct classification of about 69%.

To date, the most promising means of predicting violence are behavioral measures that use extensive interview and collateral information about past behavior, sometimes with the help of weighted formulas derived from studies of prisoners. In these studies, a history of brain injury has never been a significant enough predictor variable to require incorporation in any of the best formulas. The Revised Psychopathy Checklist (Hare et al., 1990), a specialized instrument making use of past history as behavioral data, has shown quite usefully high levels of predictive validity in predicting future dangerousness. It does not include known cerebral impairment as a powerful predictor variable.

TREATMENT

Patients with brain damage can be sorted into groups on the basis of the origin of the cerebral insult, and these groupings have differential implications for understanding the relationship between cerebral damage and violent behavior and for planning treatment. As noted earlier, in TBI most patients are male, in a ratio estimated at 2:1; within adults, the males with greatest incidence are between the ages of 16 and 30 (Boll & Barth, 1983). In many cases their damage arises from risk-taking behavior while driving or in the course of work in heavy and dangerous occupations; in many cases alcohol is involved. These correlates of TBI are associated with other premorbid biases relating to personality characteristics of impulsivity and antisocial personality disorder (Jennett, 1972; Wood, 1987). This bias in the general TBI population affects the interpretation of postinjury behavior; if there is a high incidence of problems with impulsivity (including aggression) in TBI patients, these cannot necessarily be attributed to the head injury itself. In many cases, behavioral problems of poor impulse regulation and risk taking preceded and may have contributed to the head injury. Other kinds of quickly acquired cerebral impairment arising from nontraumatic causes (e.g., tumors) are not as strongly associated with such premorbid personality and behavior correlates. Psychogeriatric populations have special features associated with their advanced age, in addition to cerebral impairment and problems with impulsivity, and these may affect the kinds of treatments that are to be used.

Physical Treatments

Drug treatments and physical restraints are commonly used to control agitated aggression during the acute posttraumatic stage following a head injury. Medications have to be chosen carefully in order to sedate without veiling the patient's neurological status, and that is a topic outside the scope of this chapter.

Once the brain-damaged patient's survival is assured, if behavior shows problems with aggression, pharmacological approaches reflecting three different aspects of the neurochemistry of aggression have been tried (Cassidy, 1990). These are drugs such as beta-adrenergic blockers, which will decrease excitatory neurotransmitters (e.g., dopamine); those that facilitate the activity/inhibit the reuptake of the main inhibitory neurotransmitters (e.g., serotonin); and anticonvulsants. Chandler, Barnhill, and Gualtieri (1988) found the dopamine agonist amantadine helpful in treating destructiveness in two patients during their recovery from coma. Beta-adrenergic blockers such as propranolol have been found useful in reducing aggressive and assaultive behavior across the lifespan, both in case reports (Jenike, 1985) and in double-blind placebo-controlled studies (Greendyke & Berkner, 1989), although results show up rather slowly and are not found in cases with premorbid personality disorder. In some case reports, lithium carbonate (a serotonin enhancer) has been found useful in providing emotional regulation (Glenn et al., 1989; Haas & Cope, 1985; Schiff et al., 1982), whereas other case studies have reported success using the antidepressant amitriptyline as a means of controlling agitation (Jackson, Corrigan, & Arnett, 1985). Antidepressants that inhibit serotonin reuptake have shown effects in some studies (Coccaro, Gabriel, & Siever, 1990). Anticonvulsants have been recommended in cases where aggression appears as an episodic dyscontrol disorder (Lewin & Sumners, 1992), and a close linkage of aggression with posttraumatic seizure disorder has been more generally discussed in instances where mania is the prominent feature of the posttraumatic behavior (Shukla, Cook, Mukherjee, Godwin, & Miller, 1987).

In association with the hormonal hypothesis, estrogen has been used to reduce chronic severe aggression in some case reports (e.g., Arnold, 1993), although it has been used more often to treat aggression specifically in sex offenders (Horn, 1987), mostly in individual case studies. Of interest in the cases reviewed by Jenike (1985) was that even after disabling rages had been mitigated in geriatric brain-damaged patients, there was no improvement in any higher cognitive functions; this finding provides support for the hypothesis that the core problem in the association between brain damage and violence association lies more in broad regulatory functions than in specific cognitive defects in reasoning or knowledge.

Anxiolytic drugs would seem to be useful in reducing tension and thus possibly the aggression shown by brain-damaged patients, although there is a recent case report with contrary findings: After alprazolam was begun, a man who had a history of head trauma had an episode of dangerously aggressive behavior (French, 1989).

Violence associated with long-standing personality disorders, in which abnormal brain chemistry such as serotonin dysfunction may provide a physiological substrate to the behavior, has not proven responsive to pharmacological treatments (Coccaro, 1993). In general, there is a paucity of well-designed controlled studies of drug treatments for brain-damage-associated violence (Yudofsky & Silver, 1987); the drugs that are being used represent a somewhat crude trial-and-error "empirical" approach because there is as yet no good model of the neurochemical mechanisms that are most central to the problem, according to Cassidy (1990a). In light of these problems, the use of psychological and especially behaviorally oriented interventions has been recommended, rather than the use of sedatives (Swartzman & Teasell, 1993).

Psychological Treatments

It has been shown that the personal experience of exposure to violence will reduce physiological reactivity in subsequent exposures (Linz & Donnerstein, 1989). This suggestion that classical conditioning might play a role in violent behavioral sequences gives rise to the possibility that the same principles might be mobilized to reverse this demonstrated desensitization effect. I am not aware of any studies that have attempted this. Although psychological treatment for aggressive behavior arising out of rapid-onset brain damage has been heavily behavioral in orientation, it has used principles derived from operant conditioning theory rather than classical conditioning. This behavioral approach reflects the recognition that it is inappropriate to look for psychodynamic etiology for a disorder with an established exogenous etiology,[1] and that it is highly appropriate to bring a very visibly troubling behavior under control relatively quickly.

An initial assessment of the level and direction of aggression can be used to guide treatment planning. With a brain-injured man, for example, a classical behavioral review of the circumstances in which temper becomes a problem will usually demonstrate that displays of temper are under considerably more control than the patient has acknowledged. The assessor can find out whether temper is a problem by directly asking the brain-damaged patient while a close family member is present, so that the patient cannot simply avoid dealing with the problem. If temper problems are identified, direct questions can then be asked about the kinds of temper behaviors the patient shows, the circumstances in which the behaviors are seen, and the people who are most likely to be the objects of these different expressions of temper.

The most typical finding in the course of such a behavioral review of temper is that the worst expressions of temper are reserved for targets within the family and for situations where the displays cannot be seen by others; the targeted individuals are those who have the least likelihood of escaping and are usually physically weaker than the patient. This revelation of the amount of control being exercised in the choice of targets provides a direct avenue through which more conscious and cognitive tactics for dealing with frustrations as they arise, in order to reduce the probability of violence, can be discussed.

Franzen and Lovell (1987) have outlined a treatment approach based on specific behavioral techniques. Social skills training and stress inoculation are recommended as a means of reducing stress that arises from social situations if these are seen as triggers to aggression. Other behavioral interventions, such as "time out," differential reinforcement of other behavior in the place of aggression, differential reinforcement of behavior incompatible with aggression (e.g., walking away), modeling, and withdrawal of positive reinforcers are all outlined, with examples provided that are specific to aggressive behavior.

Evidence from behaviorally oriented treatment has mostly consisted of individual case reports, often showing very rapid and effective results. Case studies have used stress inoculation (Lira & Carne, 1983); a point system with response costs and rewards (Wesolowski & Zencius, 1992); mixed "cooling down," behavioral rehearsal, and relaxation training techniques (Crane & Joyce, 1991); and more loosely structured social skills training (Sladyk, 1992) in successfully reducing aggressive behavior. Burke, Wesolowski, and Lane (1988), who used a broad-spectrum behavior therapy approach with five brain-injured cases, reported significant and immediate decreases in aggression. Their methods included cognitively oriented procedures (e.g., self-control training and self-monitoring), as well as more traditional environmental manipulations. Behavioral programs do not always proceed directly to success, as in a case reported by Andrewes (1989), where cognitive limitations led to problems in initial attempts to control screaming in a 32-year-old woman with diffuse cerebral damage following a suicide attempt. Treatment success was achieved after modifications to account for her cognitive limitations.

Emotional instability arising out of direct organic mechanisms cannot always be aimed by the patient toward external targets or readily brought under behavioral control. This is particularly true in the case of episodic rage disorders with associated seizures. In such cases the patient is often also a direct victim of his own emotional disinhibition, in that it may contribute to both self-destructive behavior and seizures. Despite these exceptions, most violence arising out of cerebral damage is not typically uncontrollable and random; as noted above, this can be determined in a behavioral review of the situations in which aggression occurs.

In cases where cerebral impairment and aggression are not the direct results of a well-defined physical event, but rather are associated with complex long-term personality disorders, neither psychological nor pharmacological treatment has proven to be very effective.

CONCLUSION

There are syndromes of aggression and violence that appear to be associated with brain damage, especially damage to structures deep in the temporal lobes. Despite this, much is not yet established about the general frequency of this association, or about the association of brain damage in other areas with violent behavior. There is similarly mixed evidence concerning the role of neurotransmitters and hormones in aggressive and violent behavior. In particular, there is an ongoing debate about the role of structural or electrochemical brain damage in contributing to criminal violence. The more careful research tends to suggest that brain injury is found only in a very small proportion of criminal psychopaths, and that causality is far from clear in most of these cases.

Models attempting to understand the nature of the connection between brain damage and violence have generally concluded that something other than purely cognitive inadequacies accounts for the association. Instead, a more general model of impaired regulation of emotional responsivity and of cognitive inhibition appears to be the most promising. Generally, many factors interact in such a complex behavior as violence—including premorbid aggression, premorbid personality disorder, past and present abuse of alcohol or other drugs, marital and family situation, and employment prospects, as well as brain injury. Arising from the relatively weak association between violence and brain damage, a cognitive-behavioral model for assessment and intervention in violence is recommended—one that incorporates both individual and situational factors.

NOTE

1. McCabe and Green (1987) took a rather psychodynamic approach in treating three adolescents with severe head injuries and socially disinhibited behavior, with some success; however, they did not focus so much on the dynamic origins of the disinhibition as they did on a dynamic formulation of the tasks of adolescence, and on how these brain-damaged young people could be helped to work on these tasks.

REFERENCES

Ake v. Oklahoma, 470 U.S. 68 (1985).

American Psychiatric Association. (1987). *Diagnostic and statistical manual of mental disorders* (3rd ed., rev.). Washington, DC: Author.

American Psychiatric Association. (1994). *Diagnostic and statistical manual of mental disorders* (4th ed.). Washington, DC: Author.

Andrewes, D. G. (1989). Management of disruptive behavior in the brain-damaged patient using selective reinforcement. *Journal of Behavior Therapy and Experimental Psychiatry, 20*, 261–264.

Arnold, S. (1993). Estrogen for refractory aggression after traumatic brain injury. *American Journal of Psychiatry, 150*, 1564–1565.

Berman, M., & Gladue, B. (1993). The effects of hormones, Type A behavior pattern, and provocation of aggression in men. *Motivation and Emotion, 17*, 125–138.

Berman, M., Taylor, S., & Marged, B. (1993). Morphine and human aggression. *Addictive Behaviors, 18,* 263–268.

Bolger, J. P, & Dougherty, L. M. (1993). *Inhibition and aggressive behavior in psycho-geriatric inpatients.* Paper presented at the meeting of the National Academy of Neuropsychology, Cincinnati, OH.

Boll, T. J., & Barth, J. (1983) Mild head injury. *Psychiatric Developments, 3,* 263–275.

Brooke, M. M., Questad, K. A., Patterson, D. R., & Bashak, K. J. (1992). Agitation and restlessness after closed head injury: A prospective study of 100 consecutive admissions. *Archives of Physical Medicine and Rehabilitation, 73,* 320–323.

Brooks, N. (1988). Behavioral abnormalities in head injured patients. *Scandinavian Journal of Rehabilitation Medicine,* 20(Suppl. 17), 41–46.

Brooks, N., Campsie, L., Symington, C., Beatty, S., & McKinlay, W. (1986). The five year outcome of severe blunt head injury: A relative's view. *Journal of Neurology, Neurosurgery and Psychiatry, 49,* 764–770.

Burke, W. H., Wesolowski, M. D., & Lane, I. (1988). A positive approach to the treatment of aggressive brain injured clients. *International Journal of Rehabilitation Research, 11,* 235–241.

Caplan, B., & Shechter, J. (1990). Clinical applications of the Matching Familiar Figures Test: Impulsivity vs. unilateral neglect. *Journal of Clinical Psychology, 46,* 60–67.

Carlson, N. R. (1988). *Foundations of physiological psychology.* Boston: Allyn & Bacon.

Cassidy, J. W. (1990a). Neurochemical substrates of aggression: Toward a model for improved intervention. Part 1. *Journal of Head Trauma Rehabilitation,* 5(2), 83–86.

Cassidy, J. W. (1990b). Neurochemical substrates of aggression: Toward a model for improved intervention. Part 2. *Journal of Head Trauma Rehabilitation,* 58(3), 70–73.

Chandler, M. C., Barnhill, J. L., & Gualtieri, C.T. (1988). Amantadine for the agitated head-injury patient. *Brain Injury, 2,* 309–311.

Coccaro, E. F. (1993). Psychopharmacological studies in patients with personality disorders: Review and perspective. *Journal of Personality Disorders, 7*(Spring Suppl. 1), 181–192.

Coccaro, E. F., Gabriel, S., & Siever, L. J. (1990). Buspirone challenge: Preliminary evidence for a role for central $5-HT_{1A}$ receptor function in impulsive aggressive behavior in humans. *Psychopharmacology Bulletin, 26,* 393–405.

Coccaro, E. F., & Kavoussi, R.J. (1992). Self- and other-directed human aggression: The role of the serotonergic system. *International Clinical Psychopharmacology,* 6(Suppl. 6), 70–83.

Crane, A. A., & Joyce, B. G. (1991). Cool down: A procedure for decreasing aggression in adults with traumatic head injury. *Behavioral Residential Treatment, 6,* 65–75.

Damasio, A., & Tranel, D. (1990). Individuals with sociopathic behavior caused by frontal damage fail to respond autonomically to social stimuli. *Behavioral Brain Research, 41,* 81–94.

DeFeudis, F. V., & Schauss, A. G. (1987). The role of brain monoamine metabolite concentrations in arsonists and habitually violent offenders: Abnormalities of criminals or social isolation effects? *International Journal of Biosocial Research, 9,* 27–30.

Drudge, O., & Rosen, J. (1986). Behavioral and emotional problems and treatment in chronically brain-impaired adults. *Annals of Behavioral Medicine, 8,* 9–14.

Eichelman, B. (1983) The limbic system and aggression in humans. *Neuroscience and Biobehavioral Reviews, 7,* 391–394.

Ford, C. S., & Beach, F. A. (1951). *Patterns of sexual behavior.* New York: Harper.

Fordyce, D. J., Roueche, J. R., & Prigitano, G. P. (1983). Enhanced emotional reactions in chronic head trauma patients. *Journal of Neurology, Neurosurgery and Psychiatry, 46,* 620–624.

Franzen, M. D., & Lovell, M. R. (1987). Behavioral treatments of aggressive sequelae of brain injury. *Psychiatric Annals, 17,* 389–396.

French, A. P. (1989). Dangerously aggressive behavior as a side effect of alprazolam. *American Journal of Psychiatry, 146,* 276.

Gladue, B. (1991). Aggressive behavioral characteristics, hormones, and sexual orientation in men and women. *Aggressive Behavior, 17,* 313–326.

Glenn, M. B., Wroblewski, B., Parziale, J., Levine, L., Whyte, J., & Rosenthal, M. (1989). Lithium carbonate for aggressive behavior or affective instability in ten brain-injured patients. *American Journal of Physical Medicine and Rehabilitation, 68,* 221–226.

Gorenstein, E. E. (1982). Frontal lobe functions in psychopaths. *Journal of Abnormal Psychology, 91,* 368–379.

Greendyke, R. M., & Berkner, J. P. (1989). Treatment of behavioral problems with pindolol. *Psychosomatics, 30,* 161–165.

Greer, M. K., & Lyons-Crews, M. (1989). A case study of the cognitive and behavioral deficits of temporal lobe damage in herpes simplex encephalitis. *Journal of Autism and Developmental Disorders, 19,* 317–326.

Haas, J. F., & Cope, D. N. (1985). Neuropharmacologic management of behavior sequelae in head injury: A case report. *Archives of Physical Medicine and Rehabilitation, 66,* 472–474.

Hare, R. D., Harpur, T. J., Hakstian, A. R., Forth, A. E., Hart, S. D., & Newman, J. P. (1990). The Revised Psychopathy Checklist: Reliability and factor structure. *Psychological Assessment: A Journal of Consulting and Clinical Psychology, 2,* 338–341.

Hart, S. D., Forth, A. E., & Hare, R. D. (1990). Performance of criminal psychopaths on selected neuropsychological tests. *Journal of Abnormal Psychology, 99,* 374–379.

Hebb, D. O. (1942). The effect of early and late brain injury upon test scores, and the nature of normal adult intelligence. *American Philosophical Society Proceedings, 85,* 275–292.

Horn, L. J. (1987). "Atypical" medications for the treatment of disruptive, aggressive behavior in the brain-injured patient. *Journal of Head Trauma Rehabilitation, 2,* 18–28.

House, A., Dennis, M., & Molyneux, A. (1989). Emotionalism after stroke. *British Medical Journal, 298,* 991–994.

Jackson, R. D., Corrigan, J. D., & Arnett, J. A. (1985). Amitriptyline for agitation in head injury. *Archives of Physical Medicine and Rehabilitation, 66,* 180–181.

Jenike, M. A. (1985). Propranolol as treatment for aggressive behavior in elderly brain-damaged patients. *Clinical Gerontologist, 3,* 36–39.

Jennett, B. (1972). Prognosis after severe head injury. *Clinical Neurosurgery, 19,* 200–207.

Jennett, B. (1986). Medical aspects of head injury. *Medicine North America, 36,* 5210–5238.

Joseph, R. (1990). *Neuropsychology, neuropsychiatry, and behavioral neurology.* New York: Plenum Press.

Kandel, E., & Freed, D. (1989). Frontal-lobe dysfunction and antisocial behavior: A review. *Journal of Clinical Psychology, 45,* 404–413.

Kaufman, A. S. (1990). *Assessing adolescent and adult intelligence.* Boston: Allyn & Bacon.

Kaye, K., & Grigsby, J. (1990). Prediction of independent functioning and behavior problems in geriatric patients. *Journal of the American Geriatrics Society, 38,* 1304–1310.

Kreutzer, J. S., Wehman, P. H., Harris, J. A., Burns, C. T., & Young, H. F. (1991). Substance abuse and crime patterns among persons with traumatic brain injury referred for supported employment. *Brain Injury, 5,* 177–187.

Langevin, R., & Ben-Aron, M. (1987). Brain damage, diagnosis, and substance abuse among violent offenders. *Behavioral Sciences and the Law, 5,* 77–94.

Leger, D. W. (1992). *Biological foundations of behavior.* New York: HarperCollins.

Levin, H. S., Benton, A. L., & Grossman, R. G. (1982). *Neurobehavioral consequences of closed head injury.* New York: Oxford University Press.

Levin, H. S., & Grossman, R. G. (1978). Behavioral sequelae of closed head injury: A quantitative study. *Archives of Neurology, 35,* 720–727.

Levin, H. S., & Peters, B. H. (1976). Neuropsychological testing following head injuries: Prosopagnosia without visual field defect. *Diseases of the Nervous System, 37,* 68–71.

Lewin, J., & Sumners, D. (1992). Successful treatment of episodic dyscontrol with carbamazepine. *British Journal of Psychiatry, 161,* 261–262.

Licata, A., Taylor, S., Berman, M., & Cranston, J. (1993). Effects of cocaine on human aggression. *Pharmacology, Biochemistry and behavior, 45,* 549–552.

Linnoila, V. M., & Virkkunen, M. (1992). Aggression, suicidality, and serotonin. *Journal of Clinical Psychiatry, 53,*(10, Suppl.), 46–51.

Linz, D., & Donnerstein, E. (1989). Physiological desensitization and judgments about female victims of violence. *Human Communication Research, 15,* 509–522.

Lira, F. T., & Carne, W. (1983). Treatment of anger and impulsivity in a brain damaged patient: A case study applying stress inoculation. *Clinical Neuropsychology, 5,* 159–160.

Luria, A. R. (1980). *Higher cortical functions in man* (B. Haigh, Trans.; 2nd ed.). New York: Basic Books.

Lynam, D. (1993). Explaining the relations between IQ and delinquency: Class, race, test motivation, school failure, or self-control? *Journal of Abnormal Psychology, 102,* 187–196.

Mark, V. H., & Ervin, F. R. (1970). *Violence and the brain.* New York: Harper & Row.

Martell, D. A. (1992). Estimating the prevalence of organic brain-dysfunction in maximum-security forensic psychiatric patients. *Journal of Forensic Sciences, 37,* 878–893.

Martinius, J. (1982). Homicide of an aggressive adolescent boy with right temporal lesion: A case report. *Neuroscience and Biobehavioral Reviews, 7,* 419–422.

McCabe, R. J., & Green, D. (1987). Rehabilitating severely head-injured adolescents: Three case reports. *Journal of Child Psychology and Psychiatry, 28,* 111–126.

McCaul, K. D., Gladue, B. A., & Joppa, M. (1992). Winning, losing, mood, and testosterone. *Hormones and Behavior, 26,* 486–504.

Meyers, C. A., & Berman, S. A. (1992). Case report: Acquired antisocial personality disorder associated with unilateral left orbital frontal lobe damage. *Journal of Psychiatry and Neuroscience, 17,* 121–125.

Miller, L. (1990). Major syndromes of aggressive behavior following head injury: An introduction to evaluation and treatment. *Cognitive Rehabilitation, 8,* 14–19.

Miller, J. D., & Jones, P. (1985). The clinical spectrum of head injury. *Journal of Neurology, Neurosurgery and Psychiatry, 48,* 596.

Moffitt, T. E. (1988). Neuropsychology and self-reported early delinquency in an unselected birth cohort: A preliminary report from New Zealand. In T. E. Moffitt & S. A. Mednick (Eds.), *Biological contributions to crime causation* (pp. 93–117). Dordrecht, The Netherlands: Martinus Nijhoff.

Nachshon, I. (1988). Hemisphere function in violent offenders. In T. E. Moffitt & S. A. Mednick (Eds.), *Biological contributions to crime causation* (pp. 55–67). Dordrecht, The Netherlands: Martinus Nijhoff.

Restak, R. M. (1992). See no evil: The neurological defense would blame violence on the damaged brain. *The Sciences, 32*(4), 16–21.

Rosenbaum, A., & Hoge, S. K. (1989). Head injury and marital aggression. *American Journal of Psychiatry, 146,* 1048–1051.

Rosenbaum, A., Hoge, S. K., Adelman, S. A., Warnken, W. J., Fletcher, K. E., & Kane, R. L. (1994). Head injury in partner-abusive men. *Journal of Consulting and Clinical Psychology, 62,* 1187–1193.

Sachdev, P., & Smith, J. (1992). Amygdalo-hippocampectomy for pathological aggression. *Australian and New Zealand Journal of Psychiatry, 26,* 671–676.

Santoro, J., & Spiers, M. (1994) Social cognitive factors in brain injury-associated personality change. *Brain Injury, 8,* 265–276.

Saver, J. L., & Damasio, A. R. (1991). Preserved access and processing of social knowledge in a patient with acquired sociopathy due to ventromedial frontal damage. *Neuropsychologia, 29,* 1241–1249.

Schiff, H. B., Sabin, T. D., Geller, A., Alexander, L., & Mark, V. (1982). Lithium in aggressive behavior. *American Journal of Psychiatry, 139,* 1346–1348.

Schwab, K., Grafman, J., Salazar, A. M., & Kraft, J. (1993). Residual impairments and work status 15 years after penetrating head injury: Report from the Vietnam Head Injury Study. *Neurology, 43,* 95–103.

Shukla, S., Cook, B. L., Mukherjee, S., Godwin, C., & Miller, M. G. (1987). Mania following head trauma. *American Journal of Psychiatry, 144,* 93–96.

Sladyk, K. (1992). Traumatic brain injury, behavioral disorder, and group treatment. *American Journal of Occupational Therapy, 46,* 267–270.

Spreen, O. (1981). The relationship between learning disability, neurological impairment, and delinquency. *Journal of Nervous and Mental Disease, 169,* 909–913.

Stevenson, R. W. (1995, February 19). Researchers see gene links to violence, but are wary. *New York Times,* p. 29.

Strauss, E., & Wada, J. (1991). Psychiatric and psychosocial changes associated with anterior temporal lobectomy. In O. Divinsky & W. H. Theodore (Eds.), *Epilepsy and behavior* (pp 135–149). New York: Wiley.

Susman, E., & Inoff-Germain, G. (1987). Hormones, emotional dispositions, and aggressive attributes in young adolescents. *Child Development, 58,* 1114–1134.

Swartzman, L., & Teasell, R. (1993). Psychological consequences of stroke. *Physical Medicine and Rehabilitation, 7,* 179–194.

Taylor, S. P., & Chermack, S. T. (1993). Alcohol, drugs and human physical aggression. *Journal of Studies on Alcohol, 54*(Suppl. 11), 78–88.

Tikovsky, R. S., Alavi, A., Devous, M. D., & van Heertum, R. L. (1994, December). Jury still out [Letter]. *APA Monitor,* p. 2.

Virkkunen, M., & Linnoila, V. M. (1993). Brain serotonin, type II alcoholism and impulsive violence. *Journal of Studies on Alcohol, 54*(Supp. 11), *11,* 163–169.

Volavka, J., Martell, D., & Convit, A. (1992). Psychobiology of the violent offender. *Journal of Forensic Sciences, 37,* 237–251.

Weisman, A. M., & Taylor, S. P. (1994). Effect of alcohol and risk of physical harm on human physical aggression. *Journal of General Psychology, 121,* 67–75.

Wesolowski, M. D., & Zencius, A. H. (1992). Treatment of aggression in a brain injured adolescent. *Behavioral Residential Treatment, 7,* 205–210.

Wood, R. L. (1987). *Brain injury rehabilitation: A neurobehavioral approach.* Rockville, MD: Aspen.

Yudofsky, S. C., & Silver, J. M. (1987). Pharmocologic treatment of aggression. *Psychiatric Annals, 17,* 397–407.

8

Impulsivity in Adults:
A Critical Review
of Measurement Approaches

JAMES D. A. PARKER

R. MICHAEL BAGBY

The large number of impulsivity measures that have been developed in recent years is just one sign of the growing interest in this construct. Over the years, a number of behavioral techniques have been developed for assessing impulsivity (for reviews, see Gerbing, Ahadi, & Patton, 1987; Messer, 1976), and several self-report measures have been developed specifically to assess the impulsivity construct (Barratt, 1983, 1985; Dickman, 1990; Eysenck, Pearson, Easting, & Allsopp, 1985). In addition, most omnibus measures of personality, designed to assess basic personality dimensions, include at least one impulsivity-related measure (Parker, Bagby, & Webster, 1993).

Although numerous scales and measures have been developed to assess impulsivity, there is a common observation in the literature that many of these measures do not intercorrelate very highly (Barratt, 1985; Corulla, 1987; Luengo, Carrillo-de-la-Peña, & Otero, 1991; Malle & Neubauer, 1991; Parker et al., 1993). Since there exists little consensus in the literature about what constitutes impulsivity (Parker et al., 1993), the low correlations among different impulsivity measures reflects the diversity of theoretical approaches to this construct. As a number of writers have suggested, the lack of conceptual clarity in the impulsivity construct has become a source of widespread confusion in the literature on this topic (Gerbing et al., 1987; Luengo et al., 1991; Parker et al., 1993).

Gerbing et al. (1987) and we ourselves (Parker et al., 1993) have identified many of the impulsivity-related dimensions assessed by frequently used impulsivity measures. One broad dimension included in most such measures is the tendency to engage in spontaneous behaviors or to have spontaneous thoughts. Related labels for this dimension include acting without thinking, "restlessness," "distractibility," "quick decision-making ability," and "impatience" (Gerbing et al., 1987). A second broad dimension included in many impulsivity measures is the tendency to be disorganized and unprepared in day-to-day activities. A third broad dimension, also included in many measures, has been labeled "carefree" or "happy-go-lucky" attitudes and behaviors (Gerbing et al., 1987). Researchers contemplating the use of a particular impulsivity measure should pay close attention to the types of dimensions that are assessed. Although many measures assess a cross-section of impulsivity-related dimensions, other measures assess only a narrow facet of the impulsivity construct.

This chapter is an attempt to evaluate the psychometric properties of several self-report and behavioral measures that have been developed to assess impulsivity. Whenever possible, the chapter also provides information on the theoretical approach to impulsivity used in the development of the measure. The goal of this evaluation is to provide information that will be useful to individuals who need to select a particular impulsivity measure for research or assessment purposes.

SELF-REPORT MEASURES

Impulsivity Inventories

Several self-report measures have been developed that were designed specifically to assess various features of the Impulsivity construct. One of the oldest of these measures is the Barratt Impulsiveness Scale (BIS; Barratt, 1959), originally developed as a 44-item (true–false format) self-report measure of Impulsivity. The BIS was developed with a sample of 300 individuals (no information was presented by the test developer about the identity of these subjects). It would appear that the items for the BIS were selected on the basis of face validity only. Barratt (1959) reported an excellent 4-week test–retest reliability ($r = .87$, $n = 300$) for the scale, although the limited internal-reliability information he provided suggested that the original scale had weak item homogeneity.

The original BIS was based on a unidimensional model of impulsivity. More recently, Barratt (1983, 1985) has proposed a tridimensional model of impulsivity that differentiates among "motor impulsiveness," "cognitive impulsiveness," and "nonplanning impulsiveness" dimensions. Over the years, the BIS has been revised several times to conform with Barratt's reconceptualization of the impulsivity construct. Many of the details regarding these revisions, however, have not been published. A recent version of the scale (BIS-10) has scoring that matches Barratt's tridimensional impulsivity model: The scale has an 11-item Motor Impulsiveness subscale, an 11-item Cognitive Impulsiveness subscale, and a 12-item Nonplanning Impulsiveness subscale. Unfortunately, many of the psychometric data on the revised versions of the BIS either have not been published or are cited in sources difficult to locate (see, e.g., citations in Barratt, 1983, 1985). Luengo et al. (1991), using a Spanish translation of the BIS-10 in two samples of undergraduates ($n = 307$ and $n = 264$), found poor alpha coefficients for most of the BIS-10 subscales (the median coefficient was .25), although the coefficient for the total scale was higher (.56 for the first sample and .65 for the second sample). Luengo et al. (1991) did, however, report relatively high 1-year test–retest reliabilities for the BIS-10 in 132 undergraduates; the median test–retest correlation for the three subscales was .61, while the test–retest correlation for the total scale was .60. Barratt (1994) has recently presented some preliminary factor-analytic data on a revision of the BIS-10 (BIS-11), using two small samples (151 college students and 92 psychiatric inpatients). Although these results are preliminary, they generally support Barratt's three-factor impulsivity model.

Eysenck et al. (1985) have developed a 54-item self-report scale, the I.7, that assesses two broad impulsivity dimensions: "impulsiveness" and "venturesomeness." Impulsiveness is conceptualized by Eysenck et al. (1985) as behaving without thinking and without realizing the risk involved in the behavior. Venturesomeness, on the other hand, is defined as being conscious of the risk of the behavior but acting anyway. Along with a 19-item Impulsiveness subscale and a 16-item Venturesomeness subscale, the I.7 also has a 19-item Empathy subscale. The I.7 was developed with a sample of 1,320 normal adults, and the factor structure was replicated in a sample of 589 normal adults (Eysenck et al., 1985). Each subscale was developed as a unidimensional measure.

In general, the psychometric data that have been reported on the I.7 are good. The alpha coefficient for the Impulsiveness subscale was .84 in a sample of 559 men and .83 in a sample of 761 women; the alpha coefficient for the Venturesomeness scale was .85 for men and .84 for women. Luengo et al. (1991), using a Spanish translation of the I.7 in a sample of 132 undergraduates, obtained 1-year test–retest reliabilities of .76 for the Impulsiveness scale and .80 for the Venturesomeness scale. Eysenck and Eysenck (1980) have also demonstrated that the impulsiveness and venturesomeness dimensions are relatively distinct from the basic personality dimensions of neuroticism, extraversion, and psychoticism. In a sample of 251 boys and 143 girls, impulsiveness correlated with psychoticism .37 for boys and .34 for girls, with extraversion .18 for boys and .16 for girls, and with neuroticism .44 for boys and .40 for girls. A similar low to moderate pattern of correlations was found for venturesomeness.

Dickman (1990) has differentiated between two types of impulsivity: "dysfunctional impulsivity," the tendency to act with absence of forethought when this behavior can create problems; and "functional impulsivity," the tendency to act without forethought when this behavior is beneficial. To assess these two impulsivity dimensions, Dickman (1990) has developed the Functional and Dysfunctional Impulsivity (FDI) scales. The FDI Functional Impulsivity subscale has 11 items, and the Dysfunctional Impulsivity scale has 12 items; both subscales appear to have good psychometric properties. The internal-reliability coefficient for the Dysfunctional subscale was .85, and that for the Functional subscale was .74, in a sample of 188 college students (Dickman, 1990). Although test–retest correlations have not been reported, the FDI scales have received extensive construct validation via both self-report and behavioral measures. Using a visual discrimination task with 217 undergraduates, Dickman (1990) found an "association between functional impulsivity and the speed and accuracy with which subjects carry out the processes involved in the comparison of visual stimuli" (p. 101).

Omnibus Personality Scales

Personality researchers who have devised measures to assess a broad range of basic dimensions have long had an interest in developing scales that tap impulsivity-related constructs. Downey (1923), who developed one of the first omnibus personality measures, endeavored to assess several such constructs. The omnibus personality measures that followed typically included impulsivity-related subscales (Link, 1936; Stagner, 1936). This section examines the impulsivity subscales that have been included in some of the more widely used omnibus personality measures. Unless explicitly specified otherwise, these measure were developed as unidimensional measures of impulsivity-related constructs.

The Guilford–Zimmerman Temperament Survey (GZTS; Guilford & Zimmerman, 1949; Guilford, Zimmerman, & Guilford, 1976), a 300-item self-report measure of 10 basic personality dimensions, contains a 30-item Restraint subscale relevant to the impulsivity construct. This subscale assesses the "happy-go-lucky, carefree, impulsive individual" (Guilford & Zimmerman, 1949, p. 8). In general, the psychometric properties of the various GZTS subscales are very good. The internal-reliability coefficient for the Restraint subscale was .80 in a random sample of 100 adults taken from a large sample of approximately 1,000 adults (Guilford et al., 1976). The 1-year test–retest correlation for the Restraint subscale in a sample of 322 college students was .74. Guilford et al. (1976) have presented extensive construct validity data on the Restraint subscale, using a variety of self-report (e.g., Minnesota Multiphasic Personality Inventory, studies), peer rating, and behavioral measures. For example, in a sample of 101 undergraduates, the authors reported a satisfactory correlation of .47 between the Restraint scale and peer ratings. Although the Restraint subscale was originally developed to assess impulsivity as a unidimensional construct, a confirmatory factor-analytic study (Parker et al., 1993) found it to have a replicable multidimensional structure: The subscale assesses both cautious–spontaneous and methodical–disorganized dimensions of the impulsivity construct.

Form A of the Sixteen Personality Factor Questionnaire (16PF; Cattell & Eber, 1962), a 187-item self-report measure (true–false format) of basic personality dimensions, has a subscale very relevant to the impulsivity construct: the 10-item Factor G scale ("expedient vs. conscientious"). Cattell and Eber (1962) described an individual scoring low on this unidimensional measure (high on expedience) as "unsteady in purpose. He is often casual and lacking in effort for group undertakings and cultural demands. His freedom from group influence may lead to antisocial acts, but at times makes him more effective, while his refusal to be bound by rules causes him to have less somatic upset from stress" (p. 15). The psychometric properties of the 16PF Factor G subscale are adequate. Cattell and Eber (1962) reported that 6-day test–retest reliability in a sample of 146 adults was .81 and 2-month test–retest reliability in a sample of 132 undergraduates was .84, although the internal-reliability coefficient for the measure in a sample of 218 undergraduates was only a satisfactory .57. These authors also reported extensive construct validity data on the Factor G subscale, using a variety of self-report and behavioral measures.

The California Psychological Inventory (CPI; Gough, 1975) is a 480-item self-report measure (true–false format) that assesses a variety of personality dimensions. The 50-item Self-Control subscale from the CPI is relevant to the impulsivity construct. This subscale assesses "the degree and adequacy of self-regulation and self-control and freedom from impulsivity and self-centeredness" (Gough, 1975, p. 10). The psychometric properties of the various CPI subscales are generally quite satisfactory. For example, the test–retest correlation (1 year) for the Self-Control subscale in a sample of 125 undergraduates was .68, and it was .75 in a sample of 101 adults. Gough (1975) did not report internal reliabilities for the CPI, although he presented extensive data on the construct validity of the CPI. Like the authors of the GZTS and PF16, he also presented extensive construct validity data on the Self-Control subscale, utilizing a variety of self-report and behavioral measures.

The EASI-III Temperament Survey (Buss & Plomin, 1975) is a self-report measure (5-point Likert scale format) designed to assess four basic temperament dimensions: "emotionality," "activity," "sociability," and "impulsivity." Buss and Plomin (1975) defined impulsivity as having two basic dimensions: "(1) resisting versus giving in to urges, impulses, or motivational states; and (2) responding immediately and impetuously to a stimulus versus lying back and planning before making a move" (p. 8). The 20-item Impulsivity scale (developed on a rational basis) has four 5-item subscales: Inhibitory Control, Decision Time, Sensation Seeking, and Persistence. To date, there are few published data currently available on the psychometric properties of the EASI-III. The main source of information on the EASI-III (Buss & Plomin, 1975) claims that the scale has good psychometric properties, but cites only unpublished data to support this position. Apart from correlations with the other temperament dimensions on the EASI-III, few construct validity data have been published on its Impulsivity scale (Buss & Plomin, 1975).

In one of two studies on the EASI-III, Parker and Fedoroff (1994) examined the replicability of the four-factor model for the EASI-III Impulsivity scale by testing for goodness of fit via confirmatory factor analysis in a sample of 221 normal adults. This model was found to have poor fit to the data. In the second study, the same authors were able to derive a replicable set of impulsivity dimensions from the EASI-III Impulsivity scale, using a series of exploratory factor analyses with the adults tested in the first study. A two-factor model (Spontaneous–Cautious Impulsivity and Disorganized–Methodical Impulsivity) was derived from the EASI-III Impulsivity scale and subsequently tested for its goodness of fit with a second sample of normal adults ($n = 111$) and a sample of 179 male forensic psychiatry patients. In both samples, the two-factor model was found to have good fit to the data.

The Multidimensional Personality Questionnaire (MPQ; Tellegen, 1982), a 300-item self-report measure of basic personality dimensions, has a 24-item Control/Impulsiveness subscale related to the impulsivity construct. An individual scoring high on the scale is described by Tellegen (1982) as someone who is "reflective; is cautious, careful, plodding; is rational and sensible; likes to anticipate events; likes to plan her (his) activities," while an individual scoring low on the scale is described as one who is "impulsive and spontaneous; can be reckless and careless; prefers to play things by ear" (p. 8). In general, the psychometric properties of the various MPQ scales are good. The factor structure of the entire scale has been replicated in different samples, and the subscales have excellent internal reliabilities and test–retest reliabilities. With respect to the Control/Impulsiveness subscale, for example, the 30-day test–retest reliability in a sample of 75 undergraduates was .88. The internal-reliability coefficient for this subscale was .86 in a sample of 500 female undergraduates, and it was .82 in a sample of 300 male undergraduates (Tellegen, 1982). In addition, the MPQ has received extensive construct validation (Tellegen, 1982; Zevon & Tellegen, 1982). Although the Control/Impulsiveness subscale was developed to assess a unidimensional construct, a confirmatory factor-analytic study (Parker et al., 1993) found this subscale to have a replicable multidimensional structure: The subscale assesses both cautious–spontaneous and methodical–disorganized dimensions of the impulsivity construct.

Form E of the Personality Research Form (PRF; Jackson, 1984) is a 352-item self-report scale (true–false format) with two subscales particularly relevant to the impulsivity construct: the 16-item Impulsivity subscale and the 16-item Harm Avoidance subscale. Jackson has described a high scorer on the impulsivity subscale as someone who "tends to act on the spur of the moment and without deliberation; gives vent readily to feelings and wishes; speaks freely; may be volatile in emotional expression" (p. 7). Jackson (1984) has described a high scorer on the Harm Avoidance subscale as someone who "does not enjoy exciting activities, especially if danger is involved; avoids risk of bodily harm; seeks to maximize personal safety" (p. 7). In general, the psychometric properties of all of the PRF subscales are excellent. Jackson (1984) reported 1-week test–retest correlations of .81 for the Impulsivity subscale and .90 for the Harm Avoidance subscale in a sample of 135 undergraduates. Internal-reliability coefficients of .91 for the Harm Avoidance subscale and .85 for the Impulsivity subscale were also reported by Jackson (1984) in a sample of 84 undergraduates. The various PRF subscales have also received extensive construct validation (Jackson, 1984). In a recent confirmatory factor-analytic study of the PRF Impulsivity subscale, we (Parker et al., 1993) found this subscale to be a unidimensional measure that assesses only the facet of the impulsivity construct pertaining to spontaneous behaviors or thoughts.

The Basic Personality Inventory (BPI), also developed by Jackson (1989), is a 240-item self-report scale (true–false format) that has one measure relevant to the impulsivity construct: the 20-item Impulse Expression subscale. Jackson (1989) has described a high scorer on the Impulse Expression subscale as someone who "lacks ability to think beyond the present and to consider the consequences of action; is prone to undertake risky and reckless actions; inclined to behave irresponsibly; finds routine tasks boring" (p. 9). The psychometric properties of the BPI Impulse Expression subscale appears to be very good. Holden, Fekken, Reddon, Helmes, and Jackson (1988) reported a 1-month test–retest correlation of .74 for this subscale in a psychiatric sample ($n = 112$). They also reported an internal-reliability coefficient of .90 for subscale in the same sample. The BPI, like Jackson's other scales, has received extensive construct validation (Jackson, 1989), and the inventory was developed with special care to eliminate items likely to be influenced by social desirability. Inspection of the BPI Impulse Expression items suggests that the measure assesses a broad range of facets of the impulsivity construct (spontaneous behaviors and cognitions, nonplanning of activities, and carefree impulsivity are all represented).

The Tridimensional Personality Questionnaire (TPQ; Cloninger, 1987a, 1987b) is a 100-item self-report scale (true–false format) developed to assess three broad personality dimensions: "novelty seeking," "harm avoidance," and "reward dependence." Two subscales on the dimension of novelty seeking are particularly relevant to the impulsivity construct: the 8- item Impulsiveness vs. Reflection subscale, and the 9-item Exploratory Excitability vs. Stoic Rigidity subscale. Cloninger (1987b) has defined novelty seeking as the "heritable tendency toward frequent exploratory activity and intense exhilaration in response to novel or appetitive stimuli" (p. 413). The psychometric properties of the TPQ scales are adequate. With respect to the Impulsiveness and Exploratory Excitability subscales, internal-reliability coefficients for a sample of 326 male and 350 female adults were in the mid-.50s (Svrakic, Przybeck, & Cloninger, 1991). Six-month test–retest reliabilities in a sample of 441 adults was .58 for the Impulsiveness subscale and .68 for the Exploratory Excitability subscale (Cloninger, Przybeck, & Svrakic, 1991). A number of recent construct validity studies have been reported on the TPQ scales (Cloninger, Svrakic, & Przybeck, 1993; Svrakic, Whitehead, Przybeck, & Cloninger, 1993).

The NEO Personality Inventory—Revised (NEO-PI-R; Costa & McCrae, 1992) is a 240-item self-report scale (5-point Likert scale format) that assesses the five-factor personality model (Digman, 1990). The Neuroticism scale contains an 8-item Impulsiveness subscale. An individual scoring high on the Impulsiveness subscale is described as being in control of his or her emotions and behaviors. Unlike other self-report measures discussed in this chapter, the NEO-PI-R has two different forms: a self-report version (Form S), and a rating form for peers or family members (Form R). The psychometric properties of the NEO-PI-R Impulsiveness subscale appear to be very good (for both Form S and Form R). The internal-reliability coefficient for this subscale (Form S) was above .80 in several different samples (Costa & McCrae, 1992). Test–retest correlations (6 years) for the Impulsiveness subscale were .70 for Form S in a sample of 398 adults, and .75 for Form R in a sample of 167 spouse ratings (Costa & McCrae, 1988). Although the NEO-PI-R Impulsiveness subscale has excellent psychometric properties, potential users of the scale should note that the items appear to assess a narrow facet of the impulsivity construct (e.g., the control of impulsive behaviors).

Although it was developed to be a self-report measure of various behaviors and attitudes relating to eating disorders, the Eating Disorder Inventory—2 (EDI-2; Garner, 1991), a 91-item scale (6-point Likert format), contains a subscale related to the impulsivity construct: the 11-item Impulse Regulation subscale. Garner (1991) notes that the Impulse Regulation subscale "assesses the tendency toward impulsivity, substance abuse, recklessness, hostility, destructiveness in interpersonal relationships, and self-destructiveness" (p. 6). The Impulse Regulation subscale is one of three provisional subscales Garner included when the original

EDI was revised. Much less is known about the psychometric properties of the provisional subscales than about those of the regular subscales, although a good internal-reliability coefficient was found for the Impulse Regulation subscale (Garner, 1991) in a sample of eating disorder patients (n = 107, alpha = .77) and a female college sample (n = 205, alpha = .79). No information is currently available on the test–retest reliability of the Impulse Regulation subscale, and only limited construct validity data have been published. Nevertheless, the scale may be useful in future research because it contains items related to self-regulation abilities not included in other impulsivity measures.

Another scale that may assess unique features of the impulsivity construct is the Survey of Work Styles (SWS; Jackson & Gray, 1989). The SWS is a 96-item self-report measure (5-point Likert format) developed as a multidimensional measure of the Type A behavior pattern. The 16-item Impatience subscale is relevant to the impulsivity construct and identifies individuals who are likely to act or feel impatient in their work environment. The psychometric properties of the SWS Impatience subscale are adequate. Jackson and Gray (1989) reported an internal-reliability coefficient of .82 for this subscale in a sample of 163 male middle-level managers, although they did not report test–retest correlations. The SWS has received extensive construct validation (Jackson & Gray, 1989), and the scale was developed with special care to eliminate items likely to be influenced by social desirability. The subscale may be of interest to future researchers on the impulsivity construct because it contains items that ask about behaviors in a variety of occupation-related situations.

BEHAVIORAL APPROACHES

Although there has been considerable interest in developing behavioral methods for the assessment of impulsivity, one does not find the diversity of measures found in the self-report literature. In general, two different types of behavioral measures for impulsivity have been developed. The first type of measure, which has attracted most of the attention in the literature on behavioral approaches to impulsivity, utilizes various reaction time tasks. The second type of measure, which has attracted considerably less attention in the literature, utilizes different time perception tasks.

Reaction Time Measures

A decade after its development, the Matching Familiar Figures Test (MFFT; Kagan, Rosman, Day, Albert, & Phillips, 1964) had become the most frequently used measure of impulsivity (for a review of the early literature on the MFFT, see Messer, 1976). Today, it continues to be one of the most widely used behavioral impulsivity measures. The MFFT was developed to measure the reflection—impulsivity construct, defined by Messer (1976) as "the tendency to reflect on the validity of problem solving under a very special condition, namely, when several possible alternatives are available and there is some uncertainty over which one is the most appropriate" (p. 1026). The test consists of a set of drawings, each of which contains a standard figure and eight similar figures; the respondent is asked to identify which of the eight figures is identical to the target figure (only one is identical). The MFFT generates two scores: mean elapsed time to the respondent's initial response (latency score), and the mean number of errors made before arriving at a correct response (error score). Lower latency scores and higher error scores are hypothesized to be indicators of impulsivity (Kagan et al., 1964).

Messer (1976) reviews much of the early literature on the MFFT, which found the measure to have adequate psychometric properties. Block, Block, and Harrington (1974), for example, found internal-reliability coefficients of .89 for the MFFT latency score and .62 for the MFFT error score. A review of four different studies found test–retest correlations (ranging from 1 to 8 weeks) that varied from .58 to .96 for the MFFT latency score, and from .34 to .80 for the MFFT error score (Messer, 1976). Although the measure appears to have good reliability, serious concerns have been raised in the literature regarding the MFFT's validity. The MFFT has been found to be associated with performance tests that assess impulsivity-related constructs, such as the Porteus Maze Test (Gow & Ward, 1982), the Draw-a-Line-Slowly test (Bentler & McClain, 1976), and the Walk-a-Line-Slowly test (Olson, Bates, & Bayles, 1990); however, results with observer ratings have been discouraging. Bentler and McClain (1976), for example, found low and nonsignificant correlations between MFFT scores and teacher ratings of impulsive behavior in children. A similar lack of association has also been found in other studies examining the relationship between MFFT scores and teacher ratings of classroom behavior (Sergeant, van Velthoven, & Virginia, 1979; Smith & Singer, 1977).

Reaction time tasks have been incorporated in other behavioral measures for impulsivity (Barratt & Patton, 1983; Edman, Schalling, & Levander, 1983; Gerbing et al., 1987). One of the core features of most definitions of impulsivity is that this construct reflects a tendency to make quick decisions and to act without thinking (Parker et al., 1993). One would predict, therefore, that "high impulsive subjects would have short reaction times and make many errors in a choice reaction time task" (Edman et al., 1983, p. 2). A number of different reaction time tasks have been utilized to assess impulsivity. For example, Dickman (1990) and Edman et al. (1983) used a method that required subjects to respond to various visual stimuli; Gerbing et al. (1987) used a procedure that required subjects to respond to a tone; and Malle and Neubauer (1991) used response latencies to a set of items from several personality questionnaires.

Although various of reaction time tasks have been used to assess impulsivity, sparse reliability data have been published on this method. In the only study we could locate, Edman et al. (1983) reported 1-month test–retest reliabilities of .69 for mean reaction time and .22 for the number of correct responses in a sample of 55 adolescent males. Validity studies on the relationship between reaction time tasks and other impulsivity measures have produced contradictory results. Edman et al. (1983) report correlations of –.41 between mean reaction time and a self-report measure of impulsivity, and –.40 between the number of correct responses and the same self-report measure. When Edman et al. (1983) retested subjects a month later, the correlations between reaction time tasks and the self-report impulsivity measure dropped to –.25 for mean reaction time and –.30 for the number of correct responses. Malle and Neubauer (1991) and Gerbing et al. (1987) found low or nonsignificant correlations between response time tasks and the MFFT, and between response time tasks and various self-report measures of impulsivity.

Time Perception Measures

Several time estimation (TE) and time production (TP) tasks have also been used as methods for assessing impulsivity (Barratt & Patton, 1983; van den Broek, Bradshaw, & Szabadi, 1992; Gerbing et al., 1987). This approach is based on the hypothesis (1) that impulsive individuals tend to overestimate the amount of time that has passed when a stopwatch is run for a given interval and they are asked to estimate this interval; and (2) that such individuals tend to signal sooner when they are asked to indicate that a specific interval has passed. "An impulsive individual would be likely to estimate, for example, that five minutes had elapsed when only four minutes had actually elapsed (Time Estimation) and similarly, this individual would be more likely to maintain that he or she had waited ten minutes when, in actuality, only eight minutes had elapsed (Time Production)" (Gerbing et al., 1987, p. 362).

Although time perception tasks may prove to be a useful method for studying impulsivity, few reliability and validity data have been published on TE and TP tasks. We have been unable to find a single published study that reports on the test–retest reliability of TE or TP, although Gerbing et al. (1987) reported that the correlation between the mean error of 10 TE trials and the mean error of 15 TP trials was –.82 in a sample of 243 undergraduates. Two studies that have examined the relationship between TE/TP tasks and other behavioral measures of impulsivity have not been encouraging. Both van den Broek et al. (1992) and Gerbing et al. (1987) found a nonsignificant relationship between the MFFT and time perception (TE and TP) tasks.

RELATIONSHIPS AMONG SELF-REPORT
AND BEHAVIORAL MEASURES

Problems in the Literature

It should be apparent by now that a critical problem in the impulsivity literature is the lack of association among many commonly used impulsivity measures. There are inconsistent results when self-report measures are intercorrelated with one another, or when behavioral measures are intercorrelated with one another (Gerbing et al., 1987, Luengo et al., 1991; Parker et al., 1993). When self-report and behavioral measures are intercorrelated, however, the results have been much more consistent: There appears to be little association between these two types of measures (Gerbing et al., 1987; Luengo et al., 1991; Malle & Neubauer, 1991).

The lack of association among self-report and behavioral impulsivity measures may be the result of differing theoretical conceptionalizations of the construct, as well as methodological weaknesses in some of the studies that have examined relationships among measures. Several of the investigations that have attempted to examine and clarify the empirical relationship among commonly used impulsivity scales have used measures that have not been standardized for the populations under study (Luengo et al., 1991; Malle & Neubauer, 1991). The use of small or inappropriately sized samples may have also rendered unreliable the results of several studies that have examined the factor structure of frequently used impulsivity measures (Gerbing et al., 1987; Luengo et al., 1991). To further explore the relationship between self-report and behavioral measures of impulsivity, we collected some new data on a cross-section of behavioral and self-report impulsivity measures.

New Empirical Data

The present study compared the PRF, MPQ, and GZTS self-report impulsivity subscales with several behavioral measures of impulsivity: the MFFT (Kagan et al., 1964) and tasks designed to assess TE and TP abilities (Gerbing et al., 1987). Subjects consisted of 50 undergraduate students (18 men and 32 women) attending a large Canadian university (mean age for the men, 23.05 3.83 years; for the women, 21.88 4.72 years). During the first part of the 45-minute experimental session, subjects completed the Impulsivity scale from the PRF (Jackson, 1984), the Control/Impulsiveness scale from the MPQ (Tellegen, 1982), and the Restraint scale from the GZTS (Guilford et al., 1976). Self-report measures were scored so that high scores represented high levels of impulsivity. Subjects then completed the MFFT and the TE and TP tasks (the order of the MFFT or time perception tasks was randomized for each subject). All subjects completed the TE and TP tasks in the same randomized order. For the TE task, six estimation intervals were presented: two 15-second, two 30-second, and two

60-second intervals. For the TP task, six production intervals were presented: two 15-second, two 30-second, and two 60-second intervals. TE and TP scores were calculated as the mean error (in seconds) for the various tasks.

Table 8.1 presents intercorrelations between the various self-report and behavioral impulsivity measures. The PRF, GZTS, and MPQ impulsivity subscales were found to be highly intercorrelated (ranging from .78 to .89). These results are similar to the data reported in our earlier study (Parker et al., 1993), using the same group of self-report measures. The TP and TE scores correlated −.84—a result almost identical to one reported by Gerbing et al. (1987). In both studies, individuals who overestimated the amount of time that had transpired in the TE task were also very likely to signal sooner to indicate that a specific time period had passed in the TP task.

The MFFT latency score and MFFT error score correlated −.57 in the present study—a result slightly larger than the median correlation of −.48 across the various MFFT studies reviewed by Messer (1976). Consistent with other research using the MFFT, the present study found that the more time taken by a respondent before making a first guess, the fewer errors the respondent made before arriving at a correct response. Also consistent with previous research on the relationship between the MFFT and time perception (van den Broek et al., 1992; Gerbing et al., 1987), the present study found no association between these two behavioral measures. More importantly, however, all of the correlations between the self-report and behavioral measures were low and nonsignificant in the present study.

CONCLUSION

The new data reported in this chapter (see Table 8.1), as well as many of the impulsivity studies examined in this review, suggest that researchers

TABLE 8.1. Correlations between Self-Report and Behavioral Impulsivity Measures

Impulsivity measure	1	2	3	4	5	6
1. PRF Impulsivity	—					
2. MPQ Control/Impulsiveness	.89[*]	—				
3. GZTS Restraint	.79[*]	.78[*]	—			
4. TP	−.25	−.14	−.17	—		
5. TE	.20	.12	.20	−.84[*]	—	
6. MFFT latency	.01	.05	.03	.10	.01	—
7. MFFT error	−.18	−.16	−.06	−.08	.09	−.57[*]

Note. PRF, Personality Research Form; MPQ, Multidimensional Personality Questionnaire; GZTS, Guilford–Zimmerman Temperament Survey; TP, time production; TE, time estimation; MFFT, Matching Familiar Figures Test.
[*]$p < .05$.

need to be very cautious when selecting impulsivity measures. Self-report and behavioral measures of impulsivity appear to be assessing very different constructs. In addition, there would appear to be considerable variation in the facets of the impulsivity construct measured by many self-report measures. Some impulsivity measures assess only a narrow facet of the construct, although this is not always apparent from the available literature on a specific scale. Researchers need to be cautious when generalizing across impulsivity studies that use different measurement approaches.

REFERENCES

Barratt, E. S. (1959). Anxiety and impulsiveness related to psychomotor efficiency. *Perceptual and Motor Skills, 9,* 191–198.

Barratt, E. S. (1983). The biological basis of impulsiveness: The significance of timing and rhythm disorders. *Personality and Individual Differences, 4,* 387–391.

Barratt, E. S. (1985). Impulsiveness subtraits: Arousal and information processing. In J. T. Spence & C. E. Itard (Eds.), *Motivation, emotion and personality* (pp. 137–146). Amsterdam: Elsevier/North-Holland.

Barratt, E. S. (1994). Impulsiveness and aggression. In J. Monahan & H. J. Steadman (Eds.), *Violence and mental disorder: Developments in risk assessment* (pp. 61–79). Chicago: University of Chicago Press.

Barratt, E. S., & Patton, J. H. (1983). Impulsivity: Cognitive, behavioral, and psychophysiological correlates. In M. Zuckerman (Ed.), *Biological bases of sensation seeking, impulsivity, and anxiety* (pp. 77–116). Hillsdale, NJ: Erlbaum.

Bentler, P. M., & McClain, J. (1976). A multitrait–multimethod analysis of reflection–impulsivity. *Child Development, 47,* 218–226.

Block, J., Block, J. H., & Harrington, D. M. (1974). Some misgivings about the Matching Familiar Figures Test as a measure of reflection–impulsivity. *Developmental Psychology, 10,* 611–632.

Buss, A. H., & Plomin, R. (1975). *A temperament theory of personality development.* New York: Wiley.

Cattell, R. B., & Eber, H. W. (1962). *Manual for Forms A and B: Sixteen Personality Factor Questionnaire.* Champaign, IL: Institute for Personality and Ability Testing.

Cloninger, C. R. (1987a). A systematic method for clinical description and classification of personality variants. *Archives of General Psychiatry, 44,* 573–588.

Cloninger, C. R. (1987b). Neurogenetic adaptive mechanisms in alcoholism. *Science, 236,* 410–416.

Cloninger, C. R., Przybeck, T. R., & Svrakic, D. M. (1991). The Tridimensional Personality Questionnaire: U.S. normative data. *Psychological Reports, 69,* 1047–1057.

Cloninger, C. R., Svrakic, D. M., & Przybeck, T. R. (1993). A psychobiological model of temperament and character. *Archives of General Psychiatry, 50,* 975–990.

Corulla, W. J. (1987). A psychometric investigation of the Sensation Seeking Scale Form V and its relationship to the I.7 Impulsiveness questionnaire. *Personality and Individual Differences, 8,* 651–658.

Costa, P. T., & McCrae, R. R. (1988). Personality in adulthood: A six-year longitudinal study of self-reports and spouse ratings on the NEO Personality Inventory. *Journal of Personality and Social Psychology, 54*, 853–863.

Costa, P. T., & McCrae, R. R. (1992). *Revised NEO Personality Inventory (NEO-PI-R) and NEO Five-Factor Inventory (NEO-FFI): Professional manual.* Odessa, FL: Psychological Assessment Resources.

Dickman, S. J. (1990). Functional and dysfunctional impulsivity: Personality and cognitive correlates. *Journal of Personality and Social Psychology, 58*, 95–102.

Digman, J. M. (1990). Personality structure: Emergence of the five-factor model. *Annual Review of Psychology, 41*, 417–440.

Downey, J. E. (1923). *The will-temperament and its testing.* Yonkers, NY: World.

Edman, G., Schalling, D., & Levander, S. E. (1983). Impulsivity and speed and errors in a reaction time task: A contribution to the construct validity of the concept of impulsivity. *Acta Psychologica, 53*, 1–8.

Eysenck, S. B. J., & Eysenck, H. J. (1980). Impulsiveness and venturesomeness in children. *Personality and Individual Differences, 1*, 73–78.

Eysenck, S. B. J., Pearson, P. R., Easting, G., & Allsop, J. F. (1985). Age norms for inpulsiveness, venturesomeness and empathy in adults. *Personality and Individual Differences, 6*, 613–619.

Garner, D. M. (1991). *Eating Disorder Inventory—2: Professional manual.* Odessa, FL: Psychological Assessment Resources.

Gerbing, D. W., Ahadi, S. A., & Patton, J. H. (1987). Toward a conceptualization of impulsivity: Components across the behavioral and self-report domains. *Multivariate Behavioral Research, 22*, 357–379.

Gough, H. G. (1975). *Manual for the California Psychological Inventory.* Palo Alto, CA: Consulting Psychologists Press.

Gow, L., & Ward, J. (1982). The Porteus Maze Test in the measurement of reflection–impulsivity. *Perceptual and Motor Skills, 54*, 1043–1052.

Guilford, J. P., & Zimmerman, W. S. (1949). *The Guilford–Zimmerman Temperament Survey: Manual of instructions and interpretations.* Beverly Hills, CA: Sheridan Supply.

Guilford, J. S., Zimmerman, W. S., & Guilford, J. P. (1976). *The Guilford–Zimmerman Temperament Survey handbook.* San Diego, CA: EdITS.

Holden, R. R., Fekken, G. C., Reddon, J. R., Helmes, E., & Jackson, D. N. (1988). Clinical reliabilities and validities of the Basic Personality Inventory. *Journal of Consulting and Clinical Psychology, 56*, 766–768.

Jackson, D. N. (1984). *Personality Research Form manual.* Port Huron, MI: Research Psychologists Press.

Jackson, D. N. (1989). *Basic Personality Inventory manual.* Port Huron, MI: Research Psychologists Press.

Jackson, D. N., & Gray, A. (1989). *Survey of Work Styles manual: Research edition.* Port Huron, MI: Sigma Assessment Systems.

Kagan, J., Rosman, B. L., Day, D., Albert, J., & Phillips, W. (1964). Information processing in the child: Significance of analytic and reflective attitudes. *Psychological Monographs, 78*(1, Whole No. 578).

Link, H. C. (1936). A test of four personality traits of adolescents. *Journal of Applied Psychology, 20*, 527–534.

Luengo, M. A., Carrillo-de-la-Peña, M. T., & Otero, J. M. (1991). The components of impulsiveness: A comparison of the I.7 Impulsiveness questionnaire and the Barratt Impulsiveness Scale. *Personality and Individual Differences, 12*, 657–667.

Malle, B. F., & Neubauer, A. C. (1991). Impulsivity, reflection, and questionnaire response latencies: No evidence for a broad impulsivity trait. *Personality and Individual Differences, 12,* 865–871.

Messer, S. B. (1976). Reflection–impulsivity: A review. *Psychological Bulletin, 83,* 1026–1052.

Olson, S. L., Bates, J. E., & Bayles, K. (1990). Early antecedents of childhood impulsivity: The role of parent–child interaction, cognitive competence, and temperament. *Journal of Abnormal Child Psychology, 18,* 317–334.

Parker, J. D. A., Bagby, R. M., & Webster, C. D. (1993). Domains of the impulsivity construct: A factor analytic investigation. *Personality and Individual Differences, 15,* 267–274.

Parker, J. D. A., & Fedoroff, P. J. (1994). *Conceptualizing the impulsivity construct: Toward a reliable multidimensional model.* Manuscript submitted for publication.

Sergeant, J. A., van Velthoven, R., & Virginia, A. (1979). Hyperactivity, impulsivity and reflectivity and their relationship and implications for clinical child psychology. *Journal of Child Psychology and Psychiatry, 20,* 47–60.

Smith, I. L., & Singer, S. (1977). Multitrait–multimethod analysis of measures of reflection–impulsivity. *Educational and Psychological Measurement, 37,* 929–937.

Stagner, R. (1936). The Wisconsin Scale of Personality Traits. *Journal of Abnormal and Social Psychology, 31,* 463–471.

Svrakic, D. M., Przybeck, T. R., & Cloninger, C. R. (1991). Further contribution to the conceptual validity of the unified biosocial model of personality: U.S. and Yugoslav data. *Comprehensive Psychiatry, 32,* 195—209.

Svrakic, D. M., Whitehead, C., Przybeck, T. R., & Cloninger, C. R. (1993). Differential diagnosis of personality disorders by the seven-factor model of temperament and character. *Archives of General Psychiatry, 50,* 991–999.

Tellegen, A. (1982). *Brief manual for the Multidimensional Personality Questionnaire.* Minneapolis: University of Minnesota Press.

van den Broek, M. D., Bradshaw, C. M., & Szabadi, E. (1992). Performance of impulse and non-impulsive subjects on two temporal differentiation tasks. *Personality and Individual Differences, 13,* 169–174.

Zevon, M. A., & Tellegen, A. (1982). The structure of mood change: An idiographic/nomothetic analysis. *Journal of Personality and Social Psychology, 43,* 111–122.

9

Impulsivity in Children and Adolescents

JUDY ZAPARNIUK
STEVEN TAYLOR

Impulsivity holds a central place in many theories of child development and psychopathology. Although there are no widely adopted or precise definitions of "impulsivity," several behaviors or inferred processes are commonly used to define this term. These include (1) the tendency to execute actions too quickly or in an unreasoned or unreflective manner; (2) difficulties in withholding actions or difficulties in inhibiting actions once they have been commenced; and (3) the tendency to seek out immediate gratification at the expense of longer-term goals (Schachar, Tannock, & Logan, 1993).

According to the most recent edition of the *Diagnostic and Statistical Manual of Mental Disorders* (DSM-IV; American Psychiatric Association [APA], 1994), impulsivity is a feature of some forms of attention-deficit/hyperactivity disorder (ADHD). Three types of ADHD are defined, differing in terms of whether the disorder is characterized (1) predominantly by inattention (e.g., difficulty in sustaining attention), (2) predominantly by hyperactivity–impulsivity, or (3) by a combination of inattention and hyperactivity–impulsivity. Impulsivity, as seen in the second and third types, is indicated by the tendency to blurt out answers before the questions have been finished, impatience (i.e., difficulty in waiting one's turn), and frequently intruding on or interrupting others (e.g., breaking into games or conversations) (APA, 1994).

Clinically significant impulsivity tends to be frequent and long-standing (i.e., it lasts longer than 6 months; APA, 1994), and it impairs social functioning and school performance. Although impulsivity is a feature of ADHD, it is also found in other disorders of childhood or adolescence, including conduct disorder, antisocial personality disorder (however, because most adolescents are sullen and antisocial, technically APD cannot be diagnosed until *after* age 18), and borderline personality disorder (APA, 1994; Farrington, Loeber, & van Kammen, 1990; Satter-field, 1978). Impulsivity in its milder forms may play a role as well in DSM-IV V-code conditions, such as academic problems, parent–child relational problems, and sibling (or peer) relational problems.

The frequency of impulsivity problems in children and adolescents was recently demonstrated by the DSM-IV field trials for disruptive behavior disorders (Frick et al., 1994). The sample consisted of 440 clinic-referred youths aged 4–17 years, who were consecutive referrals to a heterogeneous group of mental health clinics. Although the youths were referred for a variety of reasons, impulsive behaviors were very frequent, as assessed by Version 2.3 of the Diagnostic Interview Schedule for Children (DISC 2.3; Shaffer, Fisher, Piacentini, Schwab-Stone, & Wicks, 1992), modified for the field trials. The following findings were obtained: 67% of the sample often blurted out answers to questions before the questions were completed; over half (51%) had difficulty waiting in lines or awaiting their turn in games or group situations; and 44% frequently interrupted or intruded on others.

There are several theories of impulsivity, and it seems likely that numerous factors are involved in the etiology and maintenance of impulsive problems. Cognitive factors thought to be involved include (1) attentional functioning; (2) task comprehension; (3) processes involved in initiating and executing responses; (4) processes involved in delaying, inhibiting, or interrupting responses; and (5) mechanisms of processing feedback from the environment, including the processing of reward and punishment (Barratt & Patton, 1983; Dickman, 1990; Gray, Owen, Davis, & Tsaltas, 1983; Newman & Wallace, 1993; Schachar et al., 1993). Although these factors are reviewed elsewhere in this volume, we mention them because they provide the rationale for many measures of impulsivity.

In this chapter we review the measures of impulsivity most widely used with children and adolescents, along with some of the more recent, promising measures. In the first section we review observer-rated scales, including parent- and teacher-rated measures; this is followed by a review of the self-report measures for children and adolescents. We then examine neuropsychological tests and other cognitive processing tasks. We conclude by considering the question of how these measures are related to one another: Do they measure a unitary dimension of impulsivity, or do they assess multiple dimensions? The measures covered in this review are summarized in Table 9.1.

TABLE 9.1. Measures of Impulsivity in Children and Adolescents

Observer-rated scales

Diagnostic Interview Schedule for children, version 2.3 (DISC 2.3), and other
   diagnostic interviews
Child Behavior Checklist (CBCL)
Conners Rating Scales—Revised (CRS-R)
Self-Control Rating Scale (SCRS)
Direct observation and videotape ratings

Self-report measures

Eysenck I.6 Impulsiveness scale
Barratt Impulsiveness Scale, version 10 (BIS-10)

Neuropsychological tests and other cognitive tasks

Circle tracing and related tasks
Matching Familiar Figures Test (MFFT)
Trail Making Test
Stroop word–color test
Continuous-performance test (CPT) and Gordon Diagnostic System (GDS)
Card-playing task
Delay-of-gratification test
Stop-signal paradigm
Time perception tests

OBSERVER-RATED SCALES

Diagnostic Interviews

There are several structured interviews for the diagnosis of DSM-III-R
disorders of childhood and adolescence, such as the DISC 2.3 (Shaffer et
al., 1992). Many of these interviews have been recently revised, or are
currently under revision, to assess DSM-IV disorders (e.g., Frick et al.,
1994, revised the DISC 2.3 for the DSM-IV field trials). An advantage of
these interviews is that they can sample information from multiple
sources, including parents, teachers, and the child.

Although structured interviews can provide reliable and valid assessments of DSM-III-R and DSM-IV disorders, such measures are of limited
value in assessing impulsivity because they contain few relevant items.
To illustrate, the DISC 2.3 contains only three impulsivity items ("difficulty waiting in lines," "often interrupts or intrudes," and "often blurts
out answers").

Diagnostic interviews are useful screening devices for severe impulsivity problems. However, they provide limited coverage because they tend
to focus on school-related problems. Moreover, these measures may not be
sufficiently sensitive for detecting mild forms of impulsive problems.

Child Behavior Checklist

The Child Behavior Checklist (CBCL; Achenbach, 1991; Achenbach & Edelbrock, 1983, 1986, 1987) consists of items assessing behavior problems and social competence. There are teacher, parent, and youth versions, which are similar in format. The most recent version of Achenbach's scale (Cross-Informant Version; 1991) permits direct comparison of results among the parent, teacher, and youth ratings. Each version presents the participant with a list of behavioral problems; these are each rated according to whether a given behavior is "not true" (scored 0), "sometimes or somewhat true" (1), or "very true or often true" (2) of the subject. Factor analysis was used to derive the CBCL subscales; some subscales assess internalizing problems (e.g., somatic complaints, obsessive–compulsive symptoms), whereas other subscales assess externalizing problems (hyperactivity, aggression, delinquency).

The CBCL was carefully constructed, has extensive normative data for ages 2–16 years, and has acceptable reliability (Barkley, 1997). However, it provides a limited assessment of impulsivity. To overcome this limitation, White et al. (1994) expanded the assessment of impulsivity by combining four CBCL items with two items from the Self-Report Delinquency Scale (Elliott, Huizinga, & Ageton, 1985). All items are teacher-rated, and are as follows: "fails to finish things he starts," "impulsive or acts without thinking," "demands must be met immediately," "talks out of turn," "wants to have things right away," "impatient." (The wording for the first item reflects the fact that the scale was constructed for the assessment of males; the wording can be changed accordingly to assess both genders.) The modified scale has good internal consistency (alpha = .90: White et al., 1994). Unfortunately, norms are unavailable. Also lacking are data on test–retest reliability and interteacher reliability.

Conners Rating Scales—Revised

The Conners Rating Scales—Revised (CRS-R; Goyette, Conners, & Ulrich, 1978) can be completed by teachers or parents and is commonly used to assess ADHD. The parent version consists of 48 items, and the teacher version has 24 items. Informants are asked to rate the presence and severity of behavior on a 4-point scale (0 = "not at all," 3 = "very much"). Both the parent and teacher versions provide scores on five scales: Conduct Problems, Learning Problems, Psychosomatic Complaints, Anxiety, and Impulsive—Hyperactive Problems. Norms are available for ages 3–17 years (Barkley, 1990; Goyette et al., 1978). Interrater agreement appears adequate for research purposes, and the CRS-R can discriminate ADHD from non-ADHD children (Barkley, 1988, 1997; Breen & Altepeter, 1990). Many items overlap with the CBCL, although both versions of the

CRS-R have the advantage of being briefer and providing a more detailed assessment of impulsivity problems. Unfortunately, however, there is no separate CRS-R scale for assessing impulsivity. Thus, researchers and clinicians are required to examine the individual items from the CRS-R.

Self-Control Rating Scale

The Self-Control Rating Scale (SCRS) contains 33 items, rated by either parents or teachers, that assess a child's ability to inhibit behavior, follow rules, and control impulsive reactions (Kendall & Braswell, 1982, 1985; Kendall & Wilcox, 1979). Each item is rated on a 7-point scale (1 = "maximum self-control," 7 = "maximum impulsivity"). The scale yields an overall measure of self-control. Norms are available only from a small sample (n = 110) of students ranging from 8 to 12 years of age (Kendall & Wilcox, 1979). The scale has good internal consistency (alpha = .98) and adequate interrater (teacher–parent) reliability and test–retest reliability (Kendall & Braswell, 1982; Kendall & Wilcox, 1979). The scale can discriminate ADHD children from controls (Barkley, 1988, 1997; Breen & Altepeter, 1990). This scale appears useful for research purposes. Its limitations include the limited available norms and the fact that most of the reliability data are based on ratings from teachers rather than parents. Accordingly, findings using ratings from parents should be interpreted with caution (Breen & Altepeter, 1990).

Direct Observation and Videotape Ratings

Videotape observations can provide a direct measure of impulsive behavior. In a study of measures of impulsivity, White et al. (1994) videotaped each of their subjects for 20 minutes while they were completing other measures (e.g., other impulsivity tests or IQ tests). Tapes were rated by three trained coders on a 4-point scale for each of two dimensions: motor restlessness and impatience–impersistence. Motor restlessness was defined by the extent to which a subject showed movement and expressed physical energy (e.g., leg jiggling, rocking in the chair). Impatience–impersistence was indicated by such behaviors during the testing situation as quitting easily, refusals to guess or think more, looking at watch, and reaching for the test materials before they were presented. Mean intraclass correlations across coders were .81 to .82, indicating good intercoder agreement (White et al., 1994). Other reliability data were not reported.

Similar methods have been developed to assess ADHD, including direct observation in the classroom and other settings (e.g., Barkley, Fischer, Newby, & Breen, 1988; Jacob, O'Leary, & Rosenblad, 1978; Milich, Loney, & Landau, 1982). Unfortunately, many of these methods contain few items specifically assessing impulsivity.

Videotape ratings and related methods can be useful means of assessing impulsivity as it occurs in a child's or adolescent's environment. However, such methods are used mostly for research purposes and have several limitations that have prevented their widespread use. The methods require specially trained raters, and norms are unavailable. Furthermore, the reliability and validity of the ratings may vary with the sorts of activities that the child is completing at the time (i.e., impulsive behaviors may be less evident for some tasks than others). Reactivity may also be a problem, in that children may alter their behavior if they are aware of being observed.

SELF-REPORT MEASURES

Eysenck Impulsiveness Scale

In developing their measures of impulsiveness, the Eysencks (Eysenck & Eysenck, 1978, 1980; Eysenck & Zuckerman, 1978) distinguished "impulsiveness" (doing and saying things without thinking) from "venturesomeness" (sensation seeking and risk taking when the person is well-aware of the risks and willing to take the chance). Separate, factorially distinct scales were constructed to assess these constructs. The child and adolescent version of the Impulsiveness scale has been through several revisions. The most recent version of the Impulsiveness scale (a subscale of the I.6 questionnaire; Eysenck, Easting, & Pearson, 1984) is a self-report inventory consisting of 23 yes–no items, which are face-valid measures of impulsivity (e.g., "Do you often buy things on impulse?", "Do you generally do and say things without stopping to think?"). The number of responses indicative of impulsivity are summed to provide a total score. It was originally constructed to assess British subjects, but has been adapted for North American dialect (e.g., White et al., 1994) and translated into Spanish (Silva, Martorell, & Clemente, 1987).

Norms are available for ages 8 to 15 years (Eysenck et al., 1984). Internal consistency is generally adequate for a research scale, with alpha coefficients ranging from .68 to .97 (Eysenck et al., 1984; White et al., 1994). The scale discriminates conduct disordered children from controls and is predictive of future conduct problems (Luengo, Carrillo-de-la-Peña, Otero, & Romero, 1994).

The Eysenck Impulsiveness scale has been used in many questionnaire studies of impulsivity in normal and clinical populations (e.g., Glow, Lange, Glow, & Barnett, 1983; Luengo et al., 1994; White et al., 1994). Although the I.6 version is quick and easy to administer, it has several limitations. First, subjects with reading impairments or those below the third or fourth grade may have difficulty comprehending the questions. Second, it relies on a subject's honesty and awareness of his or her own behavior. Impulsive subjects with little awareness of their behavioral tendencies will obtain spuriously low scores on this scale.

Barratt Impulsiveness Scale

Like the Eysenck Impulsiveness scale, the Barratt Impulsiveness Scale (BIS) has been through several revisions, with version 10 being the most recent (BIS-10; Barratt, 1985). The scale consists of 34 items, each rated on a 4-point scale (1 = "rarely/never," 4 = "almost always/always"). The BIS-10 contains three subscales designed to assess three aspects of impulsivity: (1) Motor Impulsiveness (11 items; e.g., "I walk and move fast"), (2) Cognitive Impulsiveness (11 items; e.g., "I make up my mind quickly"), and (3) Nonplanning Impulsiveness (12 items; e.g., "I am more interested in the present than in the future"). Motor Impulsiveness measures the tendency to engage in spontaneous behavior (acting without thinking). Compared to the other BIS-10 subscales, this subscale is most similar to the Eysenck I.6 Impulsiveness scale. Cognitive Impulsiveness assesses the tendency to make quick decisions. Nonplanning Impulsiveness involves a lack of concern for the future or for the consequences of one's actions (Barratt, 1985).

The BIS was originally developed for use mainly with adults, although it has been used with adolescents as young as 12 years (Barratt, 1981; Carrillo-de-la-Peña, Otero, & Romero, 1993; Luengo et al., 1994). Carrillo-de-la-Peña et al. recently modified the BIS-10 to assess Spanish-speaking adolescents. For this version, the internal consistency (alpha coefficient) of the total score is .82, and that of the subscales ranges from .60 to .69 (Carrillo-de-la-Peña et al., 1993).

Barratt (1981) compared scores on the BIS with a performance measure of impulsivity (i.e., time perception) in a group of delinquent adolescent males, a group of psychiatric patients, and controls, all aged 13–16 years. Results revealed that although the three groups did not differ significantly on BIS scores, time perception among the three groups differed significantly. Time perception was best for controls and worst for the delinquent males.

The BIS-10 shares many of the advantages and disadvantages of the Eysenck I.6 Impulsiveness scale. The BIS-10 is short and easy to administer, but requires approximately a grade 3 or 4 reading level. Scores on the BIS-10 also depend on a subject's honesty and awareness of his or her behavior patterns. The BIS-10 has an advantage over the Eysenck instrument in that it provides a broader assessment of impulsivity, with separate scales for cognitive, motor, and nonplanning impulsivity. Unfortunately, the BIS-10 also has some disadvantages compared to the Eysenck scale: Norms are unavailable for children, and the reliability and validity data are confined almost entirely to the adult/adolescent version of the scale. Although the BIS-10 is a useful measure for the assessment of adults and adolescents, further studies are needed to determine whether it will make a useful addition to the assessment of impulsivity of children below the age of 12.

NEUROPSYCHOLOGICAL TESTS AND OTHER COGNITIVE TASKS

Circle Tracing and Related Tasks

The circle-tracing task was developed as a simple test of motor inhibition (Bachorowski & Newman, 1985). The subject is requested to trace over a 9-inch circle as slowly as he or she can, and the tracing time is then recorded. The start and stop positions on the circle are clearly marked in bright letters, and subjects are given five trials. The dependent variable in this task is the tracing time for the second trial.

Bachorowski and Newman (1990) conducted a study using the circle tracing task with university students and found that on the first trial, subjects classified as anxious or impulsive tended to trace quickly, relative to normal controls. On subsequent trials anxious subjects slowed to perform more similarly to normals, but the impulsive subjects sustained their relatively rapid pace. Subject were classified into groups high and low in anxiety and impulsiveness, based on their scores on the Eysenck Personality Questionnaire (EPQ; Eysenck & Eysenck, 1975). Subjects scoring above the median on the Extraversion (E) and Neuroticism (N) scales of the EPQ were placed in the impulsive group, whereas subjects scoring below the median on the E scale and above the median on the N scale were placed in the anxious group. White et al. (1994) reported that tracing times were correlated .28 with cognitive impulsivity, and −.08 with behavioral impulsivity, in boys aged 12–13 years. The authors reported a validity coefficient of .23 with cognitive impulsivity and 0 with behavioral impulsivity. Further studies are needed to determine whether circle tracing will make a useful addition to the assessment of impulsivity of children below the age of 12.

Similar tasks have been used to measure motor inhibition, such as drawing a line as slowly as possible, or walking as slowly as possible along a line (Maccoby, Dowley, Hagen, & Degerman, 1965; Olson, Bates, & Bayles, 1990; Toner, Holstein, & Hetherington, 1977).

Performance on the circle-tracing task and on related tasks may be influenced by the ability to inhibit one's actions. However, speedy performance may also be attributable to factors other than impulsivity. Subjects may complete the task quickly so that they may end the testing session, in order to pursue more interesting or rewarding activities (Sonuga-Barke, Houlberg, & Hall, 1994). A further problem is that this test may only detect the more severe forms of impulsivity; subjects with milder forms may be able to inhibit their motor responses for a short time.

Matching Familiar Figures Test

The Matching Familiar Figures Test (MFFT; Kagan, Rosman, Day, Albert, & Phillips, 1964) is probably the most widely used measure in studies of impulsivity in children. It consists of 12 match-to-sample trials. In each trial the subject is required to search an array of pictures for the one that exactly matches a criterion picture. The array contains the correct picture among eight similar foils. Performance is assessed by the time taken to respond and the number of errors. Fast, inaccurate performance on the MFFT is assumed to indicate impulsivity, as defined by lack of cognitive control over responding. It is assumed that the subject is unable to delay a response in the course of analyzing the stimuli and searching for the correct alternative.

Studies using the MFFT have found that as normal children grow older, they develop longer response latencies and greater accuracy (Salkind & Wright, 1977). In contrast, children with clinical disorders characterized by impulsivity, such as ADHD, respond more quickly and make more errors (Campbell, Douglas, & Morgenstern, 1971).

The MFFT has been through several revisions, intended to improve its reliability and criterion-related (known-groups) validity. Modifications in the type of stimuli and number of trials improved the psychometric properties of the measure, and the scale appears suitable for use with children aged 5–14 (Cairns & Cammock, 1978; Messer & Brodzinsky, 1981; Salkind, 1978). Also, a version of the MFFT, titled the Kansas Reflection–Impulsivity Scale for Preschoolers, has been developed for young children (Wright, 1973). Despite these additions and improvements, there are still problems with the MFFT. The main problem is that poor performance may be attributable to deficits unrelated to impulsivity. For example, MFFT performance varies with search strategy (Ault, Crawford, & Jeffrey, 1972) and with metacognitive awareness of the appropriateness of inhibiting the response (Brown, Bransford, Ferrara, & Campione, 1983). Thus, the MFFT can be regarded as an index of general cognitive functioning or information-processing competence, rather than strictly as a measure of impulsivity (Block, Gjerde, & Block, 1986; Breen & Altepeter, 1990).

Trail Making Test

The Trail Making Test is a neuropsychological measure of visual–conceptual and visual–motor tracking, which requires the subject to initiate, switch, and stop a sequence of actions (Lezak, 1995). The task consists of two parts. In Form A, the subject is given a sheet of randomly placed numbers and is asked to draw lines to consecutive connect consecutive numbers as quickly and accurately as possible, without lifting his or her pencil (i.e., to draw a line from 1 to 2 to 3, etc.). In Form B, the subject is given a sheet consisting of randomly placed numbers and letters. The subject is asked to connect consecutive numbers and letters in an alternating sequence, without lifting his or her pencil (i.e., to draw a line from A to 1 to B to 2, etc.). The time required to complete Form A is subtracted from that for Form B. This difference score provides an index of how much harder it is for the subject to perform a task with two sequences (numbers and letters) than a task with to one sequence (numbers only). An error score can be computed, although this measure is less useful because errors are relatively rare, especially in people who have not sustained brain injury (Lezak, 1983).

This test has several advantages. The necessary materials (consisting of only two test sheets and a pencil) can be easily assembled. Reliability coefficients are generally acceptable (see Lezak, 1995, for a review). The test is quick and easy to administer, and norms are available for ages 8–15 (Spreen & Strauss, 1991).

Unfortunately, the Trail Making Test also has several disadvantages when used as a measure of impulsivity. The main problem is that scores reflect multiple cognitive processes and abilities, including attention, short-term memory, visuomotor coordination, the ability to establish and maintain a set, and the ability to inhibit a previously learned set. Poor scores, as indicated by larger differences between the times required to complete Form A and Form B, can be obtained for a variety of reasons. They may be attributable to factors related to impulsivity (e.g., deficits in inhibiting inappropriate responses on Form B). However, poor scores may also result from factors unrelated to impulsivity. For example, Forms A and B place different demands on the subject in terms of learning and memory. Form A resembles common children's games such as "connect the dots," whereas Form B is likely to be novel to many children and adolescents. Accordingly, learning and memory deficits may be more likely to disrupt performance on Form B than on Form A, thus producing large differences in the times required to complete each form.

Stroop Word–Color Test

The Stroop word–color test (Golden, 1978; Stroop, 1935) assesses the person's ability to inhibit an overlearned response and maintain a cognitive set. The subject is presented with a card on which there is a list of the names of colors (i.e., red, green, and blue), each printed in colored ink. The subject is asked to name the color of the ink as quickly and accurately as possible, while ignoring the name of the word. Interference occurs when the color of the ink is different from the name of the word (e.g., the word "red" printed in green ink). The time required to read each card (response time) or the total number of errors can be used as measures of poor inhibitory control. White et al. (1994) reported that total errors and response times were correlated .94 in boys aged 12–13 years. White et al. argued that the error score was a preferable measure because it was more normally distributed than response time, whereas others argue for the importance of measuring interference effects (for a review, see MacLeod, 1991).

The Stroop test shares many of the advantages of the Trail Making Test: It is quick and easy to administer, it does not require elaborate materials, and norms are available (Golden, 1978). The Stroop can also be administered on a computer monitor. The test has adequate reliability as well (see Franzen, 1989, for a review). A disadvantage is that it can be unpleasant to complete, especially for subjects with concentration problems (Lezak, 1995). Also, it cannot be validly used with visually impaired (e.g., color-blind) subjects or those with reading disabilities, because such impairments alter the nature of the interference effect (Dyer, 1973). Apart from these difficulties, the Stroop would appear to be useful as an overall measure of several of the processes that appear to be related to impulsivity (e.g., attention and concentration, maintaining a set, inhibition of inappropriate responses).

Continuous-Performance Test

The continuous-performance test (CPT; Rosvold, Mirsky, Sarason, Bransome, & Beck, 1956) consists of a series of trials in which the subject is presented (e.g., on a computer screen) in rapid succession with a series of stimuli, such as letters or numbers. The subject is required to press a key whenever a target stimulus is presented, and to refrain from pressing the key when a nontarget stimulus is presented. In a given set of trials, there may be more than one target stimulus (e.g., the subject must respond whenever the letter X or B is presented). More complex variations of the task require the subject to respond only when the target item is preceded by a specified item (e.g., to press a key only when A follows X).

This task provides measures of the number of errors of omission (i.e., failing to press the key when the target is presented), errors of commission (i.e., pressing the key when a nontarget is presented), and number of correct responses. Correct number and number of omissions appear to assess sustained attention, whereas errors of commission may reflect impulse control and sustained attention (Breen & Altepeter, 1990).

In studies using the CPT, children with ADHD tend to perform more poorly than non-ADHD controls (Douglas, 1983). In the past, problems with the CPT in clinical practice have included the lack of a standardized procedure, the lack of normative data, and the fact that a special apparatus (e.g., a computer) is required to present the stimuli (Barkley, 1988, 1997). However, Gordon (1983) has developed a small, childproofed computerized device known as the Gordon Diagnostic System (GDS). This includes a version of the CPT, and norms are available for children aged 3–16. The GDS is able to discriminate ADHD children from controls (Gordon & Mettelman, 1988), and has performed well in other tests of reliability and criterion-related validity (see Breen & Altepeter, 1990, for a review). Thus, the GDS appears to be a useful measure of motor inhibition, although users of this instrument need to bear in mind that it is also sensitive to attentional abilities.

Card-Playing Task

The card-playing task is a computer game designed to measure a disinhibitory response style. The game creates a dominant response set for reward and then pairs that response with punishment (Newman, Patterson, & Kosson, 1987). The task consists of a deck of 100 playing cards, sequentially presented on a computer monitor. Cards are presented in a preprogrammed order of "face" cards and "number" cards. When the task begins, the subject receives a preset amount of money. For each trial the back of a card first appears, and the subject may choose to place a monetary bet that the card is a face card, or may choose to discontinue the game and keep the winnings. After each card is played, an experimenter adds or subtracts money from the subject's total stakes, depending on whether the subject won or lost. The first 10 trials present 9 face cards, so that a strong expectation of winning is established at the outset. The probability of a losing card (i.e., the probability of a number card's appearing) increases by 10% with every succeeding block of 10 cards. Thus, the probability of losing increases gradually from 10% to 100%. Given the increasing odds of losing, most nonimpulsive subjects discontinue playing when they are about halfway through the game (i.e., when the odds of losing are 50% or higher). The dependent measure is the number of cards played before deciding to quit.

Conduct-disordered children and adult psychopaths, compared to their corresponding controls, tend to play the game longer and to lose more money (Newman et al., 1987; Shapiro, Quay, Hogan, & Schwartz, 1988). This task has been used primarily as a research tool, and validity and reliability data are as yet unavailable. The available data indicate group differences at the .02 level with adults (Newman et al., 1987), and at the .05 level with youths 7–18 years of age (Shapiro et al., 1988). There have been no studies comparing the performance of ADHD children to that of controls, and so it is not known whether clinically impulsive children and adolescents are less able to delay gratification than are controls.

The card-playing task measures the tendency to persist in the face of increasing punishment and increasing lack of reward. Thus, the task is sensitive to inhibitory control and responsivity to reward and punishment. It may be argued that this task measures more than impulsivity. However, some theorists argue that impulsivity is determined in part by the extent to which the individual is affected by reward and punishment (Gray et al., 1983). In summary, the card-playing task can be regarded as a broad measure of some of the processes involved in impulsivity.

However, it must be kept in mind that this task was designed as a research tool, rather than as one intended for clinical practice. Thus (unlike measures such as the GDS), the card-playing test has no norms, and few data are available on its reliability or validity.

Delay-of-Gratification Task

The delay-of-gratification task is another computer game developed by Newman and colleagues. This task was designed to pit a less desirable but immediate monetary outcome against a more desirable but delayed one (Newman, Kosson, & Patterson, 1992). On each trial, the subject is presented with two choices: Option 1, which can be selected immediately and is associated with a 40% probability of winning money, or Option 2, which the subject must wait 10 seconds to select, but which is associated with an 80% probability of winning money. The subject selects the options by pushing one of two buttons, and receives 30 trials. Throughout the task, the subject's earnings are displayed on the computer monitor. The experimenter adds the monetary reward to his earnings after every win, in order to increase the salience of the reward.

Before commencing the task, the subject receives 10 practice trials with each button, to enable him or her to learn the probability of winning associated with each button. The experimenter instructs the subject to count how often he or she wins while practicing each button. The subject then goes on to complete the 30 trials of the task proper, in which he or she makes associated choices. The dependent variable is the percentage of trials for which the subject is unable to delay gratification.

Like the card-playing task, the delay-of-gratification task has been used primarily as a research tool. There have been few studies of its reliability or validity. Over the 30 trials, the internal consistency of responding is high (alpha = .88: White et al., 1994). There have been no studies comparing the performance of ADHD children and controls, and so it is not known whether clinically impulsive children and adolescents are less able to delay gratification than are controls. However, Newman et al. (1992) showed that adult psychopaths, compared to nonpsychopaths, were less able to delay gratification.

A similar task is Gordon's (1979) differential reinforcement for low-rate responding (DRL), which has been used with ADHD children. This task requires the subject to withhold responding for a fixed time interval in order to obtain reward (e.g., candy). A more complex version of this task is the DRL with limited hold, in which the subject is required to withhold responding for a fixed time interval, and must respond within a fixed interval in order to obtain reward (e.g., a 60-second hold time and a 5-second response time). Gordon (1979) used this paradigm without the hold period, placing ADHD and non-ADHD children aged 6–8 years in a situation requiring them to inhibit responding for 6 seconds in order to receive candy. Children who responded before 6 seconds had elapsed had to wait another 6 seconds before receiving another opportunity to receive the candy. Gordon found that, compared with normal children, ADHD children were significantly more likely to respond before the time interval had elapsed. This suggests that, like psychopaths, ADHD children have difficulty enduring delays required to receive rewards.

In summary, the tasks developed by Gordon (1979) and Newman et al. (1992) appear to be useful research tools for assessing the subject's ability to delay gratification. Thus, the tasks seem useful for measuring one aspect of impulsivity.

Stop-Signal Paradigm

The stop-signal paradigm assesses the subject's ability to inhibit a response that has been initiated. Subjects engage in a primary task (e.g., forced-choice letter discrimination) and are presented with an occasional stop-signal stimulus (e.g., a tone) instructing them to inhibit their response to the primary-task stimulus (Schachar & Logan, 1990). According to Logan (1984), response inhibition depends on a race between the primary-task processes and the stop-signal processes. If the former wins, a response occurs; if the latter wins, the response is inhibited. Plotting the probability of inhibition against stop-signal delay produces an inhibition function. In general, the better the inhibition process, the higher and steeper the function. If the inhibition mechanism is rarely triggered in stop-signal trials, a flat function should be produced.

Schachar and Logan (1990) used the stop-signal paradigm to investigate the development and pathology of inhibitory control in children. They found that the ability to inhibit developed little after grade 2, and that subjects with ADHD showed deficient inhibitory control. The latter finding was attributable primarily to the subgroup of ADHD subjects with pervasive hyperactivity, who had a more severe inhibitory deficit than did either the subgroup with situational hyperactivity or the normal control group. This paradigm has been used on subjects ranging in age from 7 to 12 years, and with adults (Schachar & Logan, 1990).

The stop-signal paradigm was designed to measure one aspect of impulsivity: the ability to inhibit a response once it has been initiated. Accordingly, additional tasks are needed to assesses other aspects of impulsivity. Like several other measures of impulsivity, the stop-signal paradigm has been used primarily as a research tool. Norms and further studies of reliability and validity are required before it can be used in clinical practice.

Time Perception Tests

According to Barratt and Patton (1983), the tendency to respond quickly without thinking arises from biologically determined differences in cognitive tempo. They argue that arousal level is related in part to impulsivity, and that action-oriented subjects have a fast conceptual tempo and respond more quickly in certain situations. According to Barratt and Patton, the internal clocks of impulsive individuals are faster than the internal clocks of nonimpulsive individuals.

Cognitive tempo is assessed by time estimation and time production tasks (Barratt & Patton, 1983). In the time estimation condition, a stopwatch is run for six consecutive intervals of 2, 4, 12, 15, 45, and 60 seconds. After each interval, the subject is asked to estimate how many seconds have passed. In the time production condition, the subject is asked to signal when he or she thinks that intervals of 2, 4, 12, 15, 45, and 60 seconds have passed. The dependent variable is the difference between the actual time and the subject's response in both time estimation and time production.

Internal consistencies of the conditions appear acceptable for research purposes (alpha = .67 to .79; White et al., 1994). However, White et al. reported that the 60-second time estimation task did not appear valid; no reason was stated.

Time estimation and time production are highly negatively correlated (r's = −.54 to −.82: Gerbing, Ahadi, & Pattont, 1987; White et al., 1994). That is, subjects who overestimate time intervals also tend to signal sooner in the time production condition. Accordingly, the scores on the time production task can be reflected, and the scores from the two conditions can be summed to provide a global time perception score.

Time perception tests were designed to measure one aspect of impulsivity: cognitive tempo. These tasks have met with mixed reviews regarding task validity (Gerbing et al., 1987; White et al., 1994). More research is required to examine the validity of the notion of cognitive tempo, and to assess time perception with children under the age of 10 years.

Measures of Impulsivity: How Are They Related?

As we have seen, there is a plethora of different measures of impulsivity, including neuropsychological tests, behavioral tasks, self-report scales, and observer-rated measures. The question arises as to whether they are measuring the same or different constructs.

Several studies of adults suggest that impulsivity is composed of several factors. Gerbing et al. (1987) administered a battery of self-report tests and cognitive tasks to a sample of university students. Factor analysis yielded 15 first-order factors and 3 second-order factors. The latter were labeled (1) Spontaneous (i.e., seeks thrills, makes quick decisions, avoids planning), (2) Not Persistent (i.e., is distractible, restless), and (3) Carefree (i.e., is happy-go-lucky, impatient). Self-report measures tended to have low correlations with cognitive measures.

Parker, Bagby, and Webster (1993) administered a battery of self-report measures to two samples of university students. Exploratory and confirmatory factor analyses suggested two factors: (1) a Cautious–Spontaneous dimension, and (2) a Methodical–Disorganized dimension. These factors are comparable to Buss and Plomin's (1975) distinction between the ability to resist giving in to urges or motivational states, and the ability to plan and organize before acting.

With regard to studies of children and adolescents, several studies have shown that different measures of impulsivity are often uncorrelated with one another, especially measures based on different sources of information (e.g., teacher ratings vs. performance on cognitive tasks) (Carrillo-de-la-Peña et al., 1993; Gaddis & Martin, 1989; Paulsen & Johnson, 1980; Thompson & Nichols, 1992; White et al., 1994). To illustrate, in one of the most comprehensive studies of the dimensions of impulsivity, White et al. (1994) factor-analyzed 11 of the more commonly used measures. These represented a broad range of tasks and of information sources (e.g., self-reports, parent reports, teacher ratings, computer tasks). Measures were included only if there were published data on their reliability and validity.

White et al. (1994) administered the measures to 404 adolescent boys (aged 12–13 years at the time of testing) recruited from public schools. The correlations among measures were remarkably low, with the highest *r* being .33 and the remaining *r*'s ranging from –.08 to .23. White et al. factor-analyzed these measures and obtained two factors, labeled Cognitive Impulsivity and Behavioral Impulsivity. Cognitive Impulsivity had high loadings on measures associated with effortful, planful cognitive performance (i.e., tasks requiring mental control and mental effort to switch adaptively between mental sets). Measures with high loadings on this factor included the Trail Making test, the Stroop test, time perception tasks, the number of cards played on the card-playing task, circle-tracing time, and performance on the delay-of-gratification task. The measures loading on this factor represented two different assessment methods (pencil-and-paper or oral performance tests and computer games).

The Behavioral Impulsivity factor measured impulsivity associated with parent-reported undercontrol, observer-rated motor restlessness, teacher- and self-reported impulsivity, and observer-rated impatience–impersistence. The variables loading on this factor represented four different methods of assessment (questionnaires, interviews, Q-sort procedures, and videotape ratings) and four different sources (children, parents, teachers, and videotape raters).

Results indicated that both Cognitive and Behavioral Impulsivity had similar correlations with socioeconomic status, but that Cognitive Impulsivity was more strongly related to IQ than was Behavioral Impulsivity. Behavioral Impulsivity was more strongly related to delinquency than was Cognitive Impulsivity. Behavioral Impulsivity was especially related to serious delinquency that was stable over time (i.e., present over the past 2 years).

Carrillo-de-la-Peña et al. (1993) obtained a similar factor solution when they factored responses from children aged 13 to 16 years. One factor had salient loadings on cognitive measures, such as the MFFT. The other factor had salient loadings on the Eysenck Impulsiveness scale and the subscales of the BIS-10. Although this study used a small sample size ($n = 46$), it is notable that the factor solution was very similar to that obtained by White et al. (1994).

The two factors obtained by White et al. (1994)—Cognitive Impulsivity and Behavioral Impulsivity—differed primarily in terms of method of assessment (i.e., self-report or cognitive tasks vs. observer-rated measures). Thus, the factors may have been artifactual, differing primarily in terms of method of assessment. Although White et al. (1994) acknowledged this possibility, they apparently did not attempt to correct for differences in method variance. It would have been useful to explore the factors of impulsivity further by means of interbattery factor analysis. This is a method that identifies the factors underlying two sets of batteries (Tucker, 1958). This is done by factoring the matrix of cross-correlations (i.e., between-battery correlations); thus, method variance (indicated by within-battery correlations) is excluded. In the case of the measures used by White et al., one "battery" would correspond to the self-report measures and cognitive tasks, and the other "battery" would correspond to the observer-rated measures. Although this method might shed further light on the dimensions of impulsivity, the generally low correlations among measures suggests that each measure might correspond to a unique "factor."

In summary, studies of adults, adolescents, and children show that impulsivity measures are often uncorrelated with one another, and that impulsivity is a multidimensional construct. There have been too few studies to determine the nature of the underlying factors. Available studies of children and adolescents have contributed little to this issue, apart from underscoring the importance of using multiple measures in order to obtain a comprehensive assessment of the various aspects of impulsivity.

SUMMARY AND CONCLUSIONS

Impulsivity is a common clinical problem, as demonstrated by the DSM-IV field trials (Frick et al., 1994). It is a feature of some forms of ADHD, and it is found in other disorders of childhood, adolescence, and adulthood (e.g., conduct disorder, antisocial personality disorder; APA, 1994). Impulsivity tends to be frequent and long-standing, and impairs social functioning and school performance. As we have seen, there are numerous measures of impulsivity, including neuropsychological tests, behavioral tasks, self-report scales, and observer-rated measures. Many of these measures assess different aspects or processes related to impulsivity. Some assessment techniques have been used mainly as research tools, whereas others have been developed more thoroughly for clinical purposes. The assessment techniques also differ widely in terms of their ease of use and age range of applicability.

Impulsivity is a multifactorial construct, and it requires a range of measures for a comprehensive assessment. Impulsivity research has paid little attention to underlying cognitive deficits, which may affect responding in some assessment techniques. Also, cognitive measures are infrequently used in ADHD outcome studies. There is a need to broaden the techniques used in assessing impulsivity, in order to provide a more complete picture of the construct.

Some important issues for further investigation are as follows. First, there is a need to further the development of cognitive tasks designed to assess specific processes of impulsivity (e.g.,the stop-signal paradigm). Second, there is a need to determine the relative sensitivity of global measures of impulsivity for treatment outcome effects, in order to advance our understanding of how best to treat impulsivity problems. Third, we must consider developmental issues in impulsivity measures, as many measures are aimed at individuals who are at various stages of cognitive and behavioral development (i.e., young children vs. adolescents/early teens). We also need to further examine the reliability and validity of the cognitive measures designed for younger children.

REFERENCES

Achenbach, T. M. (1991). *Manual for the Child Behavior Checklist—Cross-Informant Version*. Burlington: University of Vermont, Department of Psychiatry.

Achenbach, T. M., & Edelbrock, C. S. (1983). *Manual for the Child Behavior Checklist and Revised Child Behavior Profile*. Burlington: University of Vermont, Department of Psychiatry.

Achenbach, T. M., & Edelbrock, C. S. (1986). *Manual for the Teacher's Report Form and teacher version of the Child Behavior Profile*. Burlington: University of Vermont, Department of Psychiatry.

Achenbach, T. M., & Edelbrock, C. S. (1987). *Manual for the Child Behavior Checklist—Youth Self-Report*. Burlington: University of Vermont, Department of Psychiatry.

American Psychiatric Association (APA). (1994). *Diagnostic and statistical manual of mental disorders* (4th ed.). Washington, DC: Author.

Ault, R. L., Crawford, D. E., & Jeffrey, W. E. (1972). Visual scanning strategies of reflective, impulsive, fast-accurate, and slow-accurate children on the Matching Familiar Figures test. *Child Development, 43*, 1412–1417.

Bachorowski, J. A., & Newman, J. P. (1985). Impulsivity in adults: Motor inhibition and time estimation. *Personality and Individual Differences, 6*, 133–136.

Bachorowski, J. A., & Newman, J. P. (1990). Impulsive motor behavior: Effects of personality and goal salience. *Journal of Personality and Social Psychology, 58*, 512–518.

Barkley, R. A. (1990). *Attention-deficit hyperactivity disorder: A handbook for diagnosis and treatment.* New York: Guilford Press.

Barkley, R. A. (1997). Attention deficit/hyperactivity disorder. In E. J. Mash & L. G. Terdal (Eds.), *Assessment of childhood disorders* (3rd ed., pp. 71–129). New York: Guilford Press.

Barkley, R. A., Fischer, M., Newby, R., & Breen, M. J. (1988). Development of a multi-method clinical protocol for assessing stimulant drug responses in ADHD children. *Journal of Clinical Child Psychology, 17,* 14–24.

Barratt, E. S. (1981). Time perception, cortical evoked potentials, and impulsiveness among three groups of adolescents. In J. R. Hays, T. K. Roberts, & K. S. Solway (Eds.), *Violence and the violent individual* (pp. 87–95). New York: SP Medical & Scientific Books.

Barratt, E. S. (1985). Impulsiveness subtraits: Arousal and information processing. In J. T. Spence & C. E. Izard (Eds.), *Motivation, emotion, and personality* (pp. 137–146). Amsterdam: Elsevier/North-Holland.

Barratt, E. S., & Patton, J. H. (1983). Impulsivity: Cognitive, behavioral, and psychophysiological correlates. In M. Zuckerman (Ed.), *The biological bases of sensation seeking, impulsivity, and anxiety* (pp. 77–116). Hillsdale, NJ: Erlbaum.

Block, J., Gjerde, P. J., & Block, J. H. (1986). More misgivings about the Matching Familiar Figures Test as a measure of reflection–impulsivity: Absence of construct validity in preadolescence. *Developmental Psychology, 22,* 820–831.

Breen, M. J., & Altepeter, T. S. (1990). *Disruptive behavior disorders in children.* New York: Guilford Press.

Brown, A. L., Bransford, J. D., Ferrara, R. A., & Campione, J. C. (1983). Learning, remembering, and understanding. In J. H. Flavell & E. M. Markman (Vol. Eds.), *Handbook of child psychology* (4th ed.): *Vol. 3. Cognitive development* (pp. 77–166). New York: Wiley.

Buss, A. H., & Plomin, R. (1975). *A temperament theory of personality.* New York: Wiley.

Cairns, E., & Cammock, T. (1978). Development of a more reliable version of the Matching Familiar Figures Test. *Developmental Psychology, 5,* 555–560.

Campbell, S. B., Douglas, V. I., & Morganstern, G. (1971). Cognitive styles in hyperactive children and the effect of methylphenidate. *Journal of Child Psychology and Psychiatry, 12,* 55–67.

Carrillo-de-la-Peña, M. T., Otero, J. M., & Romero, E. (1993). Comparison among various methods of assessment of impulsiveness. *Perceptual and Motor Skills, 77,* 567–575.

Dickman, S. J. (1990). Functional and dysfunctional impulsivity: Personality and cognitive correlates. *Journal of Personality and Social Psychology, 58,* 95–102.

Douglas, V. I. (1983). Attention and cognitive problems. In M. Rutter (Ed.), *Developmental neuropsychiatry* (pp. 280–329). New York: Guilford Press.

Dyer, F. N. (1973). The Stroop phenomenon and its use in the study of perceptual, cognitive, and response patterns. *Memory and Cognition, 1,* 106–120.

Elliott, D. S., Huizinga, D., & Ageton, S. S. (1985). *Explaining delinquency and drug use.* Beverly Hills, CA: Sage.

Eysenck, H. J., & Eysenck, S. B. G. (1975). *Manual of the Eysenck Personality Questionnaire.* London: Hodder & Stoughton/San Deigo, CA: ITS.

Eysenck, S. B. G., Easting, G., & Pearson, P. R. (1984). Age norms for impulsiveness, venturesomeness and empathy in children. *Personality and Individual Differences, 5,* 315–321.

Eysenck, S. B. G., & Eysenck, H. J. (1978). Impulsiveness and venturesomeness: Their position in a dimensional system of personality description. *Psychological Reports, 43,* 1247–1255.

Eysenck, S. B. G., & Eysenck, H. J. (1980). Impulsiveness and venturesomeness in children. *Personality and Individual Differences, 1,* 73–78.

Eysenck, S. B. G., & Zuckerman, M. (1978). The relationship between sensation seeking and Eysenck's dimensions of personality. *British Journal of Psychology, 69,* 483–487.

Farrington, D. P., Loeber, R., & van Kammen, W. (1990). Long-term criminal outcomes of hyperactivity–impulsivity–attention deficit and conduct problems in childhood. In L. N. Robins & M. Rutter (Eds.), *Straight and devious pathways from childhood to adulthood* (pp. 62–81). Cambridge, England: Cambridge University Press.

Franzen, M. D. (1989). *Reliability and validity in neuropsychological assessment.* New York: Plenum Press.

Frick, P. J., Lahney, B. J., Applegate, B., Kerdyck, L., Ollendick, T., Hynd, G. W., Garfinkel, B., Greenhill, L., Biederman, J., Barkley, R. A., McBurnett, K., Newcorn, J., & Waldman, I. (1994). DSM-IV field trials for the disruptive behavior disorders: Symptom utility estimates. *Journal of the American Academy of Child and Adolescent Psychiatry, 33,* 529–539.

Gaddis, L. R., & Martin, R. P. (1989). Relationship among measures of impulsivity for preschoolers. *Journal of Psychoeducational Assessment, 7,* 284–295.

Gerbing, D. W., Ahadi, S. A., & Patton, J. H. (1987). Toward a conceptualization of impulsivity: Components across the behavioral and self-report domains. *Multivariate Behavioral Research, 22,* 357–379.

Glow, R. A., Lange, R. V., Glow, P. H., & Barnett, J. A. (1983). Cognitive and self-reported impulsiveness: Comparison of Kagan's MFFT and Eysenck's EPQ Impulsiveness measures. *Personality and Individual Differences, 4,* 179–187.

Golden, C. J. (1978). *Stroop color and word test: A manual for clinical and experimental use.* Chicago: Stoelting.

Gordon, M. (1979). The assessment of impulsivity and mediating behaviors in hyperactive and nonhyperactive boys. *Journal of Abnormal Child Psychology, 7,* 317–326.

Gordon, M. (1983). *The Gordon Diagnostic System.* Boulder, CO: Clinical Diagnostic Systems.

Gordon, M., & Mettelman, B. B. (1988). The assessment of attention: I. Standardization and reliability of a behavior-based machine. *Journal of Clinical Psychology, 5,* 682–690.

Goyette, C. H., Conners, C. K., & Ulrich, R. F. (1978). Normative data for Revised Conners Parent and Teacher Rating Scales. *Journal of Abnormal Child Psychology, 6,* 221–236.

Gray, J. A., Owen, S., Davis, N., & Tsaltas, E. (1983). Psychological and physiological relations between anxiety and impulsivity. In M. Zuckerman (Ed.), *The biological bases of sensation seeking, impulsivity, and anxiety* (pp. 181–227). Hillsdale, NJ: Erlbaum.

Jacob, R. G., O'Leary, K. D., & Rosenblad, C. (1978). Formal and informal classroom settings: Effects on hyperactivity. *Journal of Abnormal Child Psychology, 6,* 47–59.

Kagan, J., Rosman, B. L., Day, D., Albert, J., & Phillips, W. (1964). Information processing in the child: Significance of analytic and reflective attitudes. *Psychological Monographs, 78*(1 Whole No. 578).

Kendall, P. C., & Braswell, L. (1982). Cognitive-behavioral self-control therapy for children: A component analysis. *Journal of Consulting and Clinical Psychology, 50,* 672–689.

Kendall, P. C., & Braswell, L. (1985). *Cognitive-behavioral therapy for impulsive children.* New York: Guilford Press.

Kendall, P. C., & Wilcox, L. E. (1979). Self-control in children: Development of a rating scale. *Journal of Consulting and Clinical Psychology, 47,* 1020–1029.

Lezak, M. D. (1983). *Neuropsychological assessment* (2nd ed.). New York: Oxford University Press.

Lezak, M. D. (1995). *Neuropsychological assessment* (3rd ed.). New York: Oxford University Press.

Logan, G. D. (1984). On the ability to inhibit thought and action: A users' guide to the stop signal paradigm. In D. Dagenbach & T. H. Carr (Eds.), *Inhibitory processes in attention, memory, and language* (pp. 189–239). San Diego: Academic Press.

Luengo, M. A., Carrillo-de-la-Peña, M. T., Otero, J. M., & Romero, E. (1994). A short-term longitudinal study of impulsivity and antisocial behavior. *Journal of Personality and Social Psychology, 66,* 542–548.

Maccoby, E. E., Dowley, E. M., Hagen, J. W., & Degerman, R. (1965). Activity level and intellectual functioning in normal preschool children. *Child Development, 36,* 761–770.

MacLeod, C. M. (1991). Half a century of research on the Stroop effect: An integrative review. *Psychological Bulletin, 109,* 163–203.

Messer, S. B., & Brodzinsky, D. M. (1981). Three-year stability of reflection–impulsivity in young adolescents. *Developmental Psychology, 6,* 848–850.

Milich, R., Loney, J., & Landau, S. (1982). The independent dimensions of hyperactivity and aggression: A validation with playroom observation data. *Journal of Abnormal Psychology, 91,* 183–198.

Newman, J. P., Kosson, D., & Patterson, C. M. (1992). Delay of gratification in psychopathic and nonpsychopathic offenders. *Journal of Abnormal Psychology, 101,* 630–636.

Newman, J. P., Patterson, C. M., & Kosson, D. (1987). Response perseveration in psychopaths. *Journal of Abnormal Psychology, 96,* 145–148.

Newman, J. P., & Wallace, J. F. (1993). Diverse pathways to deficient self-regulation: Implications for disinhibitory psychopathology in children. *Clinical Psychology Review, 13,* 699–720.

Olson, S. L., Bates, J. E., & Bayles, K. (1990). Early antecedents of childhood impulsivity: The role of parent–child interaction, cognitive competence, and temperament. *Journal of Abnormal Child Psychology, 18,* 317–334.

Parker, J. D. A., Bagby, R. M., & Webster, C. D. (1993). Domains of the impulsivity construct: A factor analytic investigation. *Personality and Individual Differences, 15,* 267–274.

Paulsen, K., & Johnson, M. (1980). Impulsivity: A multidimensional concept with developmental aspects. *Journal of Abnormal Child Psychology, 8,* 269–277.

Rosvold, H. R., Mirsky, A. F., Sarason, I., Bransome, R. D., & Beck, L. H. (1956). A continuous performance test of brain damage. *Journal of Consulting Psychology, 20*, 343–350.

Salkind, N. J. (1978). Development of norms for the Matching Familiar Figures Test. *JSAS: Catalog of Selected Documents in Psychology, 8.* (Ms. No. 1718)

Salkind, N. J., & Wright, J. C. (1977). The development of reflection–impulsivity and cognitive efficiency. *Human Development, 20*, 377–387.

Satterfield, J. H. (1978). The hyperactive child syndrome: A precursor of adult psychopathy? In R. D. Hare & D. Schalling (Eds.), *Psychopathic behaviour: Approaches to research* (pp. 329–346). Chichester, England: Wiley.

Schachar, R., & Logan, G. D. (1990). Impulsivity and inhibitory control in normal development and childhood psychopathology. *Developmental Psychology, 26*, 710–720.

Schachar, R., Tannock, R., & Logan, G. D. (1993). Inhibitory control, impulsiveness, and attention deficit hyperactivity disorder. *Clinical Psychology Review, 13*, 721–739.

Shaffer, D., Fisher, P., Piacentini, J., Schwab-Stone, M., & Wicks, J. (1992). *Diagnostic Interview Schedule for Children, version 2.3.* New York: Columbia University.

Shapiro, S. K., Quay, H. C., Hogan, A. E., & Schwartz, K. P. (1988). Response perseveration and delayed responding in undersocialized aggressive conduct disorder. *Journal of Abnormal Psychology, 97*, 371–373.

Silva, F., Martorell, M. C., & Clemente, A. (1987). I.6 (junior) questionnaire: Spanish version. *Psychological Assessment: An International Journal, 3*, 55–78.

Sonuga-Barke, E. J. S., Houlberg, K., & Hall, M. (1994). When is "impulsiveness" not impulsive?: The case of hyperactive children's cognitive style. *Journal of Child Psychology and Psychiatry, 35*, 1247–1253.

Spreen, O., & Strauss, E. (1991). *A compendium of neuropsychological tests.* New York: Oxford University Press.

Stroop, J. P. (1935). Studies of interference in serial verbal reactions. *Journal of Experimental Psychology, 18*, 643–662.

Thompson, R. W., & Nichols, G. T. (1992). Correlations between scores on a continuous performance test and parents' ratings of attentional problems and impulsivity in children. *Psychological Reports, 70*, 739–742.

Toner, I. J., Holstein, R. B., & Hetherington, E. M. (1977). Reflection–impulsivity and self-control in preschool children. *Child Development, 48*, 239–245.

Tucker, L. R. (1958). An inter-battery method of factor analysis. *Psychometrika, 23*, 111–135.

White, J. L., Moffitt, T. E., Caspi, A., Bartusch, D. J., Needles, D. J., & Stouthamer-Loeber, M. (1994). Measuring impulsivity and examining its relationship to delinquency. *Journal of Abnormal Psychology, 103*, 192–205.

Wright, J. C. (1973). *The Kansas Reflection–Impulsivity Scale for Preschoolers (KRISP).* St. Louis, MO: CEMREL.

10

Impulsivity in Major Mental Disorders

E. MICHAEL COLES

DEFINITION OF MENTAL DISORDER

The *Diagnostic and Statistical Manual of Mental Disorders,* fourth edition (DSM-IV; American Psychiatric Association [APA], 1994) acknowledges that "although this manual provides a classification of mental disorders, it must be admitted that no definition adequately specifies precise boundaries for the concept of 'mental disorder' " (p. xxi).[1] It goes on to state, however:

> In DSM-IV, each of the mental disorders is conceptualized as a clinically significant behavioral or psychological syndrome or pattern that occurs in an individual and that is associated with present distress (e.g., a painful symptom) or disability (i.e., impairment in one or more important areas of functioning) or with a significantly increased risk of suffering death, pain, disability, or an important loss of freedom. (p. xxi)

DSM-IV's definition of "mental disorder" is consistent with my own (Coles, 1975, 1982) definition of "mental health" and "mental illness" as social value judgments that are based upon biological, sociocultural, and/or psychological data; of these two terms, the former represents a conjunctive concept and the latter a disjunctive concept. Perhaps the keys to the definitions, however, are DSM-IV's reference to "clinically significant" and my reference to "social value judgments." Moore (1975) noted:

"Insanity" and "mental illness" mean, and have historically meant "irrational"; to be insane, or to be mentally ill, is not to act rationally often enough to have the same assumption of rationality made about one as is made of most of humanity; and absent such an assumption of rationality, one cannot be fully regarded as a person. (p. 1493)

Thus, I have suggested (Coles, 1982) that not only is mental illness a social value judgment based upon biological, sociocultural, and/or psychological data; "it could also be the inference of irrationality that is made from [those] data" (p. 19).

Irrationality has traditionally been associated with emotionality, and "emotional illness" is a well-established euphemism for "mental illness." Both terms are often applied to individuals who appear to act without adequate consideration of the circumstances or the consequences—that is, to act without thinking, or "impulsively." It is not surprising, therefore, that "impulsive" should be a pejorative term.

CONSTRUCT EXPLICATION OF IMPULSIVITY

"Impulsivity" is a complex concept. It involves an impulse, the behavioral expression of that impulse, and the situation in which both occur.

Dickman (1990) has differentiated between two types of impulsivity, emphasizing the social evaluation or appraisal of the act: "functional impulsivity," the tendency to act without forethought when this tendency is optimal or beneficial; and "dysfunctional impulsivity," the tendency to act with absence of forethought when this tendency could be a source of problems. Whether an act is "optimal or beneficial" or "a source of problems" is a function of the situation, both social and physical, within which it occurs.

Athletes train themselves, and undergo endless series of repetitions of game actions and responses, in order to ensure that they can respond without thinking. But what happens if they should find themselves in a game situation in ordinary life—particularly if they are boxers or martial artists? Imagine, for example, that a martial arts expert is standing and talking in the coffee room at work when a female colleague—in a surprise move and in a dangerous sense of fun—jumps on his back, placing her arms around his shoulders and her head alongside his. Immediately he brings the back of his clenched fist into her face, breaking her nose. Is this an impulsive act? If so, is it an example of functional or dysfunctional impulsivity? There is no doubt that the act is the source of a problem for the female colleague. She receives a broken nose. It may also create social, and perhaps employment-related, problems for the martial artist. But is the consideration of those problems dependent on the circumstances?

Would that same act by our martial artist be evaluated in the same way if the attack had not been carried out by a female colleague, had not been initiated in a sense of fun, and had occurred in a dark lane late at night?

Use of the term "impulsivity" also reflects the extent to which the individual is considered to have exercised control of his or her impulses and/or actions. Both the pejorative and the control-related aspects of "impulsivity" are contained in the DSM-IV (APA, 1994) definition of "impulse-control disorders not elsewhere classified,": in which it notes: "The essential feature of Impulse-Control Disorders is the failure to resist an impulse, drive, or temptation to perform an act that is harmful to the person or to others" (p. 609).

What constitutes "harm" is clearly open to interpretation. In the situation just described, we are inclined to refer to the action of the martial artist as "reflexive behavior"—that is, to say that the individual, his reflexes honed to a fine edge, responds "instinctively." We do so because his behavior is not an instantiation of a general tendency to act without thinking, but a specific tendency to respond to certain situations in a well-rehearsed way. His "impulsivity," being limited to those specific behaviors, is given a more positive label. The example of the martial arts expert therefore introduces another important aspect of "impulsivity": the boundaries of its content domain, or, in other words, the breadth of the behavior it covers.

We all have a variety of different impulses, and we vary in the way and extent to which we are able to control them. A person who cannot control the impulse to smoke may be perfectly capable of controlling his or her sexual impulses. A person who cannot control the desire to eat, and thus cannot control his or her weight, may have no trouble staying sober and away from alcohol. Impulse control—or the lack thereof—is not typically generic. Although, as noted by Webster and Jackson in Chapter 1, some patients and even nonpatients, when under stress, may exhibit impulsive actions in more than one area at the same time, or in several areas in succession.

I was testifying in a "dangerous offender" hearing a number of years ago. The offender in this case had just been released from jail, having served a 7-year sentence for rape, when he returned to the scene of his earlier crime and reoffended several times in a very similar way before being reapprehended. He was given a battery of psychological tests, and the results contained some common indications of "impulsivity." However, when he was described to the court as an impulsive individual, the judge interjected a question. For several days this man had sat calmly in court, listening to all kinds of nasty things being said about him, without as much as a restless change in position. He had not shouted out his objections, and he had certainly not lost control of his bowel or bladder functions. What had been meant when he had been described as "impulsive"?

DEFINITION OF IMPULSIVITY AND IMPULSE CONTROL

"Impulsivity" has not been comprehensively, clearly, or even consistently defined (Fink & McCown, 1993; Milich & Kramer, 1984; Parker, Bagby, & Webster, 1993). Most definitions, however, contrast impulsive behavior to planned behavior: "We may define the term impulse for our purposes as the generally unpremeditated welling-up of a drive toward some action that usually has the qualities of hastiness, lack of deliberation, and impetuosity" (Frosch, 1977, p. 296).

A review of *Webster's Third New International Dictionary* (1976) indicates that in common usage, in order to be called "impulsive" a person may manifest one of three quite different characteristics:

1. Acting momentarily, and in a way that is inconsistent with the prevailing behavior (i.e., manifesting behavior that can be described as whimsical, capricious, and even unpredictable); in this instance, behavior seems to represent a brief pulse or surge of energy, rather than a steady, consistent drive.
2. Generally acting, or being prone to act, with little apparent intellectual consideration of the appropriateness or consequences of so acting (i.e., manifesting behavior that could be described as spontaneous, impetuous, or rash).
3. Generally acting, or being prone to act, as if driven or compelled to act in a particular kind of way (i.e., manifesting behavior that appears to be more reflexive than volitional, and manifesting what might be called an "irresistible impulse").

The professional literature reflects three basic assumptions about the nature of impulsivity (Milich & Kramer, 1984): An impulsive response is rapid, undesirable, and/or error-prone; it is likely to occur in the presence of appealing stimuli; and/or it is likely to occur in the absence of strong cognitive control. There are two problems with each of these definitions, however. The first is deciding when an impulsive response is an undesirable symptom or sign of mental disorder, or a desirable feature of personality. In addition to the example of the martial arts expert given above, we have to consider the work of Eysenck, Pearson, Easting, and Allsopp (1985), who made a distinction between "impulsiveness" and "venturesomeness"; and the work of Parker et al. (1993), who identified two distinct dimensions of impulsivity, which they described as "cautious–spontaneous" and "methodical–disorganized." The second problem is determining whether impulsivity is the result of a strong impulse or of weak impulse control (Buss & Plomin, 1975). The implications of this distinction are as much therapeutic as they are definitional and conceptual.

IMPULSIVITY IN DSM-IV

Two observations spring readily from a cursory review of the signs and symptoms of mental disorders in DSM-IV (APA, 1994): The social maladjustment of mental disorders is identified in a number of ways, each of which could be considered to manifest an aspect of impulsivity; and the primary manifestation of social maladjustment is in aggressiveness and/or hostile behavior.

These observations are consistent with Frosch's (1977) observation regarding the misuse of the term "acting out" as a pejorative rubric for all antisocial behavior, including behaviors that reflect problems with impulse control. It is also consistent with the general observation made by Zilboorg and Henry (1941) over 50 years ago that throughout history,

> Every mental patient presents some form of unwillingness or inability to accept life as it is. Every mental patient either aggressively rejects life as we like it—and he was thought of as heretic, witch, or sorcerer—or passively succumbs to his inability to accept life as we see it—and he was therefore called bewitched. In the mind of the mentally healthy man, including the medical man, a mentally ill person still appears as an adamant rebel against our cultural common sense or a weakling who gives in to forces other than our cultural common sense. (pp. 523–524)

Scott (1958) referred to these two forms of "inability to accept life as it is" as "social maladjustment" and "failure of positive striving," respectively.

The different ways in which DSM-IV appears to identify social maladjustment could reflect a failure to adequately define the concept of impulsivity, indicative of attempts to refine and provide new operational definitions without effectively disposing of the old. It could also, however, simply be attributable to the disjunctive nature of the concept of social maladjustment.

Some of the terms and phrases that are used in DSM-IV (APA, 1994), and that on initial reading appear to be describing impulsivity, in fact relate to affect, mood, or emotion. The associated behavior is a direct reflection of a psychological condition, rather than an instrumental interaction with the environment, and requiring no planning. Examples include the "affective instability" of personality change due to a general medical condition (p. 171), the "affective lability" of dementia due to head trauma (p. 148), the "mood lability" and "lability of mood" of alcohol intoxication (p. 196) and manic episode (p. 328), and the "emotional lability" that is considered an associated feature/disorder of amphetamine-related disorders (p. 210). At the other extreme, there are references to a lack of control of behavior that is a purely biological phenomenon, with minimal association with any psychological state; this is the case with the elimination disorders, encopresis and enuresis. These clearly do not qualify as examples of impulsivity in the strict sense of the term. The "irritability" of dementia due to huntington's disease (p. 149) and manic episode (p. 328); the "irritable or anxious mood" of cannabis-related disorders (p. 215); the poor/low frustration tolerance of major depressive episode, indicated by "an exaggerated sense of frustration over minor matters" (p. 321); and the behavior that is "grossly out of proportion to any provocation or precipitating psychosocial stressor" (p. 610), listed as a characteristic of intermittent explosive disorder, are all similarly outside the current definition.

There is an important conceptual distinction to be made between impulsivity and overreaction. "Impulsivity" refers to the speed of the reaction (i.e., how long it takes for the person to react). "Overreaction" refers to the strength and duration of the reaction once it occurs. Although these may often be correlated, they are distinct and can occur independently. It would therefore be a mistake to assume that because a person reacts strongly (i.e., violently), that person is impulsive.

A more difficult decision surrounds the use of the phrase "disinhibition" in DSM-IV to describe a behavioral characteristic of dementia due to Pick's disease (p. 150) and symptom of injury to the frontal lobes, referred to under personality change due to a general medical condition (p. 171). The term is also used in DSM-III-R to describe a result of severe alcohol intoxication (APA, 1987, pp. 196–197). At a theoretical level, these conditions imply an underlying biological impairment of control, whereas impulsivity implies a psychological—and moral—failure to exercise control. For example, as noted earlier, DSM-IV has a major Axis I diagnostic category entitled "impulse-control disorders not elsewhere classified." This is considered in greater detail below and in Chapter 11. For present purposes, however, it should be repeated that the essential feature of this category of disorders is *"the failure to resist"* an impulse, drive, or temptation to perform an act that is harmful to the person or others" (p. 609, emphasis added). This distinction, however, may be difficult to make in practice.

As illustrated by the earlier account of my testimony in a "dangerous offender" hearing, there is a similarly difficult distinction to be made between impulsivity as a general characteristic of the individual, and impulsivity as a failure to control specific impulses. Perhaps because behavior is invariably a reaction to the interaction of the individual with his or her environment, just as no one ever manifests complete control of all impulses in all situations, so no one can be expected to manifest a complete lack of control over all impulses in all situations.

Impulsivity in Axis I Disorders

On Axis I, DSM-IV (APA, 1994) lists 16 major diagnostic categories, encompassing 337–374 specific diagnoses, depending on the status accorded to subcategories. It is on Axis I that we find the various forms of dementia, for which it is noted:

> Disturbances in executive functioning are a common manifestation . . . and may be related especially to disorders of the frontal lobe or associated subcortical pathways. Executive functioning involves the ability to think abstractly and to plan, initiate, sequence, monitor, and stop complex behavior. . . . Some individuals with dementia show disinhibited behavior, including making inappropriate jokes, neglecting personal hygiene, exhibiting undue familiarity with strangers, or disregarding conventional rules of social conduct. (pp. 135–136)

Also on Axis I are a number of disorders that are characterized by the failure to control specific impulses. These range from a failure to control "aggressive impulses," which is listed as an associated descriptive feature of dissociative amnesia (p. 478) and dissociative fugue (p. 482), and the "failure to resist aggressive impulses" in intermittent explosive disorder (p. 609), to the "failure to resist impulses to steal" of kleptomania (p. 612), "continu[ing] to gamble despite repeated efforts to control, cut back, or stop the behavior" of pathological gambling (p. 616), and the unsuccessful "attempts to resist the urge" that characterize Trichotillomania (p. 618). Intermittent explosive disorder, kleptomania, pathological gambling, and trichotillomania are disorders under the general heading of impulse-control disorders not elsewhere classified, mentioned earlier. In the introduction to this category, DSM-IV (APA, 1994) notes:

> This section includes disorders of impulse control that are not classified as part of the presentation of disorders in other sections of the manual (e.g., Substance-Related Disorders, Paraphilias, Antisocial Personality Disorder, Conduct Disorder, Schizophrenia, Mood Disorders may have features that involve problems of impulse control). (p. 609)

In addition to the disorders just mentioned, the category includes pyromania and impulse-control disorder not otherwise specified.

Pyromania is somewhat of an anomaly in this context. Although it is identified in terms of a specific behavior (i.e., fire setting), the behavior is described as "deliberate and purposeful" (p. 614). As for the diagnosis of impulse-control disorder not otherwise specified, it is very generally defined: "This category is for disorders of impulse control that do not meet the criteria for any specific Impulse-Control Disorder or for another mental disorder having features involving impulse control described elsewhere in the manual (e.g., Substance Dependence, a Paraphilia)" (p. 621).

DSM-IV's reference to paraphilias in its description of impulse-control disorder not otherwise specified is interesting, since there is no explicit reference to impaired impulse control in the DSM-IV description of those conditions. The reference is to "recurrent, intense sexually arousing fantasies, sexual urges, or behaviors" (p. 522), which "cause clinically significant distress or impairment in social, occupational, or other important areas of functioning" (p. 523). There are references to acting out "with a nonconsenting partner in a way that may be injurious to the partner" (p. 523); to the individual's being "subject to arrest and incarceration" (p. 523); and to the possibility that "acting out the paraphiliac imagery may lead to self-injury" (p. 523). However, there is no reference to impulsivity. Perhaps this is an indication of the status of impulsivity as a primary, if not universal, criterion of every mental disorder that is clearly antisocial and/or irrational—and, as such, a criterion that does not require explicit mention.

DSM-IV includes on Axis I, under the heading "disorders usually first diagnosed in infancy, childhood, or adolescence," a group of disorders that were on Axis II in DSM-III (APA, 1980) and DSM-III-R (APA, 1987) together with mental retardation and personality disorders. In DSM-III and DSM-III-R these disorders were listed under two major subcategories (pervasive developmental disorders and specific developmental disorders), with the latter further classified as academic skills disorders, language and speech disorders, or motor skills disorders. In DSM-IV (APA, 1994), the Axis I disorders usually first diagnosed in infancy, childhood, or adolescence are classified into nine major subcategories. As might be expected, given the fact that this category is based solely on the age at which a disorder is usually first diagnosed, all the adult types of impulsivity are represented.

The failure to control basic biological functions is seen in the creation of categories for feeding and eating disorders of infancy or early childhood and elimination disorders. Uncontrolled/uncontrollable behaviors that have the appearance of a physiological reflex, and for which many clinicians are inclined to infer an underlying neurological impairment, are represented by the category of tic disorders.

Attention-deficit and disruptive behavior disorders are identified in terms of their maladaptive features. Although clinicians frequently make the theoretical presumption that an organic impairment underlies these disorders also, the authors of DSM-IV have explicitly stated that the latest APA (1994) diagnostic and classificatory schemes are atheoretical. These disorders instantiate Scott's (1958) criterion of "social maladjustment," whereas his companion criterion of "failure of positive striving" can be seen to be the basis for distinguishing one of the pervasive developmental disorders, autistic disorder. These categories illustrate the pejorative use of "impulsivity."

Impulsivity in Axis II Disorders

Although impulsivity is encountered in a wide array of psychiatric disorders, it is a prominent characteristic of the Axis II personality disorders (Lion & Penna, 1975); it is also widely considered to be a characteristic of the other major Axis II category, mental retardation.

The essential feature of a DSM-IV personality disorder is described as "an enduring pattern of inner experience and behavior that deviates markedly from the expectations of the individual's culture and is manifested in at least two of the following areas: cognition, affectivity, interpersonal functioning, or *impulse control*" (p. 630, emphasis added).

In antisocial personality disorder, "a pattern of impulsivity may be manifested by a failure to plan ahead. . . . Decisions are made on the spur of the moment, without forethought, and without consideration of the consequences to self or others" (p. 646). In borderline personality disorder, "frantic efforts to avoid abandonment may include impulsive actions such as self-mutilating or suicidal behaviors" (p. 650). In histrionic personality disorder, an associated feature is as follows: "These individuals are often intolerant of, or frustrated by, situations that involve delay of gratification, and their actions are often directed at obtaining immediate satisfaction" (p. 656). Along with narcissistic personality disorder, the antisocial, borderline, and histrionic personality disorders are referred to as Cluster B disorders, having in common the feature of "wild," exaggerated, dramatic emotionality.

The Cluster A personality disorders—paranoid, schizoid, and schizotypal—are characterized by "weird" emotional withdrawal and odd behavior. They are suggestive of a less focused impulsivity.

The Cluster C personality disorders—avoidant, dependent, and obsessive–compulsive—have been described as "wary." They are characterized by anxious, resistive, and/or submissive behavior, and suggest overcontrol rather than a lack of control. For example, the essential feature of obsessive–compulsive personality disorder is said to be "a preoccupation with orderliness, perfectionism, and mental and interpersonal control," and individuals with this disorder "attempt to maintain a sense of control through painstaking attention to rules, trivial details, procedures, lists, schedules, or form to the extent that the major point of the activity is lost" (p. 669).

Almost by definition, the behavior of persons with mental retardation is expected to be impulsive. Because of the frequent association of mental retardation with underlying biological and neurological disabilities, it is often assumed that the behavior of a person with a mental retardation is beyond control. Because of their limited ability for abstract thinking and the consideration of events beyond the present, acting without thinking is considered to be characteristic of them. It is also thought that persons with mental retardation may lack the adaptive social skills that are necessary to express their feelings and emotions in a socially appropriate manner, and that they lack the social power to adjust and control their environment in such a way as to ensure that it does not create problems for them.

Although some of these stereotypes may be true of some people with mental retardation, they may be misleading in other cases, as DSM-IV points out: "No specific personality and behavioral features are uniquely associated with Mental Retardation. Some individuals . . . are passive, placid, and dependent, whereas others can be aggressive and impulsive" (p. 42). Indeed, "behaviors that would normally be considered maladaptative (e.g., dependency, passivity) may be evidence of good adaptation in the context of particular individual's life (e.g., in some institutional settings)" (p. 40). In DSM-IV's conceptualization, therefore, a person with mental retardation may fall into either of Zilboorg and Henry's (1941, pp. 523–524) categories of mental disorder: The person "either aggressively rejects life as we like it" or "passively succumbs to his [or her] inability to accept life as we see it."

CONCEPTUAL AND RESEARCH IMPLICATIONS

A complete lack of behavior control is rarely, if ever, observed in a conscious person, regardless of whether he or she has an Axis I mental illness, a personality disorder, or mental retardation. With the obvious exceptions of delirious and comatose individuals, and possibly those with a physiologically based incontinence of bladder or bowel functions, the expression of a socially unacceptable impulse invariably reflects some control. Impulsivity is therefore a matter of degree: A person is more or less impulsive, and can only be described as "impulsive" or "not impulsive" with considerable loss of information.

DSM-IV's descriptions of mental disorders highlight another important point. Impulsivity can be an "essential feature" of a disorder, an "associated feature," or merely a reaction that some people may show to a disorder. Although DSM-IV explicitly distinguishes between the first two, it fails to explicate its recognition of the last. For example, with regard to intermittent explosive disorder, it states: "Signs of generalized impulsivity or aggressiveness *may* be present between explosive episodes. Individuals with narcissistic, obsessive, paranoid, or schizoid traits *may* be especially prone to having explosive outbursts of anger when under stress" (p. 610, emphasis added). Compare this to the more definitive statement with regard to the gender of individuals with reading disorder: "From 60% to 80% of individuals diagnosed with Reading Disorder are males. Referral procedures may often be biased towards identifying males, because they more frequently display disruptive behaviors in association with Learning Disorders" (p. 49).

In failing to fully take into account individual differences in reaction to disorders, DSM-IV illustrates its failure to develop the interactional model that its multiaxial classification demands. Recognition that people react differently to their disorders inevitably leads to clinical syndromes' being considered *the product of an interaction among* Axis I, Axis II, Axis III, and Axis IV conditions, rather than an indication of one of those conditions.

DSM-III (APA, 1980) brought us to the point where we need empirical research to determine whether, for example, intermittent explosive disorder only occurs in individuals who have an Axis II diagnosis in which narcissistic, obsessive, paranoid, and/or schizoid traits are prominent; an Axis III medical diagnosis of a neurological impairment; and an Axis IV psychosocial or environmental problem indicative of a high level of premorbid/perimorbid stress. DSM-III-R and DSM-IV have added little in this regard. However, the treatment implications of such a conceptualization are considerable.

THERAPEUTIC IMPLICATIONS

People in a patient's community, and even in society at large, usually do not care how or why the person acts in an uncontrolled and/or unpredictable manner—only that he or she does behave in such a manner. There are two basic ways in which individuals can exercise control over their impulsive behavior: internally (i.e., by using defense mechanisms such as repression, suppression, and/or reaction formation, in addition to such cognitive strategies as reframing) or externally (i.e., by putting themselves or being put in a situation in which it is very difficult to act out—either because there is little in their environment to stimulate their impulses, or because there are controlling features in the environment that cannot be overlooked or ignored, such as the proverbial "police officer at the shoulder").

The clinical emphasis is invariably on internal control—perhaps based on the premise that the only real control is self-control—and, in particular, on control through the elimination of the psychological impulse. However, for those people who, for whatever reason, cannot establish some form of internal control, external controls can fill the gap. Consider, for example, people who reinforce their "will" to diet or to abjure alcohol by putting physical distance between themselves and the physical source of their addictive substances. The dieter will study at the library, rather than at home where the refrigerator is handy. The reforming alcoholic will stay away from bars.

This is consistent with Dickman's (1990) differentiation between functional and dysfunctional impulsivity, which emphasizes the social evaluation or appraisal of the act. This distinction makes the definition of an impulsive act dependent not only upon its outcome, but also upon the situation in which the behavior occurs. In some cases, the professional therapist becomes a crucial part of that environment:

> We can point out and clarify the existence of a defect; we may try to repair it, patch it, or offer a replacement; we cannot interpret it. Therefore, in the classic mode of supportive technique, we must work within the patient's psychic apparatus, accept what he has, evaluate his resources—especially [those] that

may be brought into the service of control—and try to utilize them where possible and to strengthen them if there is sufficient time. If such resources are limited or lacking, we may have to lend the patient our own ego operations to help meet this lack; in such instances, therapists must sometimes accept such patients as a lifelong commitment. (Frosch, 1977, pp. 311)

For some disorders, the choice between internal and external control of impulsivity is absolute and categorical. Consider the example of criminal sex offenders. Prior to committing a sexual offences, individuals are allowed to have as many lascivious or licentious thoughts as they wish. Their fantasy life is their own, and as long as they do not act on it, particularly with an unwilling partner or in an inappropriate situation, it is of no concern to anybody else. But once they have acted out their fantasies in an inappropriate manner, and have been placed in a treatment facility, it is the absence of the thoughts that will determine when they can be safely returned to the community. No matter how strong their behavioral controls, and no matter how firm their resolve not to act impulsively, they will be subjected to absolute environmental control and detained in a correctional facility, away from the sources of satisfaction for their impulses, as long as they have the socially unacceptable sexual fantasies. The criteria for discharging a convicted sexual offender into the community are far higher than the criteria that a nonoffender has to meet in order to stay in the community.

A similar kind of rigidity can be seen in the approach to impulsivity that is considered to be a personality trait:

> Insofar as "impulsiveness" would appear to be a trait of personality (Eysenck, 1993), it would seem very important indeed that the therapeutic aim be established as one of "management" rather than "cure". This means that, to an extent, the therapist must undertake something of a role as teacher or model. The purpose must be one of helping persons identify sources of stress and of assisting them strengthen their tolerance to these events. This means assisting them find ways of releasing tensions that are acceptable to them and to other members of society. . . . Clients frequently need assistance in isolating the kinds of experiential and emotional states that predispose them to untoward impulsive actions. The same can be said of analysis of precipitating events, [which are] sometimes called "triggers". (Mittler, 1994, pp. 37–38)

The current attitude toward the treatment of impulsivity in sex offenders and in personality-disordered individuals reflects the old, univariate, disease-based model of causality, rather than the new, multivariate, behavioral model that is advocated by DSM-III (APA, 1980), DSM-III-R (APA, 1987), and DSM-IV (APA, 1994). When it comes to the development of an interactive, multivariate model for diagnosis and treatment, the American Association on Mental Retardation (1992) is leading the way. And it is a very optimistic way.

In cases where impulsivity is to be attributed to limited intellectual functioning, it may be beneficial to think of the persons in terms of their mental age rather than their intelligence quotient. The concept of a low intelligence quotient carries with it an implicit assumption of an underlying, irreversible, neurological impairment, with a corresponding impediment to learning and behavioral change. However, young children, even very young children, can learn and acquire simple skills if the information is presented to them at a level and in a way that they can understand.

Camp (1977) suggested that aggressive boys have problems inhibiting impulsive behavior because they have not learned the adequate use of verbal mediation processes. Camp, Blom, Herbert, and van Doornick (1977) consequently developed a training program called "Think Aloud," which is designed to help aggressive boys gain control of their impulsive response styles through verbal mediation procedures. Dodge and Newman (1981) have suggested that aggression in young boys is sometimes attributable to their responding before they have given adequate attention to available social cues; this too can be corrected through education.

A FINAL COMMENT

Consideration of the meaning of "impulsivity"—its construct explication—should not be dismissed as a purely semantic issue. There is a story of a small community in the interior of British Columbia that has two churches. The difference between them is purely semantic. One says, "There is no hell"; the other says, "The hell there ain't!" The story is probably apocryphal, but its message is not.

A solution has never been found to a problem that was never defined. One of the major purposes of classifying disorders is to facilitate their treatment. Until the concept of impulsivity is clearly defined, the APA classification of its disorder(s) cannot be clear, and the DSM guidelines for treatment will consequently range from nonexistent to confused.

ACKNOWLEDGMENT

The assistance of Donna McMillan in preparing an initial data base for this review is gratefully acknowledged.

NOTE

1. This and all other such quotations in this chapter are reprinted with permission from the *Diagnostic and Statistical Manual of Mental Disorders*, Fourth Edition. Copyright 1994 by the American Psychiatric Association.

REFERENCES

American Association on Mental Retardation. (1992). *Mental retardation: Definition, classification, and systems of supports* (9th ed.). Washington, DC: Author.

American Psychiatric Association (APA). (1980). *Diagnostic and statistical manual of mental disorders* (3rd ed.). Washington, DC: Author.

American Psychiatric Association (APA). (1987). *Diagnostic and statistical manual of mental disorders* (3rd ed., rev.). Washington, DC: Author.

American Psychiatric Association (APA). (1994). *Diagnostic and statistical manual of mental disorders* (4th ed.). Washington, DC: Author.

Buss, A. H., & Plomin, R. (1975). *A temperament theory of personality development.* New York: Wiley.

Camp, B. (1977). Verbal mediation in young aggressive boys. *Journal of Abnormal Psychology, 86,* 145–153.

Camp, B., Blom, G., Herbert, F., & van Doornick, W. (1977). "Think aloud": A program for developing self-control in young aggressive boys. *Journal of Abnormal Child Psychology, 5,* 157–169.

Coles, E. M. (1975). The meaning and measurement of mental health. *Bulletin of the British Psychological Society, 28,* 111–113.

Coles, E. M. (1982). *Clinical psychopathology: An introduction.* London: Routledge & Kegan Paul.

Dickman, S. J. (1990). Functional and dysfunctional impulsivity: Personality and cognitive correlates. *Journal of Personality and Social Psychology, 58,* 95–102.

Dodge, K. A., & Newman, J. P. (1981). Biased decision-making processes in aggressive boys. *Journal of Abnormal Psychology, 90*(4), 375–379.

Eysenck, S. B. G., Pearson, P. R., Easting, G., & Allsopp, J. F. (1985). Age norms for impulsiveness, venturesomeness and empathy with adults. *Personality and Individual Differences, 6,* 613–619.

Eysenck, H. J. (1993). The nature of impulsivity. In W. G. McCown, J. L. Johnson, & M. B. Shure (Eds.), *The impulsive client: Theory, research, and treatment.* Washington, DC: American Psychological Association.

Fink, A. D., & McCown, W. G. (1993). *Impulsivity in children and adolescents: Measurement, causes and treatment.* Washington, DC: American Psychological Association.

Frosch, J. (1977). The relation between acting out and disorders of impulse control. *Psychiatry, 40,* 295–314.

Lion, J. R., & Penna, M. W. (1975). Concepts of impulsivity: A clinical note. *Diseases of the Nervous System, 36,* 630–631.

Milich, R., & Kramer, J. (1984). Reflections of impulsivity: An empirical investigation of impulsivity as a construct. *Advances in Learning and Behavioral Disabilities, 3,* 57–94.

Mittler, G. (1994). The treatment of impulsivity. In C. D. Webster, M. A. Jackson, & D. M. Brunanski (Eds.), *Impulsivity: New directions in research and clinical practice. Proceedings of a conference.* Vancouver, British Columbia: Simon Fraser University.

Moore, M. S. (1975). Some myths about "mental illness." *Archives of General Psychiatry, 32,* 1483–1497.

Parker, J. D. A., Bagby, R. M., & Webster, C. D. (1993). Domains of the impulsivity construct: A factor analytic investigation. *Personality and Individual Differences, 15*(3), 267–274.

Scott, W. A. (1958). Research definitions of mental health and mental illness. *Psychological Bulletin, 55,* 29–45.

Webster's third new international dictionary of the English language unabridged. (1976). Chicago: Encyclopaedia Britannica.

Zilboorg, G., & Henry, G. W. (1941). *A history of medical psychology.* New York: Norton.

11

Impulsivity in DSM-IV Impulse-Control Disorders

STEPHEN J. HUCKER

A number of psychiatric disorders currently listed in the *Diagnostic and Statistical Manual of Mental Disorders,* fourth edition (DSM-IV; American Psychiatric Association [APA], 1994) are conditions in which various types of impulsive behavior are included in their definition; examples include bulimia nervosa, substance abuse, and borderline and antisocial personality disorders. There are some other specific disorders of impulse control, however, that are placed in a category of their own: "impulse-control disorders not elsewhere classified" (the 312 codes, pp. 609–621). This awkwardly titled group comprises some conditions that have been recognized by clinicians for nearly 200 years and given time-hallowed names, and yet about which surprisingly little is known. Indeed, the validity of these diagnoses remains disputed. The disorders named specifically in this section of the DSM-IV are pathological gambling, kleptomania, pyromania, trichotillomania, and intermittent explosive disorder. There is also a residual category, "impulse-control disorder, not otherwise specified," which is intended to include those conditions that do not meet the criteria for the foregoing diagnoses or for others listed elsewhere in the nomenclature. This chapter provides an overview of the specific impulse-control disorders, and briefly mentions a few apparently related disorders for which some information is available. Serious students of other conditions related to impulsivity are urged to examine the pertinent sections of the DSM-IV. (See also Coles, Chapter 10, this volume.)

PATHOLOGICAL GAMBLING

Pathological gamblers, as opposed to recreational gamblers, are characterized by an inability to resist the impulse to gamble. They are unable to refrain, whether they are winning or losing, and the problem interferes with other aspects of their lives. They risk their jobs, disrupt their personal and family relationships, and often resort to crime in order to support their habit. Furthermore, winning becomes essential to their self-esteem (Peck, 1986). The term "pathological gambling" was suggested in preference to "compulsive gambling" (Moran, 1970) as the problem is pleasurable (at least in the early stages) and is not something that the individual regards as foreign to his or her personality.

This disorder was officially recognized only as recently as the DSM-III (APA, 1980). For the diagnosis to be applied, 5 or more of a total of 10 subcriteria must be met under Criterion A. These are listed in full in DSM-IV (p. 618). For present purposes, we restate the items in the following form: The person shows a preoccupation with gambling (item 1); acts illegally to obtain money for gambling (item 8); gambles to escape from problems or from negative feelings, such as depression, anxiety, or guilt (item 5); after losing, persists in gambling in order to recover losses (item 6); asks for money from others when the position becomes desperate (item 10); betrays others by lying to them over the current predicament (item 7); loses jobs, other opportunities, and important relationships over gambling (item 9); becomes irritable and restless when trying to reduce or quit gambling (item 4); requires increasing amounts of money to gain excitement (item 2); and cannot cease gambling despite attempts to reduce or stop (Item 3). The DSM-IV then goes on to require that the condition is not better explained by a manic episode (Criterion B).

Pathological gambling has been characterized not only as a disorder of impulse control, but also as a compulsive disorder (DeCaria & Hollander, 1993) and as an addiction (Dickerson, 1984). In fact, Freud first noted the similarity to drug and alcohol dependence. Surveys in the United States suggest that 0.1–2.3% of the population are problem pathological gamblers (Volberg & Steadman, 1988, 1989), and in the United Kingdom the disorder is estimated to occur in about 1% of adult males (Dickerson, 1984). It affects 6.7% of adult psychiatric inpatients (Lesieur & Blume, 1990) and 8–25% of alcohol and other substance abusers (Lesieur, Blume, & Zoppa, 1986). Though both sexes gamble, most pathological gamblers are men. Typically they are white middle- to upper-middle-class individuals, and are aged 40–50 years by the time they come to professional attention. Although there is great variability in individual profiles, pathological gambling follows a progressive course and tends to remain out of control despite heavy financial losses. These individuals are driven by a need for arousal, develop tolerance (i.e., increase in size of debts and odds to obtain the same arousal levels), and show withdrawal symptoms when gambling is abruptly curtailed (e.g., irritability, restlessness, lowered mood, and poor concentration). In men, the problem often begins in adolescence, whereas women develop it rather later in life. Often there is a history of some specific stress or major loss that coincides with the onset.

Four phases have been described in the natural history of pathological gambling (Custer & Milt, 1985). The first of these is winning. This is seen mainly in men, a number of whom report a "big win" early in the course of the disorder; this then encourages their overconfidence. Men who are successful in this way tend to derive recognition from it. Female pathological gamblers, in contrast, tend to develop their problem in response to past or present emotional problems. The second phase is losing. Despite a run of bad luck, the gambler is unable to accept losses and tries to win them back ("chasing"). Bets become heavier and more frequent, and debts increase. Often gamblers resort to "magical practices," such as blowing on the dice or carrying a "lucky charm" (Henslin, 1967). They develop irrational beliefs in "lucky streaks," or come to the idea that after losing several bets in a row their luck will alter, although the odds remain unchanged ("the gambler's fallacy"—Wagenaar, 1988). A sense of urgency develops, and the gambler begins lying to cover up the situation; this results in job and relationship problems. At this point, the gambler runs out of money and commonly turns to friends and relatives for a "bail-out." The third phase is desperation. In this phase, the individual turns to uncharacteristic and often illegal behavior, such as writing bad checks or embezzling from work. About two-thirds of pathological gamblers "cross the line" in this way. The behavior is rationalized and becomes easier each time. Rosenthal (1992) observes that at this stage, the gambler frequently fantasizes "starting over" with a new identity. Interpersonal relationships continue to fail, and depression increases. The fourth phase, hopelessness, was added to the sequence by Rosenthal (1992). Suicide risk and stress-related ailments dramatically increase in this stage. The gambler accepts that losses will never be recovered, but nevertheless continues to gamble.

Not surprisingly, up to three-quarters of gamblers suffer from major depressive disorder and a third from bipolar disorders (Linden, Pope & Jones, 1986). More than half also have a problem with alcohol abuse (Linden et al., 1986; Smart & Ferris, 1996). From 17% to 24% attempt suicide (Ciarrocchi & Richardson, 1989). Some 60–70% of pathological gamblers report dissociative experiences such as "trances," "memory blackouts," and "feeling like another personality" while gambling (Jacobs, 1988, p. 31). Personality disorders, especially narcissistic and antisocial personality disorders, are common in pathological gamblers (Blaszczynski, McConaghy, & Frankova, 1989).

The outlook for the untreated pathological gambler is uncertain. Most clinicians report that because these individuals lack insight, and because of the frequent presence of comorbid conditions such as substance abuse, it is difficult to engage them in treatment. Yet Rosenthal (1992) claims that in experienced hands, pathological gambling is "an extremely treatable disorder" (p. 77). There are, however, few well-designed studies to support this claim. Taber, McCormick, Russo, Adkins, and Ramirez (1987) reported that 56% were abstinent 6 months after a 28-day inpatient program, especially if they attended Gamblers Anonymous meetings. Indeed, for some, attendance at Gamblers Anonymous with its Twelve-Step Approach may be sufficient to help them sustain abstinence. Behavior therapy has shown limited success. It may also be difficult to achieve positive results with psychodynamic psychotherapy aimed at dealing with gamblers' sense of omnipotence and attempting to confront their rationalizations and maladaptive behavior. It may be helpful to involve family members in therapy. Needless to say, treatment of any underlying mood disorder or substance abuse is also necessary.

TRICHOTILLOMANIA

The strange term "trichotillomania" simply refers to a chronic, maladaptive, and irresistible urge to pull out one's hair. The scalp hair is usually selected, although the patient may pluck from any part of the body, including eyebrows and eyelashes; in extreme cases, all body hair may be removed (Krishnan, Davidson, & Guajardo, 1985). Trichotillomania has been variously regarded as a simple habit (Jillson, 1983), as a symptom of major mental illness (Oguchi & Miura, 1977), or as an impulse-control disorder or a variant of obsessive–compulsive disorder (Swedo, 1993). The DSM-IV lists five criteria. These can be summarized as follows: Tension increases before the hair is pulled or when the person is trying to prevent pulling (Criterion B); relief or pleasure is obtained when hair is being pulled out (Criterion C); the problem is not better explained by an alternative mental disorder or medical condition (Criterion D); clinically meaningful complications occur in social, vocational, or other areas (Criterion E); and hair loss is noticeable (Criterion A).

Though the condition may easily be concealed and not reported, a questionnaire survey of college students (Christenson, Pyle, & Mitchell, 1991) suggests that it affects 0.6–1.5% of males and 0.6–3.4% of females. This is consistent with the fact that female patients present more often to clinicians than males do. Trichotillomania may begin very early in childhood, equally in both boys and girls, and at this age many cases respond to simple remedies (or no remedy at all) and follow a benign course. It may be accompanied by thumb sucking and may be dismissed as normal. Later onset, during the teens, affects mainly females. Many individuals with this disorder never consult a psychiatrist. Often any disfigurement is concealed by wigs, hairstyling, or cosmetics, but it may lead to avoidance of social contacts and result in impaired self-esteem. Patients may also eat the plucked hairs (trichophagia) and hairballs (trichobezoars), may cause medical complications.

The extent of hair loss is variable but may be complete. When the hair grows in again, it usually appears normal but may be coarser and curlier. Within the affected areas can be found broken hairs of various lengths. Usually hair is pulled in private, but some patients may do it in front of close family members. It may increase in times of stress or, conversely, in times of relaxation. It may be carried out in brief episodes or for hours a time. After plucking, the individual may stroke the hair against the cheek or lips or eat it, and the behavior may be quite ritualistic. Patients rarely report the process to be painful; indeed, individuals are often unaware that they are plucking. Overwhelming anxiety and tension are common if they try to inhibit it themselves. Patients and their families may strenuously deny the behavior.

Several researchers have found that trichotillomania is often accompanied by symptoms of other disorders, including major depressive disorder, generalized anxiety disorder, substance abuse, eating disorders, and obsessive–compulsive disorder (Swedo, 1993; Christenson, Pyle, & Mitchell, 1991). Although these patients may have features of a personality disorder (usually of the histrionic, borderline, or passive–aggressive type), some clinicians have observed that many trichotillomaniacs are likeable and socially successful (Winchel, 1992).

Various theories have been proposed to explain the phenomenon, but more recent research has concentrated on the possibility that it may be a variant of obsessive–compulsive disorder. However, unlike patients with obsessive–compulsive disorder, trichotillomaniacs regard their compulsion as pleasurable, are not usually contending with a condition that elaborates or progresses, do not have to deal with obsessional ruminations, and do not regard the behavior as alien to their nature. As noted above, early-onset cases may have a favorable prognosis even without treatment, but in adults the disorder tends to become chronic. Partly because of the lack of agreement as to what causes trichotillomania, many types of treatment have been proposed, including stress reduction, behavior therapy, hypnotherapy, dynamic psychotherapy, and self-help groups—all of which have had variable success (Winchel, 1992). Drugs that are used to treat depression and obsessive–compulsive disorder, such as clomipramine (Anafranil) and fluoxetine (Prozac), have been used successfully, but in some cases the underlying depression improves while the hair pulling persists (Winchel, 1992). Lithium carbonate may also be helpful (Christenson, Popkin, Mackenzie, & Realmuto, 1991).

PYROMANIA

Some authors have used the term "pyromania" to identify fire-setting behavior for which no clear motive can be determined (Koson & Dvoskin, 1982; Lewis & Yarnell, 1951). However, it is not difficult to conceal such motives as financial gain, political statement, concealment of another crime, or expression of anger or revenge. As is true of several other impulse-control disorders, the concept of pyromania dates back to the 19th century. The DSM-IV lists six defining characteristics. These can be restated briefly as follows: The person obtains relief, gratification, or pleasure obtained from setting fires, watching them, or playing a part in the aftermath (Criterion D); monetary gain is not the intent, and fires are not set for political or criminal reasons or because of poor judgment induced by a mental disorder (Criterion E); affect or tension is aroused before the act (Criterion B); the problem is not better explained by antisocial personality disorder, manic episode, or conduct disorder (Criterion F); the intent to set fires is deliberate, and it occurs more than once (Criterion A); and attraction to or fascination with fire is evident (Criterion C).

Earlier studies of arsonists suggested that pyromania was quite common. Lewis and Yarnell's (1951) classic study of 1,145 cases of fire setting identified 39% as cases of pyromania. Geller (1994), however, reviewed the literature from 1840 to 1989 and found a gradually diminishing frequency of reports, such that DSM-IV indicates that the condition appears to be rare (APA, 1994, p. 614). Most offenders are male. Typically the individual is preoccupied with and attracted to fires. Cases are described in which the arousal and pleasure are explicitly sexual. Some of the latter "fire fetishes" are rare, and persons with such conditions may be very specific in their needs; for example, they may be aroused only by fires they have set themselves (Barker, 1994; Prins, 1994). Relatively little information is available with respect to pyromaniacs as opposed to the heterogeneous group of fire setters in general. Also, in a study of 22 impulsive arsonists, Virkkunen, DeJong, Bartko, and Linnoila (1989) found that 68% met DSM-III criteria for intermittent explosive disorder, 95% for dysthymic disorder or major depressive disorder, and 95% for alcohol abuse. They also found some association with borderline, antisocial, paranoid, and passive–aggressive personality disorders.

Anger and vengeance are the commonest motives for fire setting (Prins, 1994), and as pyromania has been so rarely defined operationally in studies of arsonists, little can be said with certainty about the etiology of the disorder. Stekel (1924), Freud (1932/1964), and Fenichel (1945) all proposed that pyromania results from unresolved sexual feelings; however, apart from cases where there is an explicit sexual motivation (see above), only one study has explored this hypothesis empirically, and it obtained negative results (Quinsey, Chaplin, & Upfold, 1989).

Recent studies of biological correlates of fire setting suggest a possible relationship between low levels of 5-hydroxyindoleacetic acid (5-HIAA) in the cerebrospinal fluid (CSF) and low levels of 3-methoxy-4-hydroxyphenyl glycol (MHPG) in "impulsive arsonists," compared with violent offenders and normal controls (Roy, Virkkunen, Guthrie, & Linnoila, 1986). Recidivistic arsonists were subsequently found to have lower

CSF 5-HIAA and lower blood glucose after a tolerance test than nonrecidivists (Virkkunen et al., 1989). These findings, which thus far have not been replicated, do suggest a possible underlying serotonergic or adrenergic disturbance and may indicate that the disorder should be considered part of the "affective disorder spectrum" (McElroy, Pope, Keck, & Hudson, 1995).

Because the literature on fire setters is largely limited to single-case reports, there is no clear indication of the best approach to treatment. Psychodynamic writers have documented the difficulties in treating these patients because of their denial and lack of insight, refusal to accept responsibility, and coexistence of alcohol problems (Mavromatis & Lion, 1977). Several behavioral techniques have been used for children prone to fire setting, and these might be attempted in a case of pyromania (McGrath & Marshall, 1979; Koles & Jenson, 1985; Wolff, 1984; Cox-Jones, Lubetsky, Flutz, & Kolka, 1990). Individual and family therapy techniques have been applied with some success (Bumpass, Brix, & Preston, 1985). Formal multimodular programs have also claimed low recidivism rates of 1.4–6.3% (Kolko, 1988). Previous authors had suggested recidivism rates varying from 4–5% (Mavromatis & Lion, 1977) to 28% (Lewis & Yarnell, 1951). Though there have been no published drug treatment studies with a DSM-IV-defined population of pyromaniacs, the results of biochemical studies noted earlier suggest that impulsive fire setters with some features suggestive of the disorder might receive a trial of medications that increase levels of serotonin at brain synapses.

INTERMITTENT EXPLOSIVE DISORDER

The considerable changes that have occurred over the last 30 years in the proposed classifications of violent behavior are indications not so much of improved research as of the continuing lack of reliable data. The notion that violent outbursts, rages, temper tantrums, and the like have an organic basis is captured by earlier terms such as "episodic dyscontrol" (Menninger & Mayman, 1956; Monroe, 1970) and "dyscontrol syndrome" (Mark & Ervin, 1970). Editions of DSM from DSM-II through IV have used the term "explosive" for apparently similar conditions. Despite its official usage, many clinicians and researchers have doubted the existence of intermittent explosive disorder as an independent entity. Indeed, it was almost excluded from DSM-IV (Bradford, Geller, Lesieur, Rosenthal, & Wise, 1994), as violence is so much a part of other psychiatric and organic brain disorders. There is evidence that clinicians tend not to apply clear diagnostic criteria when diagnosing intermittent explosive disorder, but rather use the label loosely for patients with a history of several explosive outbursts (APA, 1994; Monopolis & Lion, 1983). In one of the few studies using rigorous criteria (DSM III-R) and very thorough evaluations,

Felthous, Bryant, Wingerter, and Barratt (1991) found only 13 cases. This suggests that the condition is rare. Most studies would, in fact, seem to involve a miscellaneous group of violent individuals. Individuals who exhibit episodic violence are mainly male. Out of 842 possible cases reviewed in preparation for DSM-IV, only 17 likely cases were identified (Bradford et al., 1994).

The DSM-IV lists three diagnostic criteria for intermittent explosive disorder. These can be rephrased as follows: Impulses of aggression are uncontrolled in several separate episodes, and eventuate in serious assaults or destruction (Criterion A); the episodic violence is out of proportion to whatever precipitants may have set it in motion (Criterion B); disorders listed elsewhere in the DSM-IV are insufficient to account for the episodes (e.g., antisocial or borderline personality disorder, manic episode, substance abuse, etc.) (Criterion C). It should be clear that the present DSM-IV criteria reflect the current status of this disorder as one defined essentially by exclusion of other conditions. Because a single episode is insufficient for the diagnosis, a careful longitudinal history is essential. Problems with relationships, job losses, criminal behavior, alcohol abuse, and injuries resulting from fights and accidents are commonly seen in these patients. As the diagnosis is essentially exclusionary, any possible organic factors must be carefully sought out through a full neurological and neuropsychological assessment. In cases where findings identify mainly specific organic signs, the diagnosis is more appropriately personality change due to a general medical condition, aggressive type. Intermittent explosive disorder can be diagnosed concurrently with other psychiatric disorders, though the clinician must decide whether such a patient's condition is not accounted for by another disorder alone.

Despite the long history of attempts at identifying intermittent explosive disorder, in clinical practice it is often very difficult to tease out its features from a background of antisocial or borderline personality disorder, substance abuse, or deliberate violence to achieve some specific purpose. Chronic aggressive behavior is typical of patients with borderline or antisocial personality disorder, with the result that there is an overlap with intermittent explosive disorder in a number of studies (Virkkunen, 1976; Pattison & Kahan, 1983). Furthermore, repetitive self-mutilation, pathological gambling, and attention-deficit/hyperactivity disorder have been associated with "episodic dyscontrol" (Bach-Y-Rita, Lion, Climent, & Ervin, 1971).

Psychodynamic theories of impulsive aggression have supposed such acts to be the result of "wounded narcissism." Biologically oriented researchers, in contrast and as noted earlier, have been inclined to view the disorder as originating in dysfunction of the limbic system of the brain (Mark & Ervin, 1977; Stein, Towey, & Hollander, 1995). Monroe (1970) noted the substantial numbers of intermittently violent patients who had abnormalities on neurological examinations, neuropsychological assessments, and electroencephalographic testing, as well as histories of learn-ing disabilities and attention-deficit/hyperactivity disorder. Minor or "soft" neurological abnormalities insufficient for a diagnosis of organic brain syndrome are not uncommon (Stein et al., 1995). In more recent years, great interest has been shown in apparent disturbances of seroton-ergic and adrenergic function in violence-prone individuals (Markowitz & Coccara, 1995; Brown, Goodwin, Ballenger, Goyer, & Major, 1989; Virkkunen et al., 1989).

Pharmacological, psychodynamic, behavioral, and social therapies have all been attempted with violent patients, but the populations have rarely been rigorously defined. It is usually not clear whether specifically impulsive violence is being treated. Usually treatment programs address other aspects of the problems that these patients commonly present. Although medication alone is rarely successful, drugs may have an important role to play in the management of some violent patients (see Conacher, Chapter 20, this volume).

KLEPTOMANIA

"Kleptomania" refers to the practice of an individual who yields repeat-edly to an impulse to steal when he or she has sufficient money and has no need for what is stolen. There are five currently accepted criteria outlined in DSM-IV, which can be restated as follows: The person is unsuccessful in resisting impulses to steal goods that are actually unnec-essary either for the person's own use or for their cash value (Criterion A); the person has no obvious motives (such as the expression of anger, existence of delusions, etc.) that might explain the behavior (Criterion D); various disorders or episodes can be excluded (e.g., conduct disorder, manic episode) (Criterion E); the person experiences gratification, relief, or pleasure when carrying out the theft (Criterion C); and tension in-creases immediately prior to the act of stealing (Criterion B).

It is questionable whether kleptomania is a valid disorder, as there is virtually no empirical research on the topic. The literature has in fact usually concerned shoplifters in general, most of whom would not fulfill the required DSM-IV criteria. Studies of shoplifters in general suggest that very few, usually fewer than 5%, suffer from kleptomania (APA, 1994). However, it may be more common than is generally believed, as it has been noted that sufferers tend to be exceptionally secretive about their problem (Goldman, 1991). Most reported cases of kleptomania tend to be female (McElroy, Pope, Hudson, Keck, & White, 1991).

Kleptomaniacs, although they are well aware they are committing crimes, do not steal for personal gain. They describe the feeling of increasing tension or pressure to steal, followed by immediate pleasure or relief, although often by considerable subsequent guilt and shame as well. Their previously mentioned secretiveness can sometimes lead to the development of self-control strategies, such as avoiding shopping malls or going only when accompanied. Some stop shopping altogether and become quite socially isolated. McElroy's group found kleptomania to be strongly associated with mood disorders (especially depression), as well as anxiety disorders, eating disorders, substance abuse, and other impulse-control disorders (McElroy, Pope, et al., 1991). Similarly, in a recent study of self-identified compulsive shoplifters, all of whom fulfilled DSM-IV criteria for kleptomania (Waldman, Hucker, & Foreman, 1996), it was found that 75% suffered from major depression, 25% from generalized anxiety disorder, 50% from bulimia nervosa, 75% from obsessive–compulsive disorder, and 75% from posttraumatic stress disorder. Findings of this kind have led some authorities to suggest that kleptomania, and possibly other impulse-control disorders as well, form part of a larger group of mood disorders—the "affective spectrum disorders," linked by a common pathophysiological abnormality involving low brain serotonin levels (McElroy, Hudson, Pope, Keck, & Aizley, 1992).

A number of individual case reports have been published relating compulsive stealing to various brain disorders and brain defects (see Goldman, 1991). Early psychoanalytic writers viewed compulsive stealing as a means of compensating for lack of affection in early life or as a defense against "castration anxiety." However, these elaborate speculations are very difficult to evaluate and explore empirically. In their study of otherwise noncriminal shoplifters, Cupchick and Atcheson (1983) suggested that some of these individuals steal to compensate symbolically for real or anticipated loss. In keeping with the common observation of depression in shoplifters, especially kleptomaniacs, some have argued that stealing may have an antidepressant effect by temporarily relieving feelings of tension (Fishbain, 1987; Goldman, 1991).

The course of untreated kleptomania is not known. The fact that at the time of the evaluation, many afflicted individuals have already been stealing compulsively for many years—often since adolescence—suggests a chronic course (McElroy, Pope, et al., 1991). Because so little research has been done on clearly defined kleptomaniacs as opposed to shoplifters, little can be said about the effects of treatment, other than that various approaches have been tried. Behavioral methods have been reported as successful with kleptomaniacs (Glover, 1985; Guidry, 1975; Wetzel, 1966; Marzagao, 1972). The soundest research thus far has been carried out by McElroy and her colleagues. From these studies have come promising results from the use of antidepressant medication, further supporting the notion that these patients are suffering from some variant of a mood disorder (Hudson & Pope, 1990; McElroy, Pope, et al., 1991; McElroy, Keck, Pope, Smith, & Strakowski, 1994). Serotonergic drugs in particular, such as fluoxetine and trazadone, are reported as producing at least partial (and sometimes full) remission.

IMPULSE-CONTROL DISORDER
NOT OTHERWISE SPECIFIED

In the DSM-IV (APA, 1994) classification scheme, "impulse-control disorder not otherwise specified" constitutes a residual category for those impulse-control disorders that do not fulfill either the criteria laid down for the specific disorders outlined earlier in this chapter, or those for other mental disorders with impulsive characteristics that are covered in other sections of DSM-IV. Substance abuse and paraphilias, for example, are not placed in this residual category because they are classified elsewhere in the manual.

Some authors have included compulsive masturbation, protracted promiscuity, pornography dependence, telephone sex, and other behaviors in their group of so called "nonparaphilic sexual disorders" or "paraphilia-related disorders" (Kafka, 1995; Travin, 1995). Other authors have referred to these as "sexual addictions" (Carnes, 1983, 1989) or "sexual compulsions" (Coleman, 1991, 1992; Anthony & Hollander, 1993). Still others have suggested a possible relation to mood disorders (Kafka, 1991; Kafka & Prentky, 1992). There have been encouraging case reports indicating that some of these behavioral patterns, as well as paraphilias, may respond to antidepressant medications (Kafka, 1995). Be this as it may, such disorders should be given a DSM-IV diagnosis of sexual disorder not otherwise specified (302.9) rather than the corresponding residual impulse-control disorder diagnosis (312.30).

Repetitive Self-Mutilation

Self-mutilation occurs in a wide variety of psychiatric disorders, including psychotic illness and mental retardation. It is particularly associated with borderline personality disorder, the DSM-IV criteria for which include the behavior. Some authors (Favazza, 1992, 1995) have described individuals who episodically cut, carve, or burn their skin, interfere with the healing of wounds, or the like. Such people describe tension relief and other positive affects as a result of the self-mutilation (Favazza, 1987).

The onset of the behavior is typically in early adolescence, and the self-harm often becomes the individual's habitual way of dealing with personal distress. Interspersed with the episodes of self-harm are periods of calm, as well as eating disorders, alcoholism or other substance abuse, or kleptomania. This pattern has been described as "repetitive self-mutilation syndrome" (Favazza, 1992). Patients are preoccupied with, and repeatedly fail to resist, harming themselves. They experience increasing feelings of tension immediately before hurting themselves, followed by feelings of relief or pleasure afterward. Such behavior is not intended to result in death and is not a response to psychotic experiences (Favazza, 1995). The syndrome has features in common with trichotillomania, as well as with severe forms of nail biting and skin picking.

The focus of recent research in this condition, as in research on other specific impulse-control disorders, has been on possible abnormalities in serotonin metabolism (Coccaro et al., 1989; Coccaro, Astill, Herbert, & Schut, 1990). Although psychotherapeutic approaches are central to the management of repetitive self-multilation (Walsh & Rosen, 1988), there have been encouraging antecdotal reports that fluoxetine (Prozac) may be helpful to these patients even in the absence of major depression (Markovitz, Calabrese, Schulz & Meltzer, 1991).

Compulsive Shopping

The apparently common phenonemon of "compulsive shopping" (Arthur, 1992), also referred to as "compulsive spending" or "oniomania" (Kraepelin, 1915; Bleuler, 1924), shows close affinities to kleptomania (McElroy, Keck, et al., 1994). Women are more likely than men to be compulsive shoppers (Faber, 1992; O'Guinn & Faber, 1989). As in kleptomania, there is a substantial comorbidity with mood and anxiety disorders (Christensen et al., 1994; McElroy et al., 1994; Waldman et al., 1996). Recent research on this phenomenom has found that mood regulation is a major determinant in impulse buying (Faber, 1992; O'Guinn & Faber, 1989): Shopping or buying is experienced as exciting and improves mood. This is followed, however, by regret and remorse, as are kleptomanic lapses. Though further systematic studies are needed, there is evidence to suggest that, as in kleptomania, treatment with antidepressants may be helpful in relieving the compulsion to shop excessively (McElroy, Satlin, Pope, Keck, & Hudson, 1991).

CONCLUSION

The specific impulse-control disorders currently defined and described in DSM-IV are a group of conditions that allegedly have some features in common. However, the differences between them are often as striking as the similarities. In fact, some authorities have disputed their existence as independent entities. With the exception of pathological gambling, they are believed to be quite rare. However, as interest in these conditions has increased, new reports of small groups of clearly defined patients have been published, suggesting that they may be commoner than has been thought. Furthermore, there is substantial comorbidity of these disorders with mood disorders, anxiety disorders, eating disorders, substance abuse, and personality disorders. As other aspects of these disorders may dominate the clinical picture, the impulsivity as a separate condition may be overlooked.

There appears to be as much information about some residual categories of impulse-control disorder (e.g., compulsive shopping and repetitive self-mutilation) as there is on those that have been granted status as specific disorders. Thus, as further data accumulate, there may be justification for expanding the core group of impulse-control disorders to include these by name in future editions of the DSM. The current burgeoning of research on serotonergic and adrenergic systems and their relevance to impulse control seems likely to lead to better understanding of the underlying biological substrates of these complex behaviors, as well as to the possibility of improved treatments with medication.

REFERENCES

American Psychiatric Association (APA). (1980). *Diagnostic and statistical manual of mental disorders* (3rd ed.). Washington, DC: Author.

American Psychiatric Association (APA). (1994). *Diagnostic and statistical manual of mental disorders* (4th ed.). Washington, DC: Author.

Anthony, D. T., & Hollander, E. (1993). Sexual compulsions. In E. Hollander (Ed.), *Obsessive–compulsive related disorders*. Washington, DC: American Psychiatric Press.

Arthur, C. (1992). Fifteen million Americans are shopping addicts. *American Demographics, 14,* 14–15.

Bach-Y-Rita, A., Lion, J. R., & Climent, C. E., & Ervin, F. R. (1971). Episodic dyscontrol: A study of 130 violent patients. *American Journal of Psychiatry, 127,* 1473–1478.

Barker, A. F. (1994). *Arson: A review of the literature.* London: Oxford University Press.

Blaszczynski, A., McConaghy, N., & Frankova, A. (1989). Crime, anti-social personality and pathological gambling. *Journal of Gambling Behavior, 5,* 137–152.

Bleuler, M. (1924). *Textbook of psychiatry.* (A. A. Brill, Trans.). New York: Macmillan.

Bradford, J., Geller, J., Lesieur, H., Rosenthal, R., & Wise, M. (1994). In T. A. Widiger, A. J. Frances, H. A. Pincus, M. B. First, R. Ross, & W. Davis (Eds.), *DSM-IV sourcebook.* Washington, DC: American Psychiatric Press.

Brown, G. L., Goodwin, F. K., Ballenger, J. C., Goyer, P. F., & Major, L. F. (1989). Aggression in humans: Correlates with CSF amine metabolites. *Psychiatry Research, 1,* 131–139.

Bumpass, E. R., Brix, R. J., & Preston, D. A. (1985). A community based program for juvenile firesetters. *Hospital and Community Psychiatry, 36,* 529–533.

Carnes, P. (1983). *Out of the shadows: Understanding sexual addictions.* Minneapolis: CompCare.

Carnes, P. (1989). *Contrary to love: Helping the sex addict.* Minneapolis: CompCare.

Christenson, G. A., Faber, R. J., de Zwaan, M., Raymond, N. C., Specker, S. M., Ekern, M., Mackenzie, T., Crosby, R., Crowe, S., Eckert, E., Mussell, M., & Mitchell, J. (1994). Compulsive buying: Descriptive characteristics and psychiatric comorbidity. *Journal of Clinical Psychiatry, 55,* 5–11.

Christenson, G. A., Popkin, M. K., Mackenzie, T. B., & Realmuto, G. M. (1991). Lithium treatment of chronic hairpulling. *Journal of Clinical Psychiatry, 52,* 116–120.

Christenson, G. A., Pyle, R. L., & Mitchell, J. E. (1991). Estimated lifetime prevalence of trichotillomania in college students. *Journal of Clinical Psychiatry, 52,* 415–417.

Ciarrocchi, J., & Richardson, R. (1989). Profiles of compulsive gamblers in treatment: Update and comparison. *Journal of Gambling Behavior, 5,* 53–65.

Coccaro, E. F., Astill, J. L., Herbert, J. L., & Schut, A. G. (1990). Fluoxetine treatment of impulsive aggression in DSM-III-R personality disorder patients [Letter]. *Journal of Clinical Psychopharmacology, 10,* 373–375.

Coccaro, E. F., Siever, L. J., Klar, H. M., Freidman, R. A., Moskowitz, A., & David, K. L. (1989) Serotonergic studies in patients with affective and personality disorders: Correlates with suicides and impulsive aggressive behavior. *Archives of General Psychiatry, 46,* 587–599.

Coleman, E. (1991). Compulsive sexual behavior. *Journal of Psychology and Human Sexuality, 4,* 37–52.

Coleman, E. (1992). Is your patient suffering from compulsive sexual behavior? *Psychiatric Annals, 22,* 320–325.

Cox-Jones, C., Lubetsky, M. J., Fultz, S. A., & Kolka, O. J. (1990). Inpatient psychiatric treatment of a young recidivist firesetter. *Journal of the American Academy of Child and Adolescent Psychiatry, 29,* 936–941.

Cupchick, W., & Atcheson, J. D. (1983). Shoplifting: An occasional crime of the moral majority. *Bulletin of the American Academy of Psychiatry and the Law, 11,* 343–354.

Custer, R. L., & Milt, H. (1985). *When luck runs out.* New York: Facts on File.

DeCaria, C. M., & Hollander, E. (1993). Pathological gambling. In E. Hollander (Ed.), *Obsessive–compulsive related disorders* (pp. 151–178). Washington, DC: American Psychiatric Press.

Dickerson, M. G. (1984). *Compulsive gamblers.* London: Longman.

Faber, R. J. (1992). Money changes everything: Compulsive buying from a biopsychosocial perspective. *American Behavioral Scientist, 35,* 809–819.

Favazza, A. (1987). *Bodies under siege.* Balitmore: Johns Hopkins University Press.

Favazza, A. (1992). Repetitive self-mutilation. *Psychiatric Annals, 22*(2), 60–63.

Favazza, A. (1995). Self-mutilation. In E. Hollander & D. Stein (Eds.), *Impulsivity and aggression* (pp. 185–200). New York: Wiley.

Felthous, A. R., Bryant, S. G., Wingerter, C. B., & Barratt, E. (1991). The diagnosis of intermittent explosive disorder in violent men. *Bulletin of the American Academy of Psychiatry and the Law, 19,* 71–79.

Fenichel, O. (1945). *The psychoanalytic theory of neurosis.* New York: Norton.

Fishbain, D. A. (1987). Kleptomania as risk taking behavior in response to depression. *American Journal of Psychotherapy, 41,* 598–603.

Freud, S. (1964). The acquisition and control of fire. In J. Strachey (Ed. and Trans.), *The standard edition of the complete psychological works of Sigmund Freud* (Vol. 22, pp. 183–193). London: Hogarth Press. (Original work published 1932)

Geller, J. (1994). The impulse control disorders. In T. A. Widiger, A. J. Frances, H. A. Pincus, M. B. First, R. Ross, & W. Davis (Eds.), *DSM-IV sourcebook* (Vol. 2). Washington, DC: American Psychiatric Press.

Glover, J. H. (1985). A case of kleptomania treated by covert sensitization. *British Journal of Clinical Psychology, 24,* 203–204.

Goldman, M. J. (1991). Kleptomania—making sense of the nonsensical. *American Journal of Psychiatry, 148,* 986–996.

Guidry, L. S. (1975). Use of a covert punishing contingency in compulsive stealing. *Journal of Behavior Therapy and Experimental Psychiatry, 6,* 169.

Henslin, J. M. (1967). Craps and magic. *American Journal of Sociology, 73,* 316–330.

Hudson, J. I., & Pope, H. G. (1990). Affective spectrum disorder: Does antidepressant response identify a family of disorders with a common pathophysiology? *American Journal of Psychiatry, 147,* 552–564.

Jacobs, D. F. (1988). Evidence for a common dissociative-like reaction among addicts. *Journal of Gambling Behavior, 4,* 27–37.

Jillson, O. T. (1983). Alopecia, II: Trichotillomania (trichotillohabitus). *Cutis, 31,* 383–389.

Kafka, M. P. (1991). Successful anti-depressant treatment of non-paraphilic sexual addictions and paraphilias in men. *Journal of Clinical Psychiatry, 52,* 60–65.

Kafka, M. P. (1995). Sexual impulsivity. In E. Hollander & D. Stein (Eds.), *Impulsivity and aggression* (pp. 221–228). New York: Wiley.

Kakfa, M., & Prentky, R. (1992). Fluoxetine treatment of non-paraphilic sexual addictions and paraphilias in men. *Journal of Clinical Psychiatry, 53,* 351–358.

Koles, M. R., & Jenson, W. R. (1985). Comprehensive treatment of chronic firesetting in a severely disordered boy. *Journal of Behavior Therapy and Experimental Psychiatry, 16,* 81–85.

Kolko, D. J. (1988). Community intervention for juvenile firesetters: A survey of two national programs. *Hospital and Community Psychiatry, 39,* 973–979.

Koson, D. F., & Dvoskin, J. (1982). Arson: A diagnostic study. *Bulletin of the American Academy of Psychiatry and the Law, 10,* 39–49.

Kraepelin, E. (1915). *Psychiatrie* (8th ed.). Leipzig: Barth.

Krishnan, K., Davidson, J., & Guajardo, C. (1985). Trichotillomania—a review. *Comprehensive Psychiatry, 26,* 123–128.

Lesieur, H. R., & Blume, S. B. (1990). Characteristics of pathological gamblers identified among patients on a psychiatric admissions service. *Hospital and Community Psychiatry, 41,* 1009–1012.

Lesieur, H. R., Blume, S. B., & Zoppa, R. M. (1986). Alcohol, drug abuse and gambling. *Alcoholism, 10,* 33–38.

Lewis, N., & Yarnell, H. (1951). *Pathological firesetting (pyromania).* New York: Coolidge Foundation.

Linden, R. D., Pope, H. D., & Jones, J. M. (1986). Pathological gambling and major affective disorder: Preliminary findings. *Journal of Clinical Psychiatry, 47,* 201–203.

Mark, V., & Ervin, F. (1970). *Violence and the brain.* New York: Harper & Row.

Markovitz, P. J., Calabrese, J. R., Schulz, S. C., & Meltzer, H. Y. (1991). Fluoxetine in the treatment of borderline and schizotypal disorders. *American Journal of Psychiatry, 148,* 1064–1067.

Markowitz, P. I., & Coccaro, E. (1995). Biological studies of impulsivity, aggression and suicidal behavior. In E. Hollander & D. J. Stein (Eds.), *Impulsivity and aggression* (pp. 71–90). New York: Wiley.

Marzagao, L. R. (1972). Systematic desensitization treatment of kleptomania. *Journal of Behavior Therapy and Experimental Psychiatry, 3,* 327–328.

Mavromatis, M., & Lion, J. (1977). A primer on pyromania. *Diseases of the Nervous System, 38,* 954–955.

McElroy, S. E., Hudson, S. I., Pope, H. G., Keck, P. E., & Aizley, H. G. (1992). The DSM-III-R impulse-control disorders not elsewhere classified: Clinical characteristics and relationships to other psychiatric disorders. *American Journal of Psychiatry, 149,* 318–327.

McElroy, S. L., Keck, P. E., Pope, H. G., Smith, J. N., & Strakowski, S. M. (1994). Compulsive buying: A report of 20 cases. *Journal of Clinical Psychiatry, 55,* 242–248.

McElroy, S. E., Pope, H. G., Hudson, J. I., Keck, P. E., & White, K. L. (1991). Kleptomania: A report of 20 cases. *American Journal of Psychiatry, 148,* 652–657.

McElroy, S. L., Pope, H. G., Keck, P. E., & Hudson, J. I. (1995). Disorders of impulse control. In E. Hollander & D. J. Stein (Eds.), *Impulsivity and aggression* (pp. 109–136). New York: Wiley.

McElroy, S. L., Satlin, A., Pope, H. G., Keck, P. E., & Hudson, J. I. (1991). Treatment of compulsive shopping with anti-depressants: A report of three case studies. *Annals of Clinical Psychiatry, 3,* 199–204.

McGrath, P., & Marshall, P. G. (1979). A comprehensive treatment program for a firesetting child. *Journal of Behavior Therapy and Experimental Psychiatry, 10,* 60–72.

Menninger, K., & Mayman, M. (1956). Episodic dyscontrol: A third order of stress adaptation. *Bulletin of the Menninger Clinic, 20,* 153–165.

Monopolis, S., & Lion, J. (1983). Problems in the diagnosis of intermittent explosive disorder. *American Journal of Psychiatry, 140,* 1200–1202.

Monroe, R. R. (1970). *Episodic behavioral disorders.* Cambridge, MA: Harvard University Press.

Moran, E. (1970). Varieties of pathological gambling. *British Journal of Psychiatry, 166,* 593–597.

Oguchi, T., & Miura, S. (1977). Trichotillomania: Its psychopathological aspects. *Comprehensive Psychiatry, 18,* 177–182.

O'Guinn, M., & Faber, R. J. (1989). Compulsive buying: A phenomenologocial exploration. *Journal of Consumer Research, 16,* 147–157.

Pattison, E. M., & Kahan, J. (1983). The deliberate self harm syndrome. *American Journal of Psychiatry, 140,* 867–872.

Peck, C. P. (1986). Risk taking behavior and compulsive gambling. *American Psychologist, 41,* 461–465.

Prins, H. (1994). *Fire-raising: Its motivation and management.* London: Routledge.

Quinsey, V. L., Chaplin, T. C., & Upfold, D. (1989). Arsonists and sexual arousal to fire setting: Correlation unsupported. *Journal of Behavior Therapy and Experimental Psychiatry, 20,* 203–209.

Rosenthal, R. J. (1992). Pathological gambling. *Psychiatric Annals, 22*(2), 70–72.

Roy, A., Virkkunen, M., Guthrie, S., & Linnoila, M. (1986). Indices of serotonin and glucose metabolism in violent offenders, arsonists and alcoholics. *Annals of the New York Academy of Sciences, 489,* 202–220.

Smart, R. G., & Ferris, J. (1996). Alcohol, drugs and gambling in the Ontario adult population, 1994. *Canadian Journal of Psychiatry, 41,* 36–45.

Stein, D. J., Towey, J., & Hollander, E. (1995). The neuropsychiatry of impulsive aggression. In E. Hollander & D. J. Stein (Eds.), *Impulsivity and aggression* (pp. 91–108). New York: Wiley.

Stekel, W. (1924). *Peculiarities of behavior: Wandering mania, dipsomania, cleptomania, pyromania and allied impulsive acts* (Vol. 2). New York: Livewright.

Swedo, S. E. (1993). Trichotillomania. In E. Hollander (Ed.), *Obsessive–compulsive related disorders* (pp. 93–112). Washington, DC: American Psychiatric Press.

Taber, J., McCormick, R. A., Russo, A. M., Adkins, B. J., & Ramirez, L. F. (1987). Follow-up of pathological gamblers after treatment. *American Journal of Psychiatry, 144,* 757–761.

Travin, S. (1995). Compulsive sexual behaviors. *Psychiatric Clinics of North America, 18,* 155–169.

Virkkunen, M. (1976). Self-mutilation in anti-social personality (disorder). *Acta Psychiatrica Scandinavica, 54,* 347–352.

Virkkunen, M., DeJong, J., Bartko, J., & Linnoila, M. (1989). Psychobiological concomitants of history of suicide attempts among violent offenders and impulsive firesetters. *Archives of General Psychiatry, 46,* 604–606.

Volberg, R. A., & Steadman, H. J. (1988). Refining prevalence estimates of pathological gambling. *American Journal of Psychiatry, 145,* 604–606.

Volberg, R. A., & Steadman, H. J. (1989). Prevalence estimates of pathological gambling in New Jersey and Maryland. *American Journal of Psychiatry, 146,* 1618–1619.

Wagenaar, W. A. (1988). *Paradoxes of gambling behavior.* Hillsdale, NJ: Erlbaum.

Waldman, J., Hucker, S., & Foreman, K. (1996). *Co-morbidity and demographics in self-identified oniomaniacs and kleptomaniacs.* Manuscript submitted for publication.

Walsh, B. W., & Rosen, P. (1988). *Self-mutilation.* New York: Guilford Press.

Wetzel, R. (1966). Use of behavior techniques in a case of compulsive stealing. *Journal of Consulting Psychology, 30,* 367–374.

Winchel, R. (1992). Trichotillomania: Presentation and treatment. *Psychiatric Annals, 22*(2), 84–89.

Wolff, R. (1984). Satiation in the treatment of inappropriate firesetting. *Journal of Behavior Therapy and Experimental Psychiatry, 15,* 337–340.

12

Impulsivity and Psychopathy

STEPHEN D. HART
REBECCA J. DEMPSTER

"Psychopathy" is a specific form of personality disorder with a distinctive pattern of interpersonal, affective, and behavioral symptoms. Interpersonally, psychopaths are grandiose, arrogant, callous, superficial, and manipulative; affectively, they are short-tempered, unable to form strong emotional bonds with others, and lacking in guilt or anxiety; and behaviorally, they are irresponsible, impulsive, and prone to delinquency and criminality. As is the case with all personality disorders, the symptoms of psychopathy are believed to have an early onset (first arising in childhood) and to persist well into adulthood; there is no known effective treatment for the disorder. Psychopathy is also referred to as "antisocial personality disorder," "sociopathy," or "dissocial personality disorder."

It would be impossible to discuss the clinical aspects of impulsivity without referring to psychopathy, and vice versa: Psychopathy is a broad or higher-order clinical construct, comprising an array of diverse symptoms, and impulsivity is a cardinal feature of that construct. Our goal in this chapter is to explore further the important connections between psychopathy and impulsivity. We begin by reviewing clinical conceptualizations of psychopathy, focusing on the diagnostic importance of impulsivity. Second, we discuss impulsivity as it pertains to some major etiological theories of psychopathy. Third, we examine the link between psychopathy and impulsive criminal behavior, particularly impulsive violence. Finally, we identify some important questions about the association between psychopathy and impulsivity that remain unanswered, and we suggest avenues for future research.

IMPULSIVITY IN CLINICAL DESCRIPTIONS
OF PSYCHOPATHY

Early Views

A simple historical review of the concept of psychopathy is made difficult by inconsistencies in the use of the term (Lewis, 1974; Millon, 1981; Pichot, 1978). Literally "disease of the mind," psychopathy originally referred to mental disorder in general: "During the late nineteenth century, the adjective 'psychopathic' meant 'psychopathological' and applied to *any and all forms* of mental disorder" (Berrios, 1996, p. 429; emphasis in original). Beginning at about this time, and continuing into the 20th century, descriptive psychopathologists increasingly recognized types of mental disorder. One trend was the identification of varieties of "total insanity"—illnesses that appeared to result in a general disintegration or deterioration of mental functions. Another, supported by "faculty psychology" (a theory of the human mind as made up of discrete functional units), was the identification of relatively specific impairments of intellectual, emotional, or volitional functions (Berrios, 1996). Influential alienists, including Pinel and Prichard, described cases characterized by a disturbance of emotion or volition. The terms used to refer to such conditions included *"manie sans délire," "monomanie,"* "moral insanity," and *"folie lucide"* (Millon, 1981; Pichot, 1978). Although unrelated to modern conceptions of psychopathy (Whitlock, 1967, 1982), these case descriptions reinforced the notion that mental disorder can exist even when reasoning is intact.

One condition identified at about this time is of particular relevance to the present discussion. "Impulsion" (or "impulsive insanity") was conceptualized as a volitional disturbance characterized by unreflective or involuntary aggression and the absence of other symptoms; according to Berrios (1996), it "provided the kernel around which the notion of psychopathic personality was eventually to become organised" (p. 428). It is interesting to note that part of the motivation for developing the concept of emotional or volitional disturbances in general, and more specifically the notion of impulsion, was forensic. For their testimony to be relevant, the expertise of alienists in that era had to extend beyond the realm of "total insanity" (Berrios, 1996).

In the first half of the 20th century, the concept of psychopathy was narrowed to refer to personality disorder in general. "Personality disorder" itself was defined as a chronic disturbance of emotion or volition, or a disturbance of their integration with intellectual functions, that was distinct from both psychotic and neurotic illness and that resulted in socially disruptive behavior. As Blackburn (1993) notes, this represented an interesting shift from viewing psychopaths as "psychologically damaged" to "psychologically damaging" (p. 80). Although there was little agreement among alienists in the specific variants of personality disorder they identified, or in the names given to these disorders, there was a general consensus that one important cluster was characterized by impulsive, aggressive, and antisocial behavior (Berrios, 1996). For example, Schneider described "labile," "explosive," and "wicked" psychopaths; Kahn described a cluster of "impulsive," "weak," and "sexual" psychopaths; and Henderson described a cluster of psychopaths with "predominantly aggressive" features (Berrios, 1996, pp. 431–433).

Modern Views

Over the past 50 years or so, the concept of psychopathy has been narrowed further still and now refers to a specific form of personality disorder, of which impulsivity is a key symptom. This modern view is represented in rich clinical descriptions by such authors as Arieti (1967), Cleckley (1941), Karpman (1961), and McCord and McCord (1964). It is clear now, despite occasional claims to the contrary, that these clinical descriptions are in good agreement with the views of psychiatrists, psychologists, criminal justice personnel, experimental psychopathologists, and even the lay public (Albert, Brigante, & Chase, 1959; Davies & Feldman, 1981; Fotheringham, 1957; Gray & Hutchinson, 1964; Livesley, 1986; Meloy, 1988; Rogers, Dion, & Lynett, 1992; Rogers, Duncan, Lynett, & Sewell, 1994; Stevens, 1994; Tennent, Tennent, Prins, & Bedford, 1990).

During the same period of time, the term "impulsivity" has acquired three distinct meanings in the field of descriptive psychopathology. First, impulsivity is viewed as a symptom, and is defined as a tendency to commit harmful acts without forethought or planning that results in impaired social functioning (e.g., Frosch & Wortis, 1954). Second, impulsivity is at times used to refer to a specific kind of aggression. "Impulsive aggression" is defined as a tendency, automatic in nature, to perceive environmental stimuli as threatening and to respond immediately in an aggressive manner (e.g., Barratt, 1994). Third, impulsivity is viewed as a more general personality trait that has multiple cognitive and behavioral manifestations in day-to-day life. This definition is similar to what has been called "impulsive character" (Frosch & Wortis, 1954), "impulsive style" (Shapiro, 1965), "multi-impulsive personality disorder" (Lacey & Evans, 1986), and "lifestyle impulsivity" (e.g., Prentky, Knight, Lee, & Cerce, 1994).

All three types of impulsivity have been linked to psychopathy. To illustrate, we discuss the diagnostic criteria for psychopathy contained in the fourth edition of the *Diagnostic and Statistical Manual of Mental Disorders* (DSM-IV; American Psychiatric Association [APA], 1994) and the 10th revision of the *International Classification of Diseases* (ICD-10; World Health Organization [WHO], 1992). We also discuss the items contained in two standardized psychological tests, the original Psychopathy Checklist and the Psychopathy Checklist—Revised (PCL and PCL-R; Hare, 1980, 1991), as well as the Screening Version of the PCL-R (PCL:SV; Hart, Cox, & Hare, 1995).

DSM-IV Criteria

In the DSM-IV, psychopathy is known as "antisocial personality disorder"; it is defined in terms of four specific criteria, two of which have multiple subcriteria (see Table 12.1). Impulsivity is included explicitly as one of the criteria related to adult antisocial behavior, A3. As the accompanying text notes, "Decisions are made on the spur of the moment, without forethought, and without consideration for the consequences to self or others; this may lead to sudden changes of jobs, residences, or relationships" (APA, 1994, p. 646). This appears to reflect the classic definition of impulsivity as a psychiatric symptom. Criterion A4 is directly related to impulsive aggression. Finally, two other criteria, A5 and A6, are related to more general lifestyle impulsivity.

ICD-10 Criteria

The ICD-10 labels the disorder "dissocial personality disorder" and defines it in terms of six diagnostic criteria, listed in Table 12.2. For research purposes, a diagnosis is made if three or more of the six criteria are present. There is no single criterion that reflects impulsivity as a symp-

---

TABLE 12.1. DSM-IV Criteria for Antisocial Personality Disorder

A. There is a pervasive pattern of disregard for and violation of the rights of others occurring since age 15 years, as indicated by three (or more) of the following:

  (1) failure to conform to social norms with respect to lawful behaviors as indicated by repeatedly performing acts that are grounds for arrest

  (2) deceitfulness, as indicated by repeated lying, use of aliases, or conning others for personal profit or pleasure

  (3) impulsivity or failure to plan ahead

  (4) irritability and aggressiveness, as indicated by repeated physical fights or assaults

  (5) reckless disregard for safety of self or others

  (6) consistent irresponsibility, as indicated by repeated failure to sustain consistent work behavior or honor financial obligations

  (7) lack of remorse, as indicated by being indifferent to or rationalizing having hurt, mistreated, or stolen from another

B. The individual is at least age 18 years.

C. There is evidence of Conduct Disorder (see [DSM-IV], p. 90) with onset before age 15 years.

D. The occurrence of antisocial behavior is not exclusively during the course of Schizophrenia or a Manic Episode.

Note. Reprinted with permission from the *Diagnostic and Statistical Manual of Mental Disorders,* fourth edition (pp. 649–650). Copyright 1994 by the American Psychiatric Association.

TABLE 12.2. ICD-10 Criteria for Dissocial Personality Disorder

Personality disorder, usually coming to attention because of a gross disparity between behaviour and the prevailing social norms, and characterized by:

(a) callous unconcern for the feelings of others;

(b) gross and persistent attitude of irresponsibility and disregard for social norms, rules, and obligations;

(c) incapacity to maintain intimate relationships, though having no difficulty in establishing them;

(d) very low tolerance for frustration and a low threshold for discharge of aggression, including violence;

(e) incapacity to experience guilt or to profit from experience, particularly punishment;

(f) marked proneness to blame others, or to offer plausible rationalizations for the behaviour that has brought the patient into conflict with society.

There may also be persistent irritability as an associated feature. Conduct disorder during childhood and adolescence, though not invariably present, may further support the diagnosis.

Includes: amoral, antisocial, asocial, psychopathic, and sociopathic personality (disorder)

Excludes: conduct disorders (F91.—)
            emotionally unstable personality disorder (F60.3)

Note. From *International Classification of Diseases, 10th edition* (WHO, 1992, p. 204).

tom. However, Criteria (b), (c), and (e) reflect lifestyle impulsivity, and Criterion (d) reflects impulsive aggression.

PCL and PCL-R Items

The original PCL (Hare, 1980) was a 22-item symptom construct rating scale, designed for use in adult male forensic populations. It was later revised and shortened to 20 items (PCL-R; Hare, 1991). As the two scales are highly correlated (Hare et al., 1990), we focus here on the current version. Table 12.3 lists the PCL-R items, which are defined in detail in the test manual. Each item is scored on a 3-point scale (0 = "item doesn't apply," 1 = "item applies somewhat," 2 = "item definitely applies"). Total scores can range from 0 to 40; scores of 30 or higher are considered diagnostic of psychopathy. The PCL-R has a stable internal structure comprising two oblique factors, correlated about .50; Factor 1 reflects "callous and remorseless use of others," whereas Factor 2 reflects a "chronically unstable and antisocial lifestyle" (Hare, 1991, p. 38; see also Hare et al., 1990; Harpur, Hakstian, & Hare, 1988; Harpur, Hare, & Hakstian, 1989; Templeman & Wong, 1994). Several recent reviews (e.g., Fulero, 1995; Rogers, 1995; Stone, 1995) have concluded that the PCL-R has excellent psychometric properties (see also Cooke & Michie, 1997), good criterion-related validity with respect to criminal behavior (see also Hart & Hare, 1996a, 1996b, 1997; Salekin, Rogers, & Sewell, 1996), and impressive construct-related validity with respect to experimental research (see also Hart & Hare, 1996b).

It is clear from Table 12.3 that impulsivity is well represented in the PCL-R. Item 14 reflects impulsivity as a symptom, and in fact is labeled "Impulsivity." Item 10 reflects impulsive aggression. A number of other items, primarily those that load on Factor 2 of the PCL-R, reflect lifestyle impulsivity; indeed, Lifestyle Impulsivity would be a reasonable alternative label for this factor.

PCL:SV Items

The PCL:SV (Hart et al., 1995; see also Hart, Hare, & Forth, 1994) is a 12-item scale based directly on the PCL-R (see Table 12.4). The PCL:SV was designed for two major purposes: (1) to assess and diagnose psychopathy in nonforensic populations, and (2) to screen for psychopathy in forensic populations. Its content is more general than that of the PCL-R; for example, the PCL:SV has no items that are scored specifically on the basis of formal criminal records. Consequently, scoring the PCL:SV requires less time and less detailed assessment information than scoring the PCL-R does. PCL:SV items are scored on a 3-point scale, as are PCL-R

TABLE 12.3. PCL-R Items and Factor Loadings

Item	Description	Factor loading[a]
1.	Glibness/superficial charm	1
2.	Grandiose sense of self-worth	1
3.	Need for stimulation/proneness to boredom	2
4.	Pathological lying	1
5.	Conning/manipulative	1
6.	Lack of remorse or guilt	1
7.	Shallow affect	1
8.	Callous/lack of empathy	1
9.	Parasitic lifestyle	2
10.	Poor behavioral controls	2
11.	Promiscuous sexual behavior	—
12.	Early behavioral problems	2
13.	Lack of realistic, long-term goals	2
14.	Impulsivity	2
15.	Irresponsibility	2
16.	Failure to accept responsibility for own actions	1
17.	Many short-term marital relationships	—
18.	Juvenile delinquency	2
19.	Revocation of conditional release	2
20.	Criminal versatility	—

Note. The items are from Hare (1991, p. 2). Copyright 1990, 1991 by Multi-Health Systems, Inc. Reproduced with permission of Multi-Health Systems, Inc., 908 Niagara Falls Blvd., North Tonawanda, NY 14120-2060, (800) 456-3003.
[a]Factor 1, Callous and Remorseless Use of Others; Factor 2, Chronically Unstable and Antisocial Lifestyle. A dash means that an item does not load on either factor.

items. Total scores can range from 0 to 24; scores of 13 or greater indicate possible psychopathy, and scores of 18 or greater indicate definite psychopathy. Total scores on the PCL-R and PCL:SV are highly correlated ($r = .80$). Evidence is accumulating that the PCL:SV has criterion- and construct-related validity similar to that of the PCL-R, even when used in noncriminal settings (e.g., Babiak, 1995; Cornell et al., 1996; Forth, Brown, Hart, & Hare, 1996; Hill, Rogers, & Bickford, 1996).

Despite the brevity of the PCL:SV, impulsivity is reflected directly or indirectly in a number of items. Item 7, "Impulsive," represents a combination of PCL-R items 14 and 3, and reflects impulsivity as a symptom. Item 8 of the PCL:SV is directly analogous to item 10 of the PCL-R and reflects impulsive aggression. Finally, the remaining items from Part 2 of the PCL:SV (i.e., items 9 through 12) also reflect lifestyle impulsivity.

Comment

It seems that impulsivity is, and always has been, a central or cardinal feature of psychopathy. Indeed, depending on how broadly one construes impulsivity, it may be related to about half of all psychopathic symptomatology. It is difficult even to imagine a psychopath who is not impulsive. However, it is important to emphasize here that the concept of impulsivity is not specific to psychopathy; that is, impulsivity may exist in people who are not psychopaths.

Although undoubtedly important, the conceptual association between psychopathy and impulsive behavior—especially behavior that is antisocial and aggressive—has proven distracting at times. Those untrained in psychopathology have frequently assumed, naively and incorrectly, that there is a simple, direct, causal link between psychopathy and criminality. The illogical extreme of this view is that all psychopaths commit crimes, and that anyone who routinely engages in antisocial behavior must be a psychopath. As far back as the early 19th century, critics argued that a mental disorder whose symptomatology includes

TABLE 12.4. PCL:SV Items

Part 1	Part 2
1. Superficial	7. Impulsive
2. Grandiose	8. Poor behavioral controls
3. Deceitful	9. Lacks goals
4. Lacks remorse	10. Irresponsible
5. Lacks empathy	11. Adolescent antisocial behavior
6. Doesn't accept responsibility	12. Adult antisocial behavior

Note. The items are from Hart, Cox, and Hare (1995, p. 23). Copyright 1995 by Multi-Health Systems, Inc. Reproduced with permission of Multi-Health Systems, Inc., 908 Niagara Falls Blvd., North Tonawanda, NY 14120-2060, (800) 456-3003.

antisocial behavior is simply a moral judgment or a tautology—one that can be misused dangerously in forensic contexts (Berrios, 1996; Hart & Hare, 1996b). However, psychopathologists too have been critical of conceptualizations of psychopathy that overfocus on antisocial behavior (Hare, Hart, & Harpur, 1991; Millon, 1981; Rogers & Dion, 1991) and have emphasized the crucial role of interpersonal and affective symptoms (Cleckley, 1941; Hare, 1991, 1993; Karpman, 1961; McCord & McCord, 1964). As Reid (1986) cautions, "all that is asocial, antisocial, hedonistic, narcissistic, frustrating, or refractory to treatment is not antisocial personality" (p. 253).

IMPULSIVITY IN ETIOLOGICAL THEORIES OF PSYCHOPATHY

A "good" theory of psychopathy should account for both (1) the full range of psychopathic symptomatology, as discussed previously; and (2) the major replicable findings from laboratory research. Although space permits only the most superficial of discussions, we now turn to an overview of four etiological theories: Lykken's fearlessness model; the Fowles–Gray model of a weak Behavioral Inhibition System; Newman's model of deficient response modulation; and Hare's hypoemotionality model.

Lykken's Fearlessness Model

Lykken's fearlessness model was first presented in the literature some 40 years ago (Lykken, 1957). In Lykken's view, psychopaths suffer from an innate fearlessness that renders them unable to "learn to avoid antisocial behaviors and to inhibit forbidden impulses, through punishment and the conditioned fear it leaves behind" (Lykken, 1995, p. 135). Although Lykken (1995) does not specify the cause of fearlessness, he seems to assume that it reflects an extreme variant of normal individual differences (presumably one with a substantial heritable component), rather than psychosocial stress or structural brain damage.

The fearlessness model accounts only partially for psychopathic symptomatology. That fearlessness would result in impulsive behavior, or at least in lifestyle impulsivity, seems intuitively obvious, as Lykken (1995) points out. However, his attempts to explain such symptoms as superficiality, egocentricity, and shallow emotions in terms of fearlessness are somewhat feeble; he must resort to disagreeing with clinical descriptions of psychopathy, or to extending fearlessness into something that resembles the more general hypoemotionality model. The fearlessness model itself has attracted relatively little attention from researchers since its introduction, to Lykken's (1995) dismay. As he notes, this is probably because it can be subsumed within the framework of the Fowles–Gray model.

Fowles–Gray Model of a Weak Behavioral Inhibition System

Fowles (1980; Fowles & Missel, 1994) has proposed a similar theory of psychopathy, based upon the work of Gray (e.g., Gray, 1987). According to the Fowles–Gray model, the Behavioral Inhibition System (BIS) is a neurophysiological system that controls the organism's response to signals of impending punishment or frustrative nonreward; another system, the Behavioral Activation System (BAS), controls responses to signals of impending reward. Arousal of the BIS is experienced as negative affect and results in inhibition of motoric activity that might lead to the expected punishment or nonreward. Thus, a weak BIS can result in the failure to inhibit activity that may lead to punishment or frustrative nonreward (i.e., deficits in passive avoidance learning). In this model, psychopaths are hypothesized to have a weak BIS, associated specifically with a deficit in anticipatory anxiety, that "produces impulsivity as a result of the failure of cues for potential punishment and frustration to inhibit reward-seeking behavior" (Fowles & Missel, 1994, p. 278).

There are some problems with the Fowles–Gray model, however. First, like Lykken's fearlessness model, it has difficulty accounting for many of the interpersonal and affective symptoms of psychopathy. Second, within Gray's theoretical framework, psychopaths are not truly impulsive. As discussed by Newman and Wallace (1993a), Gray's model provides several "pathways to disinhibition," including hyperresponsivity to reward because of a strong BAS, and abnormal responsivity to punishment because of a deficient BIS (hyporesponsivity resulting from a weak BIS, and hyperresponsivity resulting from a strong BIS). Gray himself linked impulsivity with a strong BAS (Newman & Wallace, 1993a). Thus, according to his model, it would be more appropriate to describe the behavior of psychopaths as "disinhibited" than as "impulsive." Third, although the Fowles–Gray model has received partial support from studies of electrodermal responsivity, fear conditioning, and passive avoidance learning in psychopaths (Fowles & Missel, 1994; Lykken, 1995), psychopaths may not be generally hyporesponsive to punishment; rather, their hyporesponsivity may be apparent only when they are faced with a competing reward contingency (Newman & Wallace, 1993a).

Newman's Model of Deficient Response Modulation

Newman and his colleagues (e.g., Newman and Wallace, 1993a, 1993b; Patterson & Newman, 1993) have developed a more sophisticated version of the Fowles–Gray model. In their view, "the 'impulsive' behavior of psychopaths appears to reflect difficulty in the automatic switching of attention which, in turn, interferes with their ability to assimilate unattended but potentially relevant information while they are engaged in the organization and implementation of goal-directed behavior" (Newman & Wallace, 1993a, p. 712). That is, disinhibition in psychopaths is not attributable simply to a weak BIS, but rather to an attentional deficit that reduces input to the BIS once the BAS is activated.

As the fearlessness model can be subsumed within the weak-BIS model, so can the latter be subsumed within the model of deficient response modulation (DRM). Thus, the DRM model accounts for psychopathic symptomatology and empirical research findings as well as or better than does the weak-BIS model. In addition, the DRM model can explain the finding that psychopaths exhibit hyporesponsivity to punishment only in specific contexts (Newman & Wallace, 1993a). Finally, it may even be possible to explain psychopathic deficits in the processing of linguistic and emotional stimuli within the DRM framework (Newman & Wallace, 1993a; see especially pp. 711–712). Perhaps its biggest weakness at the present time is that some of the experimental effects predicted by this model are not as strong or robust as one might hope (Lykken, 1995).

Hare's Hypoemotionality Model

Much of Hare's early work investigated anxiety in psychopaths (Hare, 1970). Beginning in the 1970s, however, he turned his attention to more general emotional and cognitive deficits. Most recently, he has postulated that psychopaths may suffer from global hypoemotionality—that is, a failure to experience fully both positive and negative emotions, which presumably is temperamental in nature (Hare, 1993, 1996).

The hypoemotionality model offers an explanation of the full range of psychopathic symptoms. As fearlessness and lack of anxiety are among the consequences of hypoemotionality, this model can explain the disinhibited behavior of psychopaths, as well as symptoms such as lack of remorse, lack of empathy, grandiosity, and so forth. In this respect, the hypoemotionality model is superior to the fearlessness and weak-BIS models. It also accounts for a broad range of research findings, including those related to abnormal linguistic and emotional functioning in psychopaths (see Hare, 1993, 1996; Hart & Hare, 1996a) at least as well as the DRM model does. Two excellent examples of research based on the hypoemotionality model are recent electrocortical and brain imaging studies showing that psychopaths do not differentiate, psychophysiologically or behaviorally, between neutral and emotional words (Intrator et al., in press; Williamson, Harpur, & Hare, 1989). Another example is Patrick's (1994) recent work on the blink–startle reflex in psychopath. Patrick finds that psychopaths are psychophysiologically unresponsive to emotional visual stimuli, whether these are positive or negative in valence.

Comment

The major etiological models reviewed here all posit that underlying psychopathy is a neurobiological deficit that results in reduced emotionality, and especially in low anxiety. According to the models, this deficit is what causes psychopaths to engage in "impulsive"—that is, disinhibited, irresponsible, and antisocial—behavior. Put another way, the impulsivity of psychopaths is epiphenomenal, secondary to a core deficit in emotion or attention.

Despite several decades of intriguing laboratory research, psychopathy remains a disorder in search of a truly satisfying etiological theory. There is no clear or unequivocal support for any of the models discussed above. However, in our view, the hypoemotionality and DRM models appear to be the most viable at the present time: They account more readily than do the others for the full range of psychopathic symptomatology, and they are more consistent with the full range of laboratory findings. Also, because they are more general, in many respects the Lykken and Fowles–Gray models can be subsumed entirely within their frameworks. Needed now is a program of research that simultaneously tests the hypoemotionality and DRM models.

IMPULSIVITY IN THE CRIMINAL BEHAVIOR OF PSYCHOPATHS

Psychopathy and Crime: An Overview

Psychopathy and crime are linked conceptually and empirically. Antisocial behavior is a symptom of psychopathy, and psychopathy—as assessed by the PCL, PCL-R, or PCL:SV—is an important risk factor for involvement in criminal conduct (Hart & Hare, 1996b, 1997). But consider some of the other symptoms of psychopathy: impulsivity, grandiosity, lack of remorse, lack of empathy, irresponsibility. If antisocial behavior is a symptom of psychopathy, then, in light of these other symptoms, in what *types* of antisocial behavior would we expect psychopaths to engage?

On the basis of their impulsivity, irresponsibility, and deceitfulness, it seems reasonable to expect psychopaths to engage in early-onset, persistent, high-density, and varied criminal behavior, generally of a petty nature. The picture here is one of a person who does not systematically look for trouble, but who would not think twice about committing an antisocial act should the opportunity present itself. As Newman and Wallace (1993a) note, "psychopaths are not *driven* to antisocial behavior by strong urges for money, sex, or violence but . . . given some strong inducement to respond, they have little capacity for behavioral inhibition" (p. 712, emphasis in original). Similarly, their tendency toward impulsive aggression leads one to think of psychopaths as people who are quick to see hostile intent in the actions of others and quick to react with a "preemptive strike"—perhaps the type of person who assaults other patrons in a bar while drinking, who strikes out at family members when annoyed, or who pulls out a concealed weapon during a verbal altercation. On the other hand, clinical descriptions sometimes relate the grandiosity, lack of empathy, and lack of remorse in psychopaths to deliberate, cold-blooded, predatory, and serious crime (Hare, 1993; Meloy, 1988). For example, there is speculation that psychopaths are overrepresented among groups of very violent offenders, such as serial rapists, sexual sadists, and certain types of murderers (Hare, 1993, 1996; Meloy, 1988). The picture evoked by this latter description is that of cunning, calculating offenders who will stop at nothing to get what they want.

How are we to reconcile the different images described above? Is one of them wrong, or are both perhaps wrong? Research on the criminal careers of psychopaths, reviewed in detail elsewhere (e.g., Hart & Hare, 1996b, 1997), does not give a clear answer to this question. It seems clear that psychopaths start their criminal careers earlier, commit crimes at a higher rate, and are more criminally versatile. They are also more likely to have engaged in past violence, both in the community and while incarcerated. According to prospective studies, the rate of general, violent, and sexually violent recidivism (reconviction or reincarceration) in psychopaths is significantly higher than it is in other offenders (see also Salekin et al., 1996). These findings seem consistent with the view of psychopaths as opportunistic offenders, but they do not rule out the possibility that at least some of their criminal behavior is planned and deliberate.

Several studies have examined the behavioral topography of psychopaths' offenses—that is, their victimology or *modus operandi*. For example, Williamson, Hare and Wong (1987) examined the police reports of violent offenders who had been assessed with the PCL. They found that psychopaths tended to victimize male strangers, whereas nonpsychopaths victimized female family members or acquaintances. Also, the violence of psychopaths seemed to be motivated primarily by revenge or retribution, whereas nonpsychopaths committed acts of violence while in a state of extreme emotional arousal. A similar pattern of findings has emerged from research looking at psychopathy and motivations for sexual offenses. Research using the PCL-R indicates that, among rapists, psychopaths are more likely to have "nonsexual" motivations for their crimes—motivations such as anger, vindictiveness, sadism, and opportunism (Brown & Forth, 1995; Dixon, Hart, Gretton, McBride, & O'Shaughnessy, 1995). Finally, two studies reported that psychopathy was correlated with sexual arousal to violent stimuli as assessed by penile plethysmography in adult male sex offenders (Quinsey, Rice, & Harris, 1995; Serin, Malcolm, Khanna, & Barbaree, 1994). There is a suggestion in these latter studies that at least some offenses committed by psychopaths can be considered deliberate, predatory, or sadistic.

Impulsivity, Psychopathy, and Violence

With a few exceptions, most researchers have tended to make rather crude distinctions among offenses when studying the criminal behavior of psychopaths. For example, offenses are frequently dichotomized into crimes against people and crimes against property; violent offenses may be divided into sexual and nonsexual offenses; or nonsexual violent offenses may be broken down according to the severity of harm to the victim. However, it is difficult to get a good sense of psychological factors related to offense behavior from distinctions of this sort.

Recently, Cornell and his colleagues have developed a rating scale that attempts to distinguish reliably between instrumental and reactive violence. "Instrumental" violence (also known as "predatory" or "goal-directed") is defined as violence that is committed to further some external goal, whereas "reactive" violence (also known as "hostile," "impulsive," "expressive," or "catathymic") is emotionally driven and a response to perceived provocation (e.g., Megargee, 1970; Baron & Richardson, 1994). Put simply, instrumental violence is a means to an end, and reactive violence is an end in itself. Cornell's rating scale, known as the Aggressive Incident Coding Sheet (AICS; Cornell, 1993), comprises nine items, which are listed in the first column of Table 12.5. The first reflects the fundamental distinction between instrumental and reactive violence. The remaining eight reflect offense characteristics that are frequently associated with either reactive or instrumental violence, but that are not used as a basis for making the instrumental–reactive distinction. For example, instrumental violence is typically associated with planning and the presence of an obvious goal. In contrast, reactive violence typi-

TABLE 12.5. Correlations between PCL-R Scores and AICS Ratings

	PCL-R Score		
AICS item	Total	Factor 1[a]	Factor 2[b]
Instrumentality	.30**	.26*	.11***
Planning	.00	.37***	−.38***
Goal-directedness	.26*	.21*	.12
Victim provocation	−.28**	−.28*	−.11
Emotional arousal	−.25*	−.18	−.18
Harm to victim	−.16	−.05	−.11
Acquaintanceship with victim	−.21*	.04	−.32**
Intoxication	.07	−.27*	.31**
Psychosis	—	—	—

Note. From Dempster et al. (1996).
[a] Correlations with PCL-R Factor 1, partialing Factor 2.
[b] Correlations with PCL-R Factor 2, partialing Factor 1. Correlations with psychosis were not calculated because of zero variance on this item.

cally is associated with a perception of provocation by the victim, high levels of anger and emotional arousal, severe injury to the victim, victimization of family members or acquaintances (as opposed to strangers), and intoxication or symptoms of mental illness during the commission of the offense.

Cornell et al. (1996) conducted two studies looking at the association between psychopathy and instrumental violence. In the first, they assessed the institutional files of 106 adult male offenders, using the PCL-R and AICS (but omitting the last two items in Table 12.5). About one-third of the offenders ($n = 38$) had no history of violence. Among the violent offenders, most who had committed instrumental violence also had a history of reactive violence; thus, instrumental violence appeared to be a less frequent but more serious form of violence. Consequently, Cornell et al. classified those with a history of at least one instrumentally violent offense as instrumental offenders ($n = 32$), and the remainder as reactive offenders ($n = 36$). Group comparisons indicated that instrumentally violent offenders had significantly higher PCL-R total scores than did reactively violent and nonviolent offenders, even after age and time served in prison were controlled for. The scores of reactively violent and nonviolent offenders were not significantly different. The biggest group differences were found on items from Factor 2 of the PCL-R, including Items 10 ("Poor behavioral controls") and 14 ("Impulsivity"). Differences were also found for items from Factor 1, including Items 5 ("Conning/manipulative") and 4 ("Pathological lying").

One methodological problem with Study 1 was that the PCL-R and AICS ratings were not independent, but were based on the same file information. This may have artifactually inflated the correlation between the two. Another problem is that it was not possible to interview offenders, which may have affected the validity of the ratings. For this reason, Cornell et al. (1996) conducted a second study of 50 adult men who had been charged with violent offenses and referred for pretrial forensic evaluations. Each defendant completed an extensive interview, which was videotaped. Detailed file and collateral information was also available for defendants. To keep the psychopathy and offense ratings independent, they were made on the basis of edited materials. Psychopathy was assessed with the PCL:SV. The first 10 items of the PCL:SV were rated on the basis of files and two 5-minute segments of the videotaped interview that contained no information concerning criminal history. After these items were scored, the "blinding" was broken, and the last two PLC:SV items were rated on the basis of juvenile and adult criminal history. AICS ratings were made by different researchers solely on the basis of criminal history, without access to other file or interview information. On the basis of AICS ratings of lifetime criminal history, defendants were classified as instrumentally violent ($n = 20$) or reactively violent ($n = 30$). As in Study 1, the analyses indicated that instrumentally violent defendants had significantly higher PCL:SV total, Part 1, and Part 2 scores than did reactively violent defendants, even after age was controlled for. Interestingly, the biggest group differences were found on five of six items from Part 1, including Items 4 ("Lacks remorse"), 3 ("Deceitful"), and 5 ("Lacks empathy"). Group differences were also found on five of six items from Part 2, although the differences on items 7 ("Impulsive") and 8 ("Poor behavioral controls") were among the smallest observed.

Taken together, the results of these two studies suggest that instrumentally violent offenders are reliably more psychopathic than are reactively violent offenders. This is consistent with the view that psychopaths are prone to deliberate and predatory violence. However, instrumentally violent offenders also had higher scores than did reactively violent offenders on PCL-R and PCL:SV items related to impulsivity and impulsive aggression, which is consistent with the view that psychopaths commit opportunistic or spontaneous crimes. Because the instrumental–reactive distinctions in both studies were made on the basis of lifetime history of violence, these apparently conflicting results could be attributable to the fact that psychopaths are predisposed to both predatory *and* opportunistic crime. Alternatively, it may be that psychopaths are "impulsively instrumental"—that is, that they commit goal-directed violence with little planning or forethought.

In a recent study, we (Dempster et al., 1996) attempted to address some of the issues raised by the findings of Cornell et al. (1996). We reviewed the institutional files of 75 adult male offenders attending an inpatient treatment program for violent offenders. PCL-R ratings were made by trained research assistants who were unaware of the study's hypotheses. AICS ratings (Cornell, 1993) were made on the basis of the index offense only, by raters who were unaware of the PCL-R scores. We calculated correlations between PCL-R total scores and the AICS items, as well as partial correlations between the PCL-R factors and the AICS items (i.e., correlations with Factor 1, partialing Factor 2; and correlations with Factor 2, partialing Factor 1). The results are summarized in Table 12.5.

As the table indicates, PCL-R total scores were correlated positively and significantly with ratings of instrumentality. When we examined the associated features, PCL-R total scores were also correlated positively with goal-directedness, and negatively with provocation, emotional arousal, and acquaintanceship with the victim. Given that AICS ratings in this study were based solely on the index offense, it appears that the violence of psychopaths indeed can be characterized as impulsively instrumental.

Interestingly, PCL-R factor scores were differentially associated with the AICS items. Factor 1 had positive and significant partial correlations with ratings of planning, instrumentality, and goal-directedness, and negative correlations with provocation and intoxication. Factor 2, on the other hand, had a positive partial correlation with intoxication, and negative partial correlations with planning and acquaintanceship with the victim. These results may help to clarify some of the discrepant and contradictory views of psychopathic crimes discussed earlier. In general, the cluster of psychopathic symptoms related to lifestyle impulsivity (reflected in Factor 2 of the PCL-R) is associated with opportunistic, spontaneous, and disinhibited violence. But remember that this syndrome of lifestyle impulsivity is not specific to psychopathy, and is observed frequently in many serious and persistent offenders. In contrast, psychopathic symptoms related to interpersonal and affective deficits are associated with planful, predatory violence. A prototypical psychopath—one who manifests the full range of psychopathic symptomatology—tends to be impulsively instrumental.

Comment

Psychopathy is robustly associated with criminal and violent behavior, including violence that is impulsively instrumental in nature. The exact nature and the reasons for this association are not entirely clear at the present time. Assuming that the proximal cause of most antisocial behavior is a conscious decision to commit crime, we speculate that psychopaths are at high risk for making such decisions, for at least two reasons. First, because of some neurophysiologically based deficit in emotion or attention, psychopaths are more likely than others to have antisocial cognitions. That is, psychopaths are more likely to consider the possibility of antisocial behavior, and to evaluate such behavior as potentially rewarding. More specifically, with respect to violence, psychopaths may have cognitive schemas that predispose them to perceive hostile intent in the actions of others, and thus to act violently in a self-protective manner (e.g., Blair, Sellars, et al., 1995; Patrick & Zempolich, in press; Serin, 1991). Second, also because of a neurophysiological deficit (perhaps the same one), psychopaths are less likely to inhibit antisocial cognitions. That is, affects such as empathy, guilt, and fear, which may naturally inhibit the expression of violent impulses, are notably absent in psychopaths. Psychopaths thus are less likely than others to evaluate antisocial behavior as threatening to their physical, psychological, and social well-being, and more likely to consider consciously and over a somewhat longer period of time how they might commit antisocial behavior (Blair, 1995; Blair, Jones, Clark, & Smith, 1995; Hare, 1996; Patrick & Zempolich, in press).

CONCLUSION

It is clear, even from this brief discussion, that impulsivity and psychopathy are associated strongly and on many levels. An increased understanding of the nature and reasons for this association is dependent on advances in the conceptualization and assessment of impulsivity. We hope that one important consequence of increased understanding will the development of prevention and rehabilitation programs targeted at impulsive offenders in general, and at violent psychopaths in particular.

ACKNOWLEDGMENT

Preparation of this chapter was supported in part by grants from the British Columbia Health Research Foundation and the Social Sciences and Humanities Research Council of Canada. The views expressed herein are our own and do not necessarily reflect those of the funding agencies.

REFERENCES

Albert, R. S., Brigante, T. R., & Chase, M. (1959). The psychopathic personality: A content analysis of the concept. *Journal of General Psychology, 60*, 17–28.

American Psychiatric Association (APA). (1994). *Diagnostic and statistical manual of mental disorders* (4th ed.). Washington, DC: Author.

Arieti, S. (1967). *The intrapsychic self.* New York: Basic Books.

Babiak, P. (1995). When psychopaths go to work: A case study of an industrial psychopath. *Applied Psychology: An International Review, 44*, 171–178.

Baron, R. A., & Richardson, D. R. (1994). *Human aggression* (2nd ed.). New York: Plenum Press.

Barratt, E. S. (1994). Impulsiveness and aggression. In J. A. Monahan & H. J. Steadman (Eds.), *Violence and mental disorder: Developments in risk assessment* (pp. 61–79). Chicago: University of Chicago Press.

Berrios, G. E. (1996). *The history of mental symptoms: Descriptive psychopathology since the nineteenth century.* Cambridge, England: Cambridge University Press.

Blair, R. J. R. (1995). A cognitive developmental approach to morality: Investigating the psychopath. *Cognition, 57*, 1–29.

Blair, R. J. R., Jones, L., Clark, F., & Smith, M. (1995). Is the psychopath morally insane? *Personality and Individual Differences, 19*, 741–752.

Blair, R. J. R., Sellars, C., Strickland, I., Clark, F., Smith, M., & Jones, L. (1995). Emotional attributions in the psychopath. *Personality and Individual Differences, 19*, 431–437.

Blackburn, R. (1993). *The psychology of criminal conduct: Theory, research, and practice.* Chichester, England: Wiley.

Brown, S. L., & Forth, A. E. (1995). Psychopathy and sexual aggression against adult females: Static and dynamic precursors. *Canadian Psychology, 36*, 19. (Abstract)

Cleckley, H. (1941). *The mask of sanity.* St. Louis, MO: Mosby.

Cooke, D. J., & Michie, C. (1997). An item response theory analysis of the Hare Psychopathy Checklist. *Psychological Assessment, 9*, 3–14.

Cornell, D. (1993). *Coding guide for instrumental versus hostile/reactive aggression.* Unpublished manuscript.

Cornell, D., Warren, J., Hawk, G., Stafford, E., Oram, G., & Pine, D. (1996). Psychopathy in instrumental and reactive violent offenders. *Journal of Consulting and Clinical Psychology, 64*, 783–790.

Davies, W., & Feldman, P. (1981). The diagnosis of psychopathy by forensic specialists. *British Journal of Psychiatry, 138*, 329–331.

Dempster, R. J., Lyon, D. R., Sullivan, L. E., Hart, S. D., Smiley, W. C., & Mulloy, R. (1996, August). *Psychopathy and instrumental aggression in violent offenders.* Paper presented at the annual meeting of the American Psychological Association, Toronto.

Dixon, M., Hart, S. D., Gretton, H., McBride, M., & O'Shaughnessy, R. (1995). Crime Classification Manual: Reliability and validity in juvenile sex offenders. *Canadian Psychology, 36*, 20. (Abstract)

Forth, A. E., Brown, S. L., Hart, S. D., & Hare, R. D. (1996). The assessment of psychopathy in male and female noncriminals: Reliability and validity. *Personality and Individual Differences, 20*, 531–543.

Fotheringham, J. B. (1957). Psychopathic personality: A review. *Canadian Psychiatric Association Journal, 2*, 52–74.

Fowles, D. C. (1980). The three arousal model: Implications for Gray's two-factor learning theory for heart rate, electrodermal activity, and psychopathy. *Psychophysiology, 17*, 87–104.

Fowles, D. C., & Missel, K. A. (1994). Electrodermal hyporeactivity, motivation, and psychopathy: Theoretical issues. In D. C. Fowles, P. Sutker, & S. H. Goodman (Eds.), *Special focus on psychopathy and antisocial personality disorder: A developmental perspective* (pp. 263–283). New York: Springer.

Frosch, J., & Wortis, S. B. (1954). A contribution to the nosology of the impulse disorders. *American Journal of Psychiatry, 111*, 132–138.

Fulero, S. M. (1995). Review of the Hare Psychopathy Checklist—Revised. In J. C. Conoley & J. C. Impara (Eds.), *Twelfth mental measurements yearbook* (pp. 453–454). Lincoln, NE: Buros Institute.

Gray, J. A. (1987). *The psychology of fear and stress* (2nd ed.). Cambridge, England: Cambridge University Press.

Gray, K. C., & Hutchinson, H. C. (1964). The psychopathic personality: A survey of Canadian psychiatrists' opinions. *Canadian Psychiatric Association Journal, 9*, 452–461.

Hare, R. D. (1970). *Psychopathy: Theory and research.* New York: Wiley.

Hare, R. D. (1980). A research scale for the assessment of psychopathy in criminal populations. *Personality and Individual Differences, 1*, 111–119.

Hare, R. D. (1991). *Manual for the Hare Psychopathy Checklist—Revised.* Toronto: Multi-Health Systems.

Hare, R. D. (1993). *Without conscience: The disturbing world of the psychopaths among us.* New York: Simon & Schuster.

Hare, R. D. (1996). Psychopathy: A clinical construct whose time has come. *Criminal Justice and Behavior, 23*, 25–54.

Hare, R. D., Harpur, T. J., Hakstian, A. R., Forth, A. E., Hart, S. D., & Newman, J. P. (1990). The Revised Psychopathy Checklist: Reliability and factor structure. *Psychological Assessment: A Journal of Consulting and Clinical Psychology, 2*, 338–341.

Hare, R. D., Hart, S. D., & Harpur, T. J. (1991). Psychopathy and the DSM-IV criteria for antisocial personality disorder. *Journal of Abnormal Psychology, 100*, 391–398.

Harpur, T. J., Hakstian, R. A., & Hare, R. D. (1988). Factor structure of the Psychopathy Checklist. *Journal of Consulting and Clinical Psychology, 56,* 741–747.

Harpur, T. J., Hare, R. D., & Hakstian, R. A. (1989). A two-factor conceptualization of psychopathy: Construct validity and implications for assessment. *Psychological Assessment: A Journal of Consulting and Clinical Psychology, 1,* 6–17.

Hart, S. D., Cox, D. N., & Hare, R. D. (1995). *Manual for the Hare Psychopathy Checklist—Revised: Screening Version (PCL:SV).* Toronto: Multi-Health Systems.

Hart, S. D., & Hare, R. D. (1996a). Psychopathy and antisocial personality disorder. *Current Opinion in Psychiatry, 9,* 129–132.

Hart, S. D., & Hare, R. D. (1996b). Psychopathy and risk assessment. *Current Opinion in Psychiatry, 9,* 380–383.

Hart, S. D., & Hare, R. D. (1997). Psychopathy: Assessment and association with criminal conduct. In D. M. Stoff, J. Brieling, & J. Maser (Eds.), *Handbook of antisocial behavior.* New York: Wiley.

Hart, S. D., Hare, R. D., & Forth, A. E. (1994). Psychopathy as a risk marker for violence: Development and validation of a screening version of the Revised Psychopathy Checklist. In J. Monahan & H. Steadman (Eds.), *Violence and mental disorder: Developments in risk assessment* (pp. 81–98). Chicago: University of Chicago Press.

Hill, C. D., Rogers, R., & Bickford, M. E. (1996). Predicting aggressive and socially disruptive behavior in a maximum security forensic psychiatric hospital. *Journal of Forensic Sciences, 41,* 56–59.

Intrator, J., Hare, R., Strizke, P., Brichtswein, K., Dorfman, D., Harpur, T., Bernstein, D., Handelsman, L., Schaefer, C., Keilp, J., Rosen, J., & Machac, J. (in press). Brain imaging (SPECT) study of semantic and affective processing in psychopaths. *Biological Psychiatry.*

Karpman, B. (1961). The structure of neurosis: With special differentials between neurosis, psychosis, homosexuality, alcoholism, psychopathy, and criminality. *Archives of Criminal Psychodynamics, 4,* 599–646.

Lacey, J. H., & Evans, C. D. H. (1986). The impulsivist: A multi-impulsive personality disorder. *British Journal of Addiction, 81,* 641–649.

Lewis, A. (1974). Psychopathic personality: A most elusive category. *Psychological Medicine, 4,* 133–140.

Livesley, W. J. (1986). Trait and behavioral prototypes of personality disorder. *American Journal of Psychiatry, 143,* 728–732.

Lykken, D. T. (1957). A study of anxiety in the sociopathic personality. *Journal of Abnormal and Social Psychology, 55,* 6–10.

Lykken, D. T. (1995). *The antisocial personalities.* Hillsdale, NJ: Erlbaum.

McCord, W., & McCord, J. (1964). *The psychopath: An essay on the criminal mind.* Princeton, NJ: Van Nostrand.

Megargee, E. (1970). The prediction of violence with psychological tests. In C. Spielberger (Ed.), *Current topics in clinical and community psychiatry* (pp. 97–153). New York: Academic Press.

Meloy, J. R. (1988). *The psychopathic mind: Origins, dynamics, and treatments.* Northvale, NJ: Jason Aronson.

Millon, T. (1981). *Disorders of personality: DSM-III Axis II.* New York: Wiley.

Newman, J. P., & Wallace, J. F. (1993a). Divergent pathways to deficient self-regulation: Implications for disinhibitory psychopathology in children. *Clinical Psychology Review, 13,* 699–720.

Newman, J. P., & Wallace, J. F. (1993b). Psychopathy. In P. C. Kendall & K. Dobson (Eds.), *Psychopathology and cognition* (pp. 293–349). New York: Academic Press.

Patrick, C. J. (1994). Emotion and psychopathy: Startling new insights. *Psychophysiology, 31,* 319–330.

Patrick, C. J., & Zempolich, K. A. (in press). Emotion and aggression in the psychopathic personality. *Aggression and Violent Behavior.*

Patterson, C. M., & Newman, J. P. (1993). Reflectivity and learning from aversive events: Toward a psychological mechanism for the syndromes of disinhibition. *Psychological Review, 100,* 716–736.

Pichot, P. (1978). Psychopathic behavior: A historical overview. In R. D. Hare & D. Schalling (Eds.), *Psychopathic behavior: Approaches to research* (pp. 55–70). Chichester, England: Wiley.

Prentky, R. A., Knight, R. A., Lee, A. F., & Cerce, D. D. (1995). Predictive validity of lifestyle impulsivity for rapists. *Criminal Justice and Behavior, 22,* 106–128.

Quinsey, V. L., Rice, M. E., & Harris, G. T. (1995). Actuarial prediction of sexual recidivism. *Journal of Interpersonal Violence, 10,* 85–105.

Reid, W. H. (1986). Antisocial personality. In A. M. Cooper, A. J. Frances, & M. H. Sacks (Eds.), *The personality disorders and neuroses* (pp. 251–261). New York: Basic Books.

Rogers, R. (1995). *Diagnostic and structured interviewing: A handbook for psychologists.* Odessa, FL: Psychological Assessment Resources.

Rogers, R., & Dion, K. (1991). Rethinking the DSM-III-R diagnosis of antisocial personality disorder. *Bulletin of the American Academy of Psychiatry and the Law, 19,* 21–31.

Rogers, R., Dion, K. L., & Lynett, E. (1992). Diagnostic validity of antisocial personality disorder: A prototypical analysis. *Law and Human Behavior, 16,* 677–689.

Rogers, R., Duncan, J. C., Lynett, E., & Sewell, K. W. (1994). Prototypical analysis of antisocial personality disorder: DSM-IV and beyond. *Law and Human Behavior, 18,* 471–484.

Salekin, R., Rogers, R., & Sewell, K. (1996). A review and meta-analysis of the Psychopathy Checklist and Psychopathy Checklist—Revised: Predictive validity of dangerousness. *Clinical Psychology: Science and Practice, 3,* 203–215.

Sartorius, N., Jablensky, A., Cooper, J. E., & Burke, J. D. (Eds.). (1988). Psychiatric classification in an international perspective. *British Journal of Psychiatry, 152*(Suppl. 1).

Serin, R. C. (1991). Psychopathy and violence in criminals. *Journal of Interpersonal Violence, 6,* 423–431.

Serin, R. C., Malcolm, P. B., Khanna, A., & Barbaree, H. E. (1994). Psychopathy and deviant sexual arousal in incarcerated sexual offenders. *Journal of Interpersonal Violence, 9,* 3–11.

Shapiro, D. F. (1965). *Neurotic styles.* New York: Basic Books.

Stevens, G. F. (1994). Prison clinicians' perceptions of antisocial personality disorder as a formal diagnosis. *Journal of Offender Rehabilitation, 20,* 159–185.

Stone, G. L. (1995). Review of the Hare Psychopathy Checklist—Revised. In J. C. Conoley & J. C. Impara (Eds.), *Twelfth mental measurements yearbook* (pp. 454–455). Lincoln, NE: Buros Institute.

Templeman, R., & Wong, S. (1994). Determining the factor structure of the Psychopathy Checklist: A converging approach. *Multivariate Experimental Clinical Research, 10,* 157–166.

Tennent, G., Tennent, D., Prins, H., & Bedford, A. (1990). Psychopathic disorder: A useful clinical concept? *Medicine, Science, and the Law, 30,* 38–44.

Whitlock, F. A. (1967). Prichard and the concept of moral insanity. *Australian and New Zealand Journal of Psychiatry, 1,* 72–79.

Whitlock, F. A. (1982). A note on moral insanity and psychopathic disorders. *Bulletin of the Royal College of Psychiatry, 6,* 57–59.

Williamson, S. E., Hare, R. D., & Wong, S. (1987). Violence: Criminal psychopaths and their victims. *Canadian Journal of Behavioural Science, 19,* 454–462.

Williamson, S. E., Harpur, T. J., & Hare, R. D. (1991). Abnormal processing of affective words by psychopaths. *Psychophysiology, 28,* 260–273.

World Health Organization (WHO). (1992). *The ICD-10 classification of mental and behavioural disorder: Clinical descriptions and diagnostic guidelines.* Geneva: Author.

13

A Conceptual Model for the Study of Violence and Aggression

JEREMY JACKSON

In recent research on the prediction of violence, the need to raise the level of methodological sophistication has become a central issue (Rice & Harris, 1995; Monahan & Steadman, 1994; Menzies, Webster, & Hart, 1993; Mulvey & Lidz, 1985). Although methodological concerns have occupied prediction researchers for some time (Monahan, 1981), recent pressures on the criminal justice system have increased the need for more accurate predictions of dangerousness and violence. Results of recent studies indicate that prediction accuracy can be improved if careful attention is paid to defining terms and refining data collection and analysis (Menzies & Webster, 1995). In this vein, Monahan and Steadman (1994) have provided a comprehensive assessment of the means by which future "risk" research should attempt to improve prediction accuracy. Recently, Menzies and Webster (1995) have supported Monahan and Steadman's (1994) call for researchers and clinicians to work together in an attempt to improve prediction accuracy through enriched theory and more sophisticated methods.

In the attempt to enhance methodological sophistication, the majority of risk research has focused on improving research design and data-analytic techniques, and on incorporating enriched theory. However, there is relatively little work on the definitional issues upon which design, analysis, and theory are premised. In this chapter I attempt to remedy this situation by reviewing a powerful technique for clarifying research problems and constructing conceptual frameworks through which to view research questions. In addition, an initial attempt is made to apply the technique to the problems encountered in risk research.

CLARIFYING RESEARCH PROBLEMS

Although data-analytic and statistical techniques are extremely important in the prediction of dangerousness and violence, their application is predicated on a clear understanding of the initial research question (Guttman, 1957). Without a clear *a priori* specification of the problem and criterion for a solution, it is not possible to determine whether the chosen design or analytic methodology is appropriate, or even whether it is capable of providing a solution. In this chapter I argue that risk research can benefit from attempts to improve the clarity of its concepts. Specifically, it is suggested that benefits can accrue from (1) a clarification of research questions and scientific constructs, (2) the provision of a definitional framework for risk research, and (3) a separation of statistical inference and data-analytic problems from definitional problems. It is not, however, the purpose of this chapter to provide a strong defense of the claim that definitional issues play a crucial role in science, or that they are distinct from empirical issues in important respects. The extent to which empirical investigations involving such techniques as factor analysis or construct validity address definitional questions is similarly deferred. Readers interested in these issues can, however, find detailed treatments in several sources (Jackson, 1996; Jackson & Maraun, 1996a, 1996b; Baker & Hacker, 1980, 1982; Ter Hark, 1990; and Wittgenstein, 1953). For the moment, however, the following quotation from Baker and Hacker (1982) is sufficient to summarize the spirit of this work: "The endemic sin of the experimental psychologist, the sin which explains and justifies Wittgenstein's remark that 'problem and method pass one another by,' is to neglect conceptual investigations which are preconditions for fruitful, intelligible experiments" (p. 228). In the following sections, the technique of "facet analysis" (FA) is introduced and applied to some important definitional problems pertinent to risk research.

FACET ANALYSIS

There are numerous ways for clinicians attempting to predict impulsive, dangerous, or violent behavior to phrase the fundamental problem: "What factors provide information about who is going to do it again?" These ways depend on exactly how each of the basic units of this problem are specified. For example, the unit "factors" may refer to a clinical variable, theoretically derived predictor, demographic correlate, and so on. The unit "is going" also has numerous possible specifications. For example, "is going" might mean at any time in the future, within the next year, once within the next 6 months, or more than once this week.

The specification of the basic facets of a problem and the clarification of the elements of those facets have been formalized in Guttman's technique of FA (Guttman, 1957, 1971; Schlesinger & Guttman, 1969; Van den Wollenberg, 1978; Levy, 1985). Guttman developed FA to deal with the difficult definitional problems that arise in constructing item sets to measure psychological concepts. The emphasis in FA is on placing restrictions on the domain of inquiry by specifying the phenomena of interest and their logical relationships. For example, the use of FA and a data-analytic technique for representing a set of correlated variables in the smallest possible dimensional space ("smallest-space analysis") has led to a substantively meaningful and replicable structure of intelligence test items (Guttman, 1971). Although FA is not well known to psychologists, it does provide an extremely useful framework for developing precise research questions and empirical predictions.

In FA the problem is stated in the form of a "mapping sentence." In the case of predictions of violence and dangerousness, a mapping sentence serves the purpose of specifying the logical relationships between and clarifying the content of, the basic units of the problem: "What factors provide information about who is going to do it again?" The mapping sentence (MS1) set forth in Figure 13.1 is an initial attempt to apply Guttman's FA to the problem of predicting dangerousness and violence.

MS1 consists of six conceptually (but not necessarily empirically) independent facets. The first facet is a risk factor facet; the second specifies the extent of determination; the third distinguishes the population of interest; the fourth specifies the legal status of the act; the fifth specifies the type of act; and the sixth specifies the time of offense. The elements of each facet restrict the domain of inquiry by specifying the phenomena of interest. This formalization is helpful because it allows the researcher to specify the research problem by combining elements from each of the facets into a single sentence. For example, combining the first element of each of the six facets results in the question: "What clinical judgment factors are thought to index which individual will be accused of a parole violation within the parole period?"

It is often useful to view the mapping sentence as a method for constructing a multidimensional conceptual space. The dimensionality of the space is determined by the number of facets, and the range of the dimensions is given by the elements of each of the facets. For example, MS1 shows that the problem of predicting dangerousness and violence can be represented in a six-dimensional conceptual space. Each of the dimensions of the space represents a logically distinct aspect of the risk research problem. I now provide a description of each of the six facets of MS1.

	Facet 1		Facet 2
What	clinical judgment theoretical aftercare situational historical demographic	*factors*	are thought to index predict are related to explain cause
	Facet 3		Facet 4
which/an	individual type of person member of a group	*will/to*	be accused of be convicted of commit
	Facet 5		Facet 6
a	parole violation criminal act violent act dangerous act aggressive act impulsive act	*within*	the parole period no specified period a period following parole time period X

FIGURE 13.1. Mapping sentence for violence prediction (MS1).

Facet 1: Risk Factors

Facet 1 specifies a set of six major risk factors that have been considered in dangerousness research. Risk factors as yet unknown, or others not considered in Facet 1, belong conceptually to this dimension. In general, any measurable or clinically derivable characteristic of a person's situation or history belongs to Facet 1. It is notable that much previous research has emphasized the need to enrich the elements of this facet (Steadman et al., 1994). Monahan and Steadman (1994), for example, argue that the application of psychological theory to the search for potentially relevant risk factors may provide considerably more useful prediction results. Recent research in psychopathy has shown that an increased emphasis on enriching the elements of this facet may be of considerable value (Hart, Kropp, & Hare, 1988).

Facet 2: Extent of Determination

The elements of Facet 2 can be loosely ordered with respect to the strength of evidence they provide for a scientific case. Clearly, from a scientific point of view, the ideal is to develop a causal understanding of the connection between risk factors and violent behavior. However, other levels of determination are widely sought and can be of tremendous practical and scientific value.

Facet 3: Population of Interest

The elements of Facet 3 distinguish among undifferentiated randomly sampled individuals (element 1); specific types of individuals who are distinguishable on the basis of some psychological syndrome or personality characteristic (element 2); and individuals who are members of fixed groups (element 3), such as prison inmates or Canadians. Although the varying base rates associated with distinct populations can provide predictive information about future violence, the logical distinction between population membership and predictor variables is important to maintain.

Facet 4: Legal Status of the Act

Although most academic researchers are interested in predicting the occurrence of a violent act, there may be important empirical differences between the factors that predict the occurrence of a violent act and those that predict the eventual conviction for committing a violent criminal act. In addition, there may be important empirical distinctions between the types or groups of people who commit violent acts and those who are convicted for committing them. Knowledge of these distinctions may be extremely useful to researchers attempting to understand the means by which violent criminal behaviors are detected and convictable.

Facet 5: Type of Violent Behavior

The elements of Facet 5 have recently been brought under scrutiny in the risk literature. Monahan and Steadman (1994), for example, make numerous recommendations concerning the changes that should be made to current conceptions of violent behavior. Mulvey and Lidz (1993) have also provided a series of suggestions for improving the measurement of violence. In the majority of this research, the focus has been on increasing the richness of information obtained from the original violent act and on increasing the amount of this information in the coded data set. However, little attention has been paid to clarifying the definitional components of the violent behavior that risk researchers wish to predict. The elements of Facet 5 represent an initial attempt to provide an admittedly crude taxonomy of some of the criterion behaviors of interest to risk researchers. Later in this chapter, an initial attempt is made to employ the mapping-sentence methodology in a conceptual/definitional analysis of the elements of Facet 5.

Facet 6: Time of Offense

The latency to reoffense has also recently become an issue of concern for risk researchers. It has been noted that such techniques as survival analysis can significantly enrich our understanding of the occurrence of violent events (Morita, Lee, & Mowday, 1989). Although the incorporation of such techniques is certainly useful for risk research, this analysis of reoffense latency answers to a prior aim. It is simply suggested that prior to data collection, the element(s) of Facet 6 that are of substantive interest to the research must be clearly specified. It is salutary to note that without a clear *a priori* specification of the elements of this facet (or any other facet), it cannot be determined what the predictions derived from the research do in fact predict.

THE VALUE OF MAPPING SENTENCES
FOR RISK RESEARCHERS

The power of the mapping-sentence methodology can be seen in its ability to incorporate previous attempts to address the methodological, conceptual, and definitional problems encountered in the prediction of dangerousness and violence. For example, a graphic representation of previous approaches to risk research (see Figure 13.2) and the methodological recommendations made by Monahan and Steadman (1994) can be readily incorporated into the framework provided by MS1. Inspection of MS1 shows that Monahan and Steadman's (1994) "risk factors" are represented in Facet 1, "clinical prediction" is represented in element 1 of Facet 2, and their criterion variable "violent behavior" is represented in element 3 of Facet 5. MS1 is an improvement over the representation provided by Monahan and Steadman, because it provides a richer and more comprehensive picture of the definitional problems encountered in risk research. In addition, the mapping sentence can be used to distinguish between various types of apparently similar research problems. For example, in their treatment of the problem of "impoverished predictor variables," Monahan and Steadman (1994) raise concern over the failure of re-

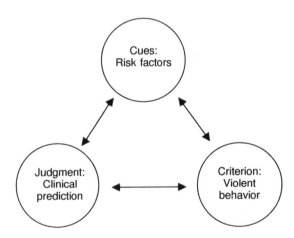

FIGURE 13.2. Approaches to the study of risk. Adapted from Monahan and Steadman (1994, p. 3). Copyright 1994 by the University of Chicago Press. Adapted by permission.

searchers to include clinical predictor variables and over the woeful inadequacy of patient classifications. MS1 is helpful here because it draws a logical distinction between the "impoverished predictor variables" problem (Facet 1) and the "patient classification" problem (Facet 3). That is, it distinguishes between the types of *people* under consideration and the *variables* that are predictive of violence. Such distinctions are useful because they emphasize the potential for research on the extent to which the predictive value of various *variables* depends on the *population* under consideration.

Measurement criteria are also an important part of the specification of the initial question. For example, Gottfredson and Gottfredson (1988) argue that researchers should scale "harm" in terms of seriousness, rather than employing a simple dichotomy (harm vs. no harm). The seriousness "scale" sought by Gottfredson and Gottfredson (1988) presupposes the logical possibility for an ordering of harm/seriousness. Among the pervasive concerns of mental health experts have been the problem of establishing such measurement scales (Mulvey & Lidz, 1993) and the lack of consistency among studies regarding the choice of a measurement scale and cutoff points (Monahan, 1988). Although some of these concerns are addressed later in this chapter, let us consider for a moment the relevance of these problems to the specification of the initial question.

Suppose that an investigator is interested in assessing risk factors related to harm/seriousness. The elements of the fourth and fifth facets specify some relevant indices of potentially harmful/serious behavior. Since some of the elements are fundamental dichotomies (e.g., parole violation vs. no parole violation, accused vs. not accused), they do not admit of the logical possibility for an ordered scale. However, since some of the elements of the fourth and fifth facets are not fundamental dichotomies (e.g., violence, dangerousness), the issue of how they should be scaled remains open to investigation. This example illustrates that conceptual/definitional issues are important considerations in determining the measurement criteria for harm. Once these are uncovered, further FAs may help shed some light on the complex, multifaceted natures of measurement claims involving harm, violence, and dangerousness (see MS2, presented later in Figure13.3).

MS1 also helps to clarify the possible consequences of varying and unclear specifications of harm. Specifically, it can be seen in MS1 that since the facets of the sentence are logically independent, ambiguity in the elements of the "harm" facets (i.e., unclear specifications of the index of harm) guarantees unclarity in the specification of the initial problem. This is not desirable because, regardless of how clearly the other elements of the question are specified or how well the empirical research addresses the initial problem, ambiguity will always remain about what problem the data addresses. This shows that the problem for research areas in which different measurement instruments and different cutoff points are employed is simply that the various studies address different questions. This is important to recognize because it rules out solutions that are based on research designs, data analysis, or statistical methods.[1]

It is important to note that "exploratory" research is not excused from a clear specification of the initial problem. In exploratory research it is still necessary to specify the phenomena of interest before the investigation begins. This is nothing more than a clear statement of where an investigator intends to look and what he or she is looking for. An example may help to illustrate the necessity for such prior clarification. Suppose that an investigator is interested in finding new predictors of impulsive behavior. Since the researcher has no *a priori* expectations concerning which variables will be predictive of impulsivity, the investigation is appropriately termed "exploratory." It has been argued that decisions concerning how an empirical investigation of such a question should be conducted depend on how the facets "predictors of" and "impulsive behavior" are specified. For example, if "predictor of" is intended to mean "theoretically derived explanatory variable," some form of theoretically guided analysis of impulsivity prediction should be conducted prior to data collection. However, if mere predictive power is of interest, any factor could be considered.

It is also important to note that clear and precise specifications of the initial problem do not rule out the possibility for unexpected discoveries. This is because the discovery that something unexpected has happened can only be made if there were prior expectations. A precise specification of prior expectations is advantageous because it sensitizes the investigator to results that appear out of place. It should also be recognized that conceptual investigations are an ongoing part of scientific research. MS1 is provisional in the sense that further clarification, new discoveries, or the potential for a more useful taxonomy may necessitate refinements or additions. Just as the *Diagnostic and Statistical Manual of Mental Disorders* has undergone restructuring from one edition to the next, so too it is expected that MS1 will require further clarification and explication.

The mapping-sentence methodology also sensitizes researchers to the potential problems associated with conflating design-related, analytic, or statistical issues with the specification of the initial problem. Although various problems indicate various different research designs and data-analytic strategies, there is an important logical distinction between a design-related or analytic question and the initial research problem. For example, in a discussion of the problems concerning the measurement of patient violence, Mulvey and Lidz (1993) suggest that a simple sum of the number of violent episodes does not provide an exact way to conceptualize violent behavior, because it does not account for the variability in patients' opportunities to be violent. However, they conflate conceptual and empirical issues when they suggest that the "conceptualization of violence" problem could be dealt with through a variety of statistical methods, such as analysis of covariance and loglinear regression (see, e.g., Jackson & Maraun, 1996b). It is important to note that conceptual/definitional problems require conceptual/definitional solutions. In this case, for example, no appeal to empirical evidence could address the conceptual issue of what we *mean* when we say that a particular behavior is violent. Addressing such questions via data analysis (i.e., empirical means) serves only to disguise the fundamental definitional issues involved in the conceptualization of harm. Such tactics are potentially dangerous because they tend to minimize the perceived importance of coming to terms with the basic definitional issue: What is the index of violence that denotes the behavior of interest?

In this section I have reviewed a potentially useful method for dealing with definitional/conceptual problems, applied the method to the problem of predicting dangerousness and violence, and provided some examples of the potential utility of the method. In addition, I have argued briefly in support of placing greater emphasis on the prior clarification of definitional issues. In this argument, I have agreed with Wittgenstein (1953) that conceptual/definitional investigations logically precede empirical scientific work, and as such provide the foundation upon which to build coherent, fruitful research programs. With this in mind, let us now turn to an analysis of the conceptual and definitional issues relevant to the concept of violence.

THE CONCEPTUAL CONTOURS OF VIOLENCE

The fifth facet of MS1 includes a number of elements that are of interest to risk researchers. Although violence is a fundamental criterion variable of interest, it is also important to be able to predict the occurrence of the other elements of Facet 5. Therefore, a conceptual framework that is limited to violent behavior must necessarily provide only partial coverage of the criterion variables of interest to risk researchers. In this section a more sophisticated form of mapping sentence is employed, in an initial attempt to apply FA to the broad array of relevant criterion variables. This conceptual framework is provided by the mapping sentence (MS2) set forth in Figure 13.3.

The basic structure of MS2 differs from that of MS1. MS2 is a function in which the domain is specified before the arrow and the range is specified after the arrow. In this case the domain is a simple set (Facet 1), while the range is a six-dimensional Cartesian set (Facets 2 through 7). As in any mathematical function, the elements of the domain set are mapped by MS2 onto the elements of the range set. The purpose of this form of mapping sentence is to provide a basis in the range for discriminating and drawing comparisons between the elements of a domain set of interest. In MS2 the six facets of the Cartesian range represent the dimensions that

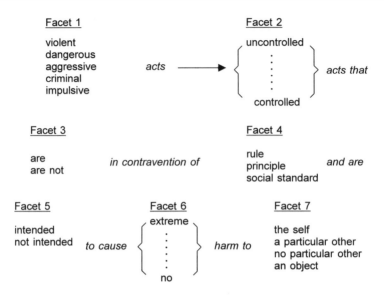

FIGURE 13.3. Mapping sentence for violence (MS2).

span the conceptual space occupied by the elements of the domain. Thus, the criterion variables of interest to risk researchers (the elements of the domain) can be denoted, compared, and contrasted on the basis of the extent of control exhibited during the action (Facet 2), the conformity or nonconformity of the action (Facet 3) with some social standard (Facet 4), the existence of intention (Facet 5), the extent of harm caused by the action (Facet 6), and the object of the action (Facet 7).

MS2 includes a second characteristic not found in MS1. Specifically, Facets 2 and 6 consist of elements defined on a continuum. Facet 2 characterizes elements of the domain as varying on a continuum of control, whereas Facet 6 characterizes elements of the domain as differing with respect to the extent of harm they cause. I now provide a more detailed description of the facets of MS2 in an analysis of their elements and logical interconnections.

Facet 1: The Domain Set of Criterion Variables

The elements of Facet 1 are five fundamental criterion behaviors of interest to risk researchers. Collectively, they represent the scope of the subject matter mapped in the Cartesian set of six facets given in MS2. The elements of this facet are to be distinguished from their empirical correlates, underlying causal mechanisms, or predictors. Although anger, for example, may be present in the majority of violent events, anger itself is not considered here to be a criterion variable of interest. Similarly, although physiological arousal has been considered to be a necessary component of aggression (Novaco, 1994), the concept of physiological arousal does not belong to the domain set. This is simply because physiological arousal is at best a necessary precondition, accompaniment, or empirical correlate of aggression, rather than a fundamental criterion variable of direct interest to risk researchers.

Similarly, the relationship between the facets of the range set and the elements of the domain set are not determined by their empirical association, theoretical connections, or causal links. It should be emphasized that the mapping-sentence methodology serves the purpose of clarifying the conceptual/logical/definitional contours of a construct. It is not the purpose of MS2 to document possible empirical/theoretical/causal links between the domain set and range set (or between elements of any of the seven facets). For example, the claim in MS2 is that, by definition, criminal acts (element 4 of Facet 1) are necessarily acts that are in contravention of a rule (element 1 of Facet 4). This is not a hypothesis or theory, but a definitional fact that could never be overturned by empirical evidence.

The elements chosen for Facet 1 represent only an initial suggestion to researchers in the field. The intent is not to defend these suggestions as the only subject matter of interest. On the contrary, it is for the field to decide which phenomena should be subsumed under its name. This particular choice of criterion variables is based merely on a survey of the criterion variables of past and present interest to risk researchers.

Facet 2: Control

The domain behaviors differ on the extent to which they contain a control component. Impulsive behaviors, for example, are uncontrolled. Aggressive behaviors, on the other hand, can be located anywhere on a continuum between uncontrolled and controlled. Whereas some forms of aggression contain an uncontrolled component (e.g., a riot), others are thought of as controlled aggression (e.g., torture). In slight contrast to violence and aggression, dangerous behavior and criminal behavior do not have strong conceptual ties to control.

Facets 3 and 4: Accordance with Standards

Violent, aggressive, dangerous, criminal, and impulsive behaviors differ on the extent to which they are in contravention of certain cultural norms, principles, or rules. With the exception of criminal behavior, however, there are no clear conceptual links between the domain behaviors and the elements of Facet 4. Consider, for example, an aggressive tackle in football or a violent blow in boxing. Often, in fact, dangerous or aggressive behaviors are applauded in Western culture. Consider Gilles Villeneuve's heroic but dangerous drives in his Formula 1 Ferrari, or Batman's aggressive and violent confrontations in the *Batman* films. Similarly, Ian Fleming's James Bond is licensed to kill, but a hero to his country. Criminal behaviors, on the other hand, are clearly defined by their relationship to a system of legal rules.

Although the domain constructs are not clearly tied to the elements of this facet, risk researchers may have considerable interest in distinguishing among and identifying behaviors that differ with respect to the elements of Facet 4. This is because violent, aggressive, dangerous, and impulsive behaviors that are not in contravention of a legal rule or moral principle are hardly in need of a remedy. The necessity for a distinction between criminal and moral violations and violations of norms is therefore a direct result of the particular sociocultural goals of risk prediction research.

Facet 5: Intention

The domain actions, whether criminal, violent, aggressive, or dangerous, may or may not be intended to cause harm. However, impulsive behaviors lack an intentional component. Although an impulsive action is not instantiated on the extent to which it is intended to cause harm, impulsive behaviors are, by definition, not carefully considered or premeditated. To the extent that premeditation is conceptually linked to intentionality, impulsivity has links with Facet 5.

Facet 6: Extremity of Harm

The concept of harm is linked closely to the concepts of dangerousness and criminal. What makes a behavior dangerous is that there exists the potential for significant harm. Without such consequences, the behavior cannot properly said to be dangerous. Similarly, the potential for harm is a fundamental component of criminal actions. In this regard, recent discoveries in the social sciences have served to widen the scope of criminal behaviors to include such offenses as impaired driving or possession of an unregistered firearm.

In contrast to the links between harm on the one hand and dangerousness and criminality on the other, the connections between harm and violence, aggression, and impulsivity are not as strong. For example, violent outbursts, although lacking control, do not necessarily contain a harm component. Violent behaviors that are directed toward an object or person, on the other hand, do contain a harm component. Of the five domain elements, impulsivity perhaps has the weakest links with harm. Although it is certainly true that there is an *empirical* relationship between harm and impulsivity, impulsive actions are not instantiated by the extent to which they involve the consequence of harm. Impulsive behaviors are not preceded by consideration of the potential consequences or pitfalls. They are carried out without reflection or premeditation. To this extent, one might expect harmful consequences to result—but just as correctly, a positive result may also obtain.

It is important here to avoid the temptation to construct empirical hypotheses about, theories of, or possible causal explanations for impulsive behavior. In a discussion of the "definition" of impulsivity, for example, Barratt (1994) draws a link between impulsivity and executive functions of the brain. Such considerations are not relevant to the definition of impulsivity, however, because they speak only to possible empirical preconditions or correlates of impulsivity. The aim of MS2 is not to contribute to this empirical web of findings, but to explore what is *meant* by the term "impulsive" (see, e.g., Baker & Hacker, 1982). It is salutary to note that without a clear prior specification of what is denoted by the term "impulsive," it will not be possible to discover which brain functions, for example, do in fact play a role in its control.

Facet 7: The Object of Action

Although harm to the objects that constitute the elements of Facet 7 can result from any of the domain actions, the object of harm is logically linked only to criminal and dangerous acts. Criminal acts, for example, cannot logically be intended to do harm to the self (except for suicide). Although a criminal act may certainly result in harm to the self (e.g., jail, injury, etc.), it is not correct to characterize criminal acts as conducted for the purpose of harming the self. It is the potential for harm to others or objects that is logically related to criminality. Similarly, although dangerous acts can result in harm to any of the elements of this facet, it is not logically correct to say that acts are dangerous if there is only the potential for harm to an object. Actions that have only the potential for harm to objects are impulsive, risky, careless, irresponsible, or clumsy, but not dangerous.

CONCLUSION

This chapter constitutes an initial attempt to address the prior definitional/logical question of what risk researchers mean by their "violence" vocabulary. However, as the mapping sentences given here indicate, the definitional issues pertaining to risk research are too complex to be surveyed completely in a single brief chapter. Risk researchers are therefore encouraged to engage in a continuing dialogue on the issues raised here. It is hoped that this dialogue will result in a concerted effort to provide a working taxonomy for risk research terms.

NOTE

1. This is a much-debated and contentious issue in modern measurement theory. A proper treatment of this claim is well beyond the scope of this chapter. The claim, however, should not be taken lightly, since at its root are arguments that undermine the logical coherence of construct validity and axiomatic measurement theory. Interested readers can find a comprehensive treatment of the relevant issues in Jackson (1996).

REFERENCES

Baker, G., & Hacker, P. (1980). *Meaning and understanding.* Chicago: University of Chicago Press.

Baker, G., & Hacker, P. (1982). The grammar of psychology: Wittgenstein's *Bemerkungen über die Philosophie der Psychologie. Language and Communication, 2(3),* 227–244.

Barratt, E. S. (1994). Impulsiveness and aggression. In J. Monahan & H. J. Steadman (Eds.), *Violence and mental disorder: Developments in risk assessment* (pp. 61–79). Chicago: University of Chicago Press.

Gottfredson, D., & Gottfredson, S. (1988). Stakes and risks in the prediction of violent criminal behavior. *Violence and Victims, 3,* 247–267.

Guttman, L. (1957). Empirical verification of the radex structure of mental abilities and personality traits. *Educational and Psychological Measurement, 17,* 391–407.

Guttman, L. (1971). Measurement as structural theory. *Psychometrika, 36(4),* 329–347.

Hart, S. D., Kropp, P. R., & Hare, R. D. (1988). Performance of male psychopaths following conditional release from prison. *Journal of Consulting and Clinical Psychology, 56,* 227–232.

Hart, S. D., Webster, C. D., & Menzies, R. J. (1993). A note on portraying the accuracy of violence predictions. *Law and Human Behavior, 17(6),* 695–700.

Jackson, J. S. H. (1996). *A critique of measurement theory in modern psychology: The case of the Sensation Seeking Scale.* Unpublished doctoral dissertation, Simon Fraser University, Burnaby, British Columbia.

Jackson, J. S. H., & Maraun, M. (1996a). The conceptual validity of empirical scale construction: The case of the Sensation Seeking Scale. *Journal of Personality and Individual Differences, 21,* 103–110.

Jackson, J. S. H., & Maraun, M. (1996b). Whereof one can not speak thereof one must remain silent. *Journal of Personality and Individual Differences, 21,* 115–118.

Levy, S. (1985). Lawful roles of facets in social theories. In D. Canter (Ed.), *Facet theory approaches to social research* (pp. 59–96). New York: Springer-Verlag.

Menzies, R. J., & Webster, C. D. (1995). Construction and validation of risk assessments in a six-year follow-up of forensic patients: A tridimensional analysis. *Journal of Consulting and Clinical Psychology, 63,* 766–778.

Menzies, R. J., Webster, C. D., & Hart, S. D. (1993). *Risk assessment and dangerousness: Theoretical and methodological issues considered.* Unpublished manuscript, Simon Fraser University, Burnaby, British Columbia.

Monahan, J. (1981). *The clinical prediction of violent behavior: An assessment of clinical techniques.* Beverly Hills, CA: Sage.

Monahan, J. (1988). Risk assessment of violence among the mentally disordered: Generating useful knowledge. *International Journal of Law and Psychiatry, 11,* 249–257.

Monahan, J., & Steadman, H. J. (1994). Toward a rejuvenation of risk assessment research. In J. Monahan & H. J. Steadman (Eds.), *Violence and mental disorder: Developments in risk assessment* (pp. 1–17). Chicago: University of Chicago Press.

Morita, J. G., Lee, T. W., & Mowday, R. T. (1989). Introducing survival analysis to organizational researchers: A selected application to turnover research. *Journal of Applied Psychology, 74*(2), 280–292.

Mulvey, E. P., & Lidz, C. W. (1985). Back to basics: A critical analysis of dangerousness research in a new legal environment. *Law and Human Behavior, 9,* 209–219.

Mulvey, E. P., & Lidz, C. W. (1993). Measuring patient violence in dangerousness research. *Law and Human Behavior, 17*(3), 277–288.

Novaco, R. W. (1994). Anger as a risk factor for violence among the mentally disordered. In J. Monahan & H. J. Steadman (Eds.), *Violence and mental disorder: Developments in risk assessment* (pp. 21–59). Chicago: University of Chicago Press.

Rice, M. E., & Harris, G. T. (1995). Violent recidivism: Assessing predictive validity. *Journal of Consulting and Clinical Psychology, 63*(5), 737–748.

Schlesinger, I. M., & Guttman, L. (1969). Smallest space analysis of intelligence and achievement tests. *Psychological Bulletin, 71*(2), 95–100.

Steadman, H. J., Monahan, J., Appelbaum, P. S., Grisso, T., Mulvey, E. P., Roth, L. H., Robbins, P. L., & Klassen, D. (1994). Designing a new generation of risk assessment research. In J. Monahan & H. J. Steadman (Eds.), *Violence and mental disorder: Developments in risk assessment* (pp. 297–318). Chicago: University of Chicago Press.

Ter Hark, M. (1990). *Beyond the inner and the outer.* Dordrecht, The Netherlands: Kluwer Academic.

Van den Wollenberg, A. L. (1978). Nonmetric representation of the radex in its factor pattern parameterization. In S. Shye (Ed.), *Theory construction and data analysis in the behavioral sciences* (pp. 327–349). San Francisco: Jossey-Bass.

Wittgenstein, L. (1953). *Philosophical investigations.* Oxford: Blackwell.

III

PRACTICE: ASSESSMENT

"By the sun, moon, and stars, by the clouds, the winds, the trees, and grass, the candleflame and swallows, the smell of the herbs; likewise by the cat's eyes, the ravens, the leeches, the spiders, and the dungmixen, the last fortnight in August will be—rain and tempest."

"You are not certain, of course?"

"As one can be in a world where all's unsure. 'Twill be more like living in Revelations this autumn than in England. Shall I sketch it out for 'ee in a scheme?"

—THOMAS HARDY, *The Mayor of Casterbridge* (1886/1981, p. 182)

By the way, leafing through my dictionary I am struck by the poverty of the language when it comes to naming or describing badness. Evil, wickedness, mischief, these words imply an agency, the conscious or at least active doing of wrong. They do not signify the bad in its inert, neutral self-sustaining state. Then there are the adjectives: dreadful, heinous, execrable, vile, and so on. They are not so much description as judgmental. They carry a weight of censure mingled with fear. Is this not a queer state of affairs? It makes me wonder. I ask myself if perhaps the thing itself—*badness*—does not exist at all, if these strangely vague and imprecise words are only a kind of ruse, a kind of elaborate cover for the fact that nothing is there. Or perhaps the words are an attempt to make it be there? Or, again, perhaps there *is* something, but the words invented it.

—JOHN BANVILLE, *The Book of Evidence* (1989, pp. 54–55)

I began to think seriously of killing myself. It was my first thought now when I awoke every morning, my last before I slept; it was the shadow behind all thoughts during the day. I'd often thought of my suicide before, had a thousand times planned out its every detail, taking a strange solace from the idea of it; but there was something different in me now, a sick sense of its inevitability.

—NINO RICCO, *In a Glass House: A Novel* (1993, p. 202)

14

Assessing Risk of Violence to Others

CHRISTOPHER D. WEBSTER
KEVIN S. DOUGLAS
DEREK EAVES
STEPHEN D. HART

Impulsivity is not just a construct embedded in the specific disorders of impulse control (as discussed by Hucker, Chapter 11, this volume, and as laid out in the six 312 codes of the *Diagnostic and Statistical Manual of Mental Disorders*, fourth edition [DSM-IV] by the American Psychiatric Association, 1994). It is also a key element in a large range of psychiatric disorders (as described by Coles, Chapter 10, this volume, and as earlier pointed out by Woodcock, 1986). Moreover, the concept is rooted in law, as Ogloff has noted in Chapter 4 of this volume.

Most contemporary Western statutes concerning involuntary certification require that an individual exhibit the prospect of imminent danger to self or others before detention can be forced. There is usually concern that the person will act before he or she can be stopped from so doing. Another example of the way the law contrives to take advantage of the notion of impulsivity comes from existing "dangerous offender" (DO) provisions (Moore, Estrich, McGillis, & Spelman, 1984). DO provisions (Part XXIV) of the *Criminal Code of Canada* (1985) offer a particularly clear example. This law was patterned on statutes enacted earlier in most of the United States. The idea is that convicted persons can be detained indefinitely on commission of a "serious personal injury offence" (sec.

752), provided that they can be shown to meet the DO standard. The law is applied mainly but not exclusively to those convicted of sexual crimes (Jakimiec, Porporino, Addario, & Webster, 1986). This is perhaps not surprising, since the current provisions emerged from a "dangerous sexual offender" statute (Webster, Dickens, & Addario, 1985). What is instructive is the extent to which the definition of dangerousness is reliant on the notion of impulsivity. There are references in Part XXIV of the *Criminal Code* to such ideas as "failure in the future to restrain his behaviour" (sec. 753(a)(i)). Restraint seems related to items 7 ("Immediate gratification") and 16 ("High explosivity") of the Impulsivity Checklist (ICL), outlined in Chapter 1. Another sample phrase in the *Criminal Code* is "substantial degree of indifference on the part of the offender respecting the reasonably foreseeable consequences to other persons of his behaviour" (sec. 753(a)(ii)). This seems to be associated with ICL items 5 ("Lack of plans") and 10 ("Causes of action unknown"), and possibly with item 18 ("Entitled"). Yet another phrase is "a likelihood of his causing injury, pain or other evil to other persons through failure in the future to control his sexual impulses" (sec. 753(b)). This phrase has some connection to ICL items 14 ("Aggressive to family/friends/others") and 19 ("Rejection of norms").

Part XXIV of the *Criminal Code of Canada* requires that at least two psychiatrists—one for the prosecution and one for the defense—testify in the formal DO hearings, which take place before a judge sitting without a jury. These examinations and cross-examinations of psychiatrists, and psychologists and criminologists who may also be qualified by the court to testify as expert witnesses, can be very instructive. Not only is the offender on trial, but so too are the clinicians (Webster, 1984, 1985). With well-informed expert witnesses, these hearings can provide an ideal forum in which to learn about the state of the literature on dangerousness and risk assessment. They can also provide an opportunity to understand how inadequate testimony, based on improper examinations, can adversely affect an individual whose case is before the court. Chapter 18 of this volume provides a list of points that some readers may find helpful as they try to assess the value of opinions proffered by colleagues.

It is our conviction that risk of violence should be assessed in a systematic way and in light of what is now known about the topic. We exclude in this chapter consideration of violence perpetrated by seemingly mentally healthy individuals as they pursue crime careers. In addition, we leave out the prediction of general criminal recidivism as a topic. This is perhaps just as well, because clinicians in fact seem to do singularly poorly at the task (Menzies, Webster, McMain, Staley, & Scaglione, 1994). The key question, then, is this: What variables might clinicians and administrators consider as they attempt evaluations of risk in cases where psychiatric disorders are thought to be involved?

In the recent past, one of us (C. D. W.) has been involved in two major risk assessment projects. The first of these entailed the publication of the so-called Violence Prediction Scheme (VPS; Webster, Harris, Rice, Cormier, & Quinsey, 1994). The second venture culminated in the presentation of the 20-item Historical/Clinical/Risk Management (HCR-20) scheme for the assessment of dangerousness and risk (Webster, Eaves, Douglas, & Wintrup, 1995), which has since been followed by Version 2 (Webster, Douglas, Eaves, & Hart, 1997). We have chosen here to emphasize the HCR-20—largely because the VPS is easily available as a short book in its own right, and also because the most central aspect of it, the Violence Risk Assessment Guide (VRAG), was earlier published separately by the authors who actually conceived the actuarial instrument and collected the data in its support (Harris, Rice, & Quinsey, 1993). Borum (1996) has recently described these instruments in some detail.

Readers anxious to cast light on how best to predict violence in mentally and personality disordered men confined to forensic psychiatric (and perhaps correctional) settings, as a result of having committed at least one serious violent act, may be better off consulting the VPS than the HCR-20. This is because the VRAG aspect of the VPS is based on actual data from over 600 men followed for 10 years, whereas the HCR-20 has to this point received only a small amount of in-depth examination for reliability and validity. The HCR-20 is conceived as a "broad-band" prediction instrument with potential application to persons with mental disorders. Although the HCR-20 is ready for testing, it is likely that over time it will be necessary to evolve specific instruments for predicting such matters as suicide, domestic assault, and sexual offending (see Chapters 15, 16, and 17, this volume). Fortunately, the concept of psychopathy, integral to both the VPS and the HCR-20, now rests on a well-researched base (see Hare, 1991, 1993, 1996; Hart, Cox, & Hare, 1995; and Hart & Dempster, Chapter 12, this volume). Before we turn to the main substance of the chapter, though, it is first necessary to outline why the present topic of risk assessment has come to be so important.

THE PAST

Until the mid-1960s, little attention was directed to the question of how well psychiatrists and other mental health professionals can predict future violence in persons with mental disorders. Assessing potential for violence was simply part of the job expected of them by courts, review boards, and various tribunals. The role was (and remains) largely enshrined in case law, statutes, statements by professional governing bodies, and the like.

The New York case of Johnny Baxstrom was to change this seemingly comfortable state of affairs (*Baxstrom v. Herald*, 1966). Baxstrom had been serving a prison sentence but, on being deemed mentally ill, was transferred to New York's state hospital for the criminally insane. He appealed this extension of restriction to liberty, and the case was eventually decided in his favor by the U.S. Supreme Court. As a result of the ruling, not only was Baxstrom let go, but 966 other persons were also released or transferred to conditions of reduced security. To Henry Steadman, a sociologist with the New York State Department of Mental Hygiene at the time, the *Baxstrom* ruling represented a remarkable opportunity to answer an important question—namely, how accurate had been the predictions of future violence previously made by mental health workers on behalf of the *Baxstrom* patients?

Steadman and Cocozza, in their 1974 book *Careers of the Criminally Insane*, explain how they came to take advantage of this naturally occurring field experiment and to answer at least partially the question of how well clinicians predict future violence. Although the study would lack the kinds of experimental and procedural controls that should ideally be present in research of this sort, it would nonetheless enable researchers to estimate the actual rather than presumed level of violence during a set follow-up period. Nearly 1,000 persons had been detained in large measure on account of their perceived dangerousness. How violent would they prove to be?

The former *Baxstrom* patients exhibited a remarkably low level of violence during a 4-year follow-up period, at least as measured by official arrest rates. Steadman and Cocozza (1974, p. 187) found that, although nearly half of the former patients were rehospitalized between 1966 and 1970, only 20% of the released *Baxstrom* patients were rearrested. Almost all of the arrests were for "nuisance" crimes, such as intoxication and vagrancy.

Of course, objections to the *Baxstrom* study could be, and were, raised. Few administrators and officials would wish to believe that all or most of these persons had been held for inordinate periods of time for no sound reason. It prompted the question, not only of the unwarranted expense in housing and supervising so many people, but of possible violation to their civil liberties. There is no need here to chronicle the objections to Steadman and Cocozza's findings—largely because a similar study based on the case of Donald Dixon in Pennsylvania (*Dixon v. Attorney General of Pennsylvania*, 1971) yielded remarkably similar findings a few years later (Thornberry & Jacoby, 1979). These two studies together, in concert with another "release against advice" study by Kozol, Boucher, and Garofalo (1972), drove home the point that there is a general tendency on the part of mental health workers to overpredict violence. The studies also made it plainly evident that clinicians' decisions concerning dangerousness appear to be made in unsystematic ways.

The *Baxstrom, Dixon,* and other studies were carefully reviewed by John Monahan in his 1981 book *Predicting Violent Behavior: An Assessment of Clinical Techniques.* Monahan set out with the notion that accurate prediction of violence in mentally disordered patients and prisoners is almost an impossibility. Yet, as he explained in his preface to the text, his mind gradually changed as he wrote the book. He came to believe, as he went through the literature in full detail, not only that mental health professionals should undertake assessment and prediction tasks in certain instances, but that they have a positive duty to do so. His book, though now dated, remains a repository of good scholarship and advice. In essence, he drew attention to how predictions in this area should be formed. Clinicians were enjoined to establish clearly the purposes of evaluations and the use to which reports will be put before the assessment process is begun (so as to ensure that the scope of assessment is restricted at the outset, and to guard against transmitting unnecessary or irrelevant information); to avoid "laundering" information (i.e., passing on to courts and other bodies as fact data about individuals that would not meet basic evidentiary standards); to take account of the important and time-honored distinction in psychology between actuarial/statistical data on the one hand and clinically derived information on the other (since the former have generally been shown to possess greater predictive power than the latter); to give weight to situational variables as well as personality factors (so that behavior can be not only predicted, but altered and managed, through paying attention to the physical and social precipitants of violence); and to establish predictions squarely on a knowledge of the "base rate" occurrence of particular kinds of violent acts (on the assumption that prediction accuracy will be enhanced if it is guided by statistical information about the frequency with which aberrant behaviors occur in the pertinent subsamples).

Monahan's 1981 book, and several of his subsequent publications (e.g., Monahan, 1984, 1988), had the effect of sparking interest in this topic of vital importance to practitioners and researchers in the forensic mental health field. He argued that future "second-generation" studies should be concerned with relatively short-term predictions made under fairly restricted circumstances (e.g., in psychiatric emergency wards), and that altogether more attention needs to be paid than previously to the precise definitions of predictor and outcome variables. These general ideas and principles lie behind the so-called "MacArthur project." This study, evidently the biggest and most thorough of its kind yet to be conducted, is being carried out simultaneously in Pittsburgh, Pennsylvania; Worcester, Massachusetts; Kansas City, Kansas; and other cities (Steadman et al., 1994). The logic behind the study is explained carefully, and preliminary data are presented in the 1994 book edited by Monahan and Steadman. It seems appropriate in the section below to review the basic points made in their text, since (to an extent, at any rate) it is "setting the agenda" not just for the MacArthur project itself, but for all current research on this topic.

THE PRESENT

We have noted above that Monahan's 1981 book continues as a sound introduction to the present topic and offers much valuable advice to clinicians and researchers. Yet it is also worth noting that Monahan himself has made one major retraction from his earlier position. He proposed in the 1981 text that mental illness is *not* a correlate of violence. Since that time Monahan (1992) and many others (Douglas & Hart, 1996; Krakowski, Volavka, & Brizer, 1986; Link & Stueve, 1994; Mulvey, 1994; Torrey, 1994; Wessely, 1993) have concluded, on the basis of literature published since the early 1980s, that mental disorders of various kinds *do* correlate with actual violence as measured during follow-up studies. His position, maintained in the 1994 book, is that there is not much point in considering "mental disorder" globally. Rather, it is necessary to examine the links between particular disorders and particular types of outcomes. At the same time, he and his colleagues stress that psychiatric diagnosis by itself is *not* a strong predictor (e.g., as compared to substance abuse— see Swanson, 1994). What does seem to be important, however, is *current* psychiatric symptomatology. It is vital to know about *present* delusions (Link & Stueve, 1994) and hallucinations (McNiel, 1994), and it is necessary in some cases to be able to address specific effects of insults to the brain (see Bowman, Chapter 7, this volume).

Another point to be drawn from the recent thinking of Monahan and Steadman (1994)—one already mentioned at the beginning of this chapter—is that the time has now probably come for increased attention to certain theoretical variables, such as psychopathy, impulsivity, and anger control. Although Monahan and others (e.g., Harris et al., 1993) have consistently argued for increased attention to such historical variables as age at time of first violent offense, sex, previous violent offenses, and the like, it remains the case that the potential value of theory-driven constructs may be far from being exhausted (see, in particular, the chapters in Monahan & Steadman, 1994, by Novaco; Barratt; and Hart, Hare, & Forth). This can be said despite the fact that previous attempts to operationalize clinical constructs—such as Megargee's (1976) hostility scheme—and other schemes for such constructs as anger, rage, guilt, and empathy, have yielded mainly very modest and only occasional medium correlational returns (e.g., Menzies, Webster, & Sepejak, 1985a; Menzies et al., 1994; Menzies & Webster, 1995).

Our position here is that, given our present state of knowledge, historical variables deserve a position of primacy in any scheme used in attempts to assess violence potential in persons with psychiatric disorders. The evidence is overwhelmingly in favor of this state of affairs. It is why we accord such historical/static/actuarial variables a large weight in our 20-item HCR-20. Nonetheless, there is evidence that clinical predictions, when made reliably, ought to be given due consideration (Lidz,

Mulvey, & Gardner, 1993). Similarly, such clinical constructs as psychotic symptoms (Douglas & Hart, 1996; Link & Stueve, 1994), anger (Novaco, 1994) and impulsivity (Barratt, 1994) have quite strong evidence behind them concerning their links to violence.

Before we launch into a description of static variables, it is first necessary here to offer a few words of caution. This is not intended to nullify the importance of these variables; it is merely to invite the reader to consider some of the practical and ethical matters associated with them. Of necessity, this is a brief discussion. We raise four points. The first point is that whenever researchers face the problem of coding information from files or other sources, they are obliged to define precisely what is meant by each item. There has to be some kind of agreement about definitions. Such definitions should accord reasonably with those of other researchers who work in the area, without restricting researchers' freedom to investigate new variables, or new combinations or versions of established variables. Such items as height, weight, and eye color are typically easy to code. Yet seemingly simple characteristics such as marital status can sometimes prove problematic, especially as society itself continues to alter its view of what constitutes marital conjunction. It is also sometimes difficult to agree on what is a violent offense and what is not. Even gender can be difficult to establish in assessing transsexuals, depending upon the various stages of surgery. In the VRAG (Harris et al., 1993), different scores are allotted depending on whether the victim is male or female. This works easily enough most of the time. Yet some thought would be necessary before coding a male bank teller as the victim in a robbery if there happened to be any women employees within the premises at the time. Trying to establish, with certainty, the age at which a male incest perpetrator committed his first predatory act can also require close attention, since it is necessary to know about extent and type of fondling or other untoward conduct that might have preceded other, more easily identified acts.

A second difficulty is that it is sometimes hard to distinguish between historical and clinical variables. Consider, for example, the notion of psychopathy. This construct has had a long history in psychiatry and clinical psychology. It was the psychiatrist Hervey Cleckley who first clearly described the condition in his 1941 book *The Mask of Sanity*. He emphasized the glibness, superficial charm, callousness, lack of empathy, irresponsibility, and various other characteristics of psychopathy. Many years later, Robert Hare and colleagues decided to score the components in a consistent manner; thus they created and standardized a psychopathy scale, the current version of which is the Psychopathy Checklist—Revised (PCL-R; Hare, 1991). This originally clinical concept now has an actuarial status because it can be quantified. Although in practical terms it may not much matter whether psychopathy is considered one type of variable or the other, it needs to be noted that the broad clinical domain is apt to be reduced as concepts succumb to the metric. This should not be construed as a threat to mental health and correctional professionals, since the challenge of identifying and refining pertinent assessment variables remains so large.

A third set of difficulties can arise from ethical considerations. One advantage, we would argue (Webster & Polvi, 1995), of an actuarial approach to risk assessment over a clinical approach is that the items become "transparent" (Baker, 1993). This means that the subjects of the assessment or their legal representatives can "see," as they presumably should be able to, what variables have entered the prediction equation and how they have been scored. Instead of relying on global clinical judgments (the bases for which are not usually specified or even specifiable), the risk evaluator using a scheme such as the HCR-20 is obliged to follow a routine that identifies each specific item. Under such a procedure, it can then reasonably be asked whether it is "fair" to base opinions on such characteristics as previous violence, young age, relationship instability, employment instability, alcohol or drug abuse, major mental disorder, and so on. It can be argued that persons under assessment run the risk of being confined on the basis of characteristics that they cannot avoid possessing and that they cannot alter. Strong legal, constitutional, and ethical arguments against reliance on these types of items can be anticipated. There are no easy solutions to these issues. To dispense with the static items in favor of clinical judgment is no solution, for the simple reason that there is ample evidence to suggest the existence of sometimes deplorable bias in the course of routine assessments of risk in individuals with Axis I mental disorders (Menzies, 1989; Pfohl, 1978) and individuals with personality disorders (Lewis & Appleby, 1988). It is also worth noting that when it comes to sentencing, the law places enormous weight on one historical variable—prior record of offending. In part, the challenge for researchers over the next 20 years is not so much one of demonstrating which actuarial variables *do* have predictive power, but which ones do not. Only recently, for example, have we come to understand that what counts is not the fact that the individual has at some time been a patient in a mental hospital, but that he or she is at the moment experiencing particular types of psychiatric symptoms (Douglas & Hart, 1996; Link & Stueve, 1994; Monahan, 1992, p. 519).

A fourth difficulty with actuarial approaches is that, given the present state of knowledge, actuarial variables—no matter how well defined and how ingeniously analyzed statistically—do not account for enough of the inevitable variability in the data. If some combination of predictor variables like those in the HCR-20 or other such systems could be shown to predict with *complete* certainty (i.e., with a probability or correlation of 1.0 or close to it), then society might have a good argument for invoking the scheme as a way of protecting itself from potentially violent persons with current mental disorders. The problem, as readers will realize, is that such complete certainty is nowhere close to being attained. In fact, if base rates of violence in a sample diverge from 50%, as they typically do, correlations of 1.0 are *literally* impossible for statistical reasons. Researchers in the are of risk assessment and prediction sometimes argue that it is in fact all but impossible to surpass a "forensic sound barrier" of a probability or correlation near .40 (Menzies, Webster, & Sepejak, 1985b). Although in recent years others have seemed able to penetrate this barrier (e.g., Harris et al., 1993; Hill, Rogers, & Bickford, 1996; Kay, Wolkenfeld, & Murrill, 1988), it remains the case that prediction–outcome correspondences in large-scale studies are at present far from perfect. Unfairness may thus ensue when the results from large-scale averages are applied specifically to individual cases. The argument can be made that such applications from general data to specific instances are not only unwarranted but improper. Perhaps the best way of putting such arguments to rest is to concede that there can indeed be difficulties with the notion of correlation as applied in a particular context, but to go on to point out the value of using other methods (e.g., receiver–operator) characteristics that are much less dependent statistically on such factors as "base rates," and so give a more accurate estimate of a scheme's performance (Mossman, 1994; Rice & Harris, 1995).

The considerations above notwithstanding, there are arguments in favor of approaches to risk assessment based on a consideration of actuarial factors. It is a simple fact, but one worth noting, that such information has long served the insurance industry very well. Actuaries devote their professional lives to calculating risk under various conditions (which, importantly, will sometimes include human error and willful wrongdoing on the part of others). Life insurance premiums are calculated largely on the basis of "static" factors (e.g., present age, age of parents at death, present medical condition, etc.). They are also "individualized" to an extent by present habits (e.g., tobacco consumption). Weather forecasting is another area with parallels to the present topic. The fact that weather predictions have become increasingly accurate in recent years is the result of a variety of factors—for instance, the availability of large data sets giving base rate outcomes for various weather conditions; increased attention to definitions of the elements of weather; and improved training of forecasters (see Monahan & Steadman, 1996). It can be argued, following Monahan and Steadman, that attention to factors that parallel those in weather forecasting would greatly improve the reliability and accuracy of violence prediction (e.g., predictions should be for specified periods of time and should indicate the degree of uncertainty, either through the use of some probabilistic numeric or through carefully defined words and phrases).

At the risk of overstatement perhaps, it would seem that, at their worst, clinical assessments of risk of violence depend less on the principles employed by meteorologists and more on those employed by fortunetellers. Even though it is unlikely that these "professionals" spend their evenings imbibing the latest literature in psychology or psychiatry, there can be no doubt that they employ useful psychological principles with great effectiveness. In the first place, they set out to predict in rather "soft" areas, such as romance; they also know that, if offered in the right way, their predictions can become self-fulfilling prophecies. Telling people that they will meet a tall, good-looking stranger in the next week carries with it a near-certainty of success, at least for urban dwellers. Once "primed" in this way, those receiving such prophecies will be apt to engineer conversations in ways that they might not otherwise have done. In addition, fortunetelling thrives on the very vagueness that actuaries would wish to disallow. With "outcome" in the crucial areas of love and money so ill defined, the fulfillment of predictions is given the maximum opportunity to succeed.

Our general position is that the assessment of risk for violence in mentally disordered persons has the maximum chance of success if the following conditions are met. First, some effort should be made to conduct the assessment according to a well-defined and published scheme. Second, individual assessors should take the trouble to be fully cognizant of the agreed-upon scheme and to ensure that their ratings are similar to those of other colleagues. Third, the actual prediction should be made for a defined type of violent behavior over a set period. This entails having knowledge of "base rate" data for similar populations. Fourth, steps should be taken to ensure that the violent act, if and when it occurs, is detected and recorded. This requires thorough knowledge of the physical and social environment in which the subject of the evaluation will be living. Fifth, an actuarial estimate of risk should be determined after a complete search of file and other background material known to be correct and substantiated. This should be expressed in probabilistic terms and will serve to anchor the eventual prediction. Sixth, the actuarial estimate should be adjusted only if there is sufficient justification to take account of current clinical factors. Our advice has been that such adjustments should be made sparingly (Webster et al., 1994, p. 57; Webster et al., 1995, pp. 20, 47). Seventh, assessors should be at pains to identify future risk management factors. This attempt to isolate the conditions apt to promote or mitigate violent acts may help suggest the means by which such occurrences may be attenuated or eliminated in the future. It helps shift interest from risk estimation to risk management.

DESCRIPTION OF THE HCR-20

Recently we set out to establish a new scheme for the prediction of violent behavior. This we did with some trepidation, since an earlier attempt in this direction, the so-called Dangerous Behavior Rating

Scheme (DBRS), has met with only very limited success (Menzies et al., 1985a, 1994; Menzies & Webster, 1995; Webster & Menzies, 1993). However, the DBRS was based on a literature much more sparse than that of today. We wanted a new scheme that would (1) be reasonably straightforward for professionals in a variety of mental health and correctional disciplines to use; (2) possess scientific integrity, in that it would take account of what is now known about the topic; (3) be defined with enough precision that it could be tested in actual practice; (4) permit at least some applicability to a broad range of risk assessment issues (e.g., civil certification, parole assessments, release of persons deemed not guilty by reason of insanity, etc.); (5) be compatible with existing administrative arrangements and practices; (6) allow for efficiency in its use; (7) minimize evident bias in the assessment process; and (8) serve as a basis for other, more specific evaluations that might be conducted subsequently (e.g., evaluations for risk of self-harm, youthful offenses, sexual offenses, or domestic assault).

In what follows, we offer a summary of the 20 items included in the HCR-20. There are 10 historical (H) variables; these are drawn from a reading of the literature, especially Monahan (1981) and Harris et al. (1993). Mental health colleagues suggested five clinical (C) items and five future risk management (R) variables that correspond with the scientific literature. The conceptual basis is quite straightforward, then, and is based on three temporal periods—past, present, and future. Each of these variables is explained in a separate, easily available manual (Webster et al., 1995, for the original HCR-20, and Webster et al., 1997, for Version 2) and in more detail elsewhere (Douglas & Webster, in press). Here we can offer only a brief note or two about each of them.

Historical Variables

"Previous violence" (item H1 of the HCR-20) is generally found to correlate with violence in the future. This is a fairly dependable finding in most studies that have tried to find such a link (e.g., Klassen & O'Connor, 1994, p. 233). The relationship has been observed in studies for decades (Convit, Jaeger, Lin, Meisner, & Volavka, 1988; Kozol et al., 1972; McNiel & Binder, 1994a, 1994b). The same can be said of "young age at first violent incident" (item H2): The younger the individual at the time of the first serious violent incident, the greater the likelihood that a pattern will persist into the future (e.g., Harris et al., 1993; Harris, Rice, & Cormier, 1991; Lattimore, Visher, & Linster, 1995; Swanson, 1994, Table 6, p. 121). "Early maladjustment" (at home, at school, or in the community; item H8 is included on the basis of the Harris et al. (1993) study, and others by Klassen and O'Connor (1989), Convit et al. (1988), and Smith and Thornberry (1995); moreover, the importance of this factor is stressed by most authorities (see, e.g. Farrington, 1995, pp. 297–301).

"Relationship instability" (item H3) has also been found to have some definite association with violence in the future (e.g., see Harris et al., 1993, who examined "never married" as a variable and found it to correlate, albeit weakly, with subsequent violence). "Employment problems" (item H4), though again not a strong correlate of violence, is probably a factor of some importance (Harris et al., 1993). Klassen and O'Connor (1988a) have noted that unemployment bears a relationship to violence. In a group of accused persons previously referred by the courts for psychiatric evaluation, unemployment at time of index arrest was one of four demographic variables (out of a total of 11) that predicted violent recidivism (beta = .18; Menzies & Webster, 1995). "Substance use problems" (item H5) merits inclusion in the HCR-20 or any similar scheme. Swanson (1994) found this factor to be quite strong in a recently published report from the Epidemiologic Catchment Area study in the United States. In fact, in this study, the presence of substance abuse increased the probability of having acted violently in the past by about 10-fold. Many others have noted this relationship (Hoffman & Beck, 1985; Haywood et al., 1995; Hodgins, 1990; Klassen & O'Connor, 1988b; Taylor, 1986).

Based on Swanson's (1994) study, any diagnosis of "Major mental illness" (item H6), particularly psychotic or mood-disorders, would seem to warrant inclusion, although it was a less potent variable in that study than was substance abuse. Several studies have noted that major mental illnesses are overrepresented in groups of violent offenders, compared to either nonviolent offenders or members of the general population (Feder, 1991; Cote & Hodgins, 1992; Taylor, 1986; Teplin, 1990; Yarvis, 1990). In a meta-analysis of the literature on psychosis and violence, Douglas and Hart (1996) found that, in general, the association is appreciable.

"Psychopathy" (item H7) is increasingly thought to be a strong variable on the historical side. Of a dozen actuarial items examined by Harris et al. (1993), it was the most powerful. Once released from confining institutions, psychopaths have been found to reoffend violently from three and a half times (Harris et al., 1991) to five times (Serin & Amos, 1995) as often as nonpsychopaths. The psychopathy construct also predicts violence in young offenders (Forth, Hart, & Hare, 1990) and in sex offenders (Quinsey, Rice, & Harris, 1995). Psychopaths may be more likely than nonpsychopaths to use weapons and threats (Serin, 1991) and to perpetrate instrumental or calculated violence (Serin, 1991; Williamson, Hare, & Wong, 1987). For these reasons, a chapter on psychopathy is included not just in Monahan and Steadman's 1994 book, but in this one as well (see Hart & Dempster, Chapter 12, where the elements of psychopathy are described in some detail). On the basis of Harris et al.'s (1993) work, any diagnosis of "Personality disorder" (item H9) gains a place in the HCR-20, though it is recognized that there will be overlap between some of these disorders and "Psychopathy" (item H7). Links between violence and antisocial (Bland & Orn, 1986; Hodgins & Cote, 1993; Robins,

Tipp, & Przybeck, 1991; Yarvis, 1990) and borderline (Snyder, Pitts, & Pokorny, 1986; Yarvis, 1990) personality disorders (or traits, in the case of Snyder et al., 1986) provides additional support for this HCR-20 item. It does, however, need to be borne in mind that DSM-IV now lists 10 main personality disorders and that some of these (e.g., avoidant and dependent) do not have much obvious connection to violence. "Prior supervision failure" (item H10)—that is, breach of release, conditions, or escape from detention—completes the list of 10 historical variables. Harris et al. (1993) found this factor to have some predictive value, as did Cooper and Werner (1990) and Hoffman and Beck (1985), though it is clear that it will not be applicable in all instances (i.e., because a person has never been detained).

Clinical Variables

By "clinical variables" we refer to states that affect a person in the present. They are intended to capture the dynamic, fluctuating violence risk markers that ought to be assessed repeatedly and regularly. "Lack of insight" (item C1) is a factor that most clinicians take into account as they assess risk for future violence. By this they mean the extent to which subjects are able rationally to comprehend why they behave the way they do, whether they have a mental disorder, the degree to which they may act violently and appreciate the consequences thereof, and the like (Amador et al., 1993). This extends to the appreciation of the importance of taking prescribed medications in cases where it is deemed prudent to do so. Misperceptions of others' behavior or intentions, too, may relate to violence (Dodge, Price, Bachorowski, & Newman, 1990). "Negative attitudes" (item C2) are assessed in the HCR-20 according to the extent to which they are antisocial, hostile, angry, or the like. Angry states and dispositions bear quite a consistent and fairly strong link to violent behavior (Kay et al., 1988; Novaco, 1994; Selby, 1984; Welsh & Gordon, 1991), as does hostility (Menzies & Webster, 1995).

"Active symptoms of major mental illness" (item C3) likewise receive attention in the HCR-20. Active and florid psychosis seems to account for the observed connection between psychosis and violence (Link, Andrews, & Cullen, 1992). Douglas and Hart (1996), in their meta-analysis of the literature, determined that studies investigating precise psychotic symptomatology (e.g., delusions, hallucinations, etc.), as opposed to those coding psychosis in general (i.e., "psychotic–not psychotic") and/or diagnostic terms, were more likely to find an association between psychosis and violence, and more likely to observe a large relationship. Others have found that so-called "threat/control-override" psychotic symptoms—which are symptoms that either override a person's sense of self-control, such as thought insertion, or threaten a person's sense of safety, such as feeling that others are out to inflict harm—are particularly strongly related to violence (Link & Stueve, 1994; Swanson, Borum, Swartz, & Monahan, 1996). Assessors will want also to be attentive to such factors as sadistic fantasies (MacCulloch, Snowden, Wood, & Mills, 1983) and homicidal ideation. Suicidality may elevate a person's likelihood of acting violently toward others (Asnis, Kaplan, van Praag, & Sanderson, 1994; Hillbrand, 1995).

"Impulsivity" (item C4) is also rated in the HCR-20, on the grounds that individuals who appear reasonably consistent in their day-to-day demeanor generally appear to present less risk of violence than those whose emotions and behaviors are highly labile (though it is recognized that exceptions to such a statement are not hard to find). Barratt (1994) has demonstrated that impulsivity, as measured by his Barratt Impulsiveness Scale, may often precipitate violence. Prentky, Knight, Lee, and Cerce (1995) found that their construct of "lifestyle impulsivity" could distinguish recidivistic from nonrecidivistic offenders. "Unresponsive to treatment" (item C5) is included to take account of the likely unwillingness or other reluctance of individuals to accept help and assistance. It is a measure not only of their capacity to be helped, but of the amount of effort they are likely to apply on their own behalf and the behalf of others. In a sample of psychiatric patients, those who failed to comply with medication regimens were at elevated risk of being hospitalized, compared to patients who complied with medication schedules (Haywood et al., 1995).

Risk Management Variables

Assessors using the HCR-20 are invited to consider the likely future circumstances of the individuals they are evaluating. It is recognized that performance in more than one set of conditions may need to be projected (e.g., an appraisal that assumes continued detention on a hospital ward, and a separate estimate of the possible effects of supervised release to a halfway house).

Whether the plans for the future lack feasibility (item R1, "Plans lack feasibility") is likely to be an important consideration for assessors. Of obvious interest are the extent and number of safeguards introduced into a plan, as well as delineation of procedures to be followed in the suspected or actual violation of agreements and conditions. In correctional circles, some authors have proposed the "risk–needs responsivity" principle, which holds that release plans must be more intensive for high-risk than for low-risk offenders, and that plans must target individual needs (Andrews et al., 1990). Andrews, Kiessling, Robinson, and Mickus (1986) have garnered empirical support for this construct. "Exposure to destabilizers," item R2, is considered vital for obvious reasons. It is clearly important to hold risk to a minimum by reducing as much as possible the likelihood of "inadvertent" recidivism or relapse. Estroff and Zimmer

(1994) noted that among a group of released psychiatric patients, higher levels of violence were related to contact with fewer, rather than more, mental health professionals. In addition, patients who experience difficulties in such social areas as housing, meals, daily activities, and finances may be at higher risk for violence than those who have these basics well managed (Bartels, Drake, Wallach, & Freeman, 1991).

"Lack of personal support" (item R3) is intended to give assessors an opportunity to gauge how much help from friends and relatives is ideally required for persons to avoid endangering their own lives or the lives of others. Klassen and O'Connor (1988a, 1988b, 1989) have found that strife within a patient's family, including frequent arguments and dissatisfaction with parents and siblings, predicts violence.

"Noncompliance with remediation attempts" (item R4) is intended to cover not just unwillingness to take prescribed medications, but failure to follow an agreed plan of action. Bartels et al. (1991) observed that treatment noncompliance was a clear predictor of violence in a sample of schizophrenic outpatients. "Stress" (item R5) is included to give evaluators a chance to indicate an impression of how able people are to deal in competent fashion with unexpected, and perhaps unfortunate, events in their lives and the lives of people close to them. Heightened levels of stress may overburden a person's coping resources and predispose him or her to react in violent ways (Felson, 1992; Guerra, Huesmann, Tolan, Van Acker, & Eron, 1995; Klassen & O'Connor, 1994).

Scoring the Items

The Appendix to this chapter provides a scoring key for the HCR-20 (Version 2). Although formal norms have yet to be developed, we have had no difficulty obtaining cases scoring 40. Under the scheme, each of the 20 items is scored 0, 1, or 2. This follows the procedure used by Hare and colleagues for the PCL-R (Hare, 1991) and is explained in more detail in Chapter 12 by Hart and Dempster.

For the R items, two scoring options are provided. Typically, the HCR-20 will be completed for persons expected to be returning soon to the community. Yet there may be times when the scheme is completed for individuals who are likely to remain detained for some time. In this latter situation, raters may opt to code the R items as they apply to institutional risk management. We describe in Version 2 of the HCR-20 (Webster et al., 1997) how the items may be adapted for this task. For such cases, the assessor should mark the "In" box located above the R items on the scoring sheet (see the Appendix). On the other hand, if the individual being assessed is soon to be released to the community, the "Out" box should be marked. Of course, both options may be chosen. That is, assessors may code the R variables *as if* the person were to be released (Out), and may also code them with respect to further detention

(In). In such cases, there will be two separate scorings of the R variables to account for either eventuality.

Some readers will perhaps argue that 20 is an insufficient number of items for reaching such a complex decision. Others may say that the system places inordinate weight on fixed, static, historical factors. A few may think that the entire scheme is suspect because it does not allow for inclusion or adequate weighting of what, to them, appear crucial variables (e.g., physical or sexual abuse as a child, or the "traditional triad" of fire setting, enuresis, and cruelty to animals—see Hellman & Blackman, 1966). The occasional critic will argue with some possible justification that *any* scheme that accords a fixed range of response (i.e., 0, 1, 2) to all items can never take account of a case in which, only one or a very few items are critical for a particular individual (Roesch, Webster, & Eaves, 1984). In such cases, it can be argued, the one or two variables are so vital that they alone should properly account for most if not all the usual total score. For example, a person may lead a perfectly ordinary and satisfactory personal and professional life, aside from an occasional single, fixed, highly encapsulated, and acted-upon violent delusion.

These considerations notwithstanding, our conviction has been and remains that assessors should place the greatest emphasis on historical/static factors. Yet we allow that clinicians and others may need in some cases to "tailor" the scores slightly in light of present and future considerations. At least so far as its present development is concerned, we are anxious that assessors use the scale (or one like it) as a checklist to ensure that evaluations are conducted in a systematic and standard fashion. This may be more important than obtaining an actual score (though this may be valuable, at least for research purposes).

Our insistence on an orderly approach to assessments derives from a wish not only to ensure that key variables are not left out of the analysis, but to reduce the chance of confirmatory bias. All that is meant by "confirmatory bias" is that, unchecked, evaluators have an inclination to seek out information that fits a hypothesis and to exclude material that does not accord with it (Borum, Otto, & Golding, 1993, p. 47). It is also the case that unless appropriate steps are taken to counter the tendency, clinicians are apt to place overreliance on aspects of a case that are seemingly unique, rather than to place weight on familiar factors (Borum et al., 1993, p. 58).

RESEARCH WITH THE HCR-20 AND PCL-R

Douglas (1996) coded the files of 200 involuntarily committed civil psychiatric patients from a large psychiatric hospital for information relevant to the scoring of the HCR-20 and PCL:SV, as well as demographic and diagnostic information, psychiatric and criminal history and so on. The mean for follow-up evaluation was 690 days, and postrelease violence in the community was coded from correctional records, and from readmissions to the original psychiatric hospital as well as to the psychiatric units of 14 general hospitals in the area. Violence was coded according to whether it was physical or nonphysical. Violence that led to arrest also was coded separately to allow for separate analyses. To estimate the strength of the relationship between the predictors and community violence, the primary statistical procedures were receiver operating characteristics (ROC) analyses and the areas under their curves (AUCs). AUCs range from 0 (perfect negative prediction) to .5 (chance prediction) to 1 (perfect prediction). The value of an AUC is taken to represent the probability that a randomly chosen, actually violent person will score above a cut-off on the predictive instrument, and that a randomly chosen, actually nonviolent person will score below the cutoff. Regression analyses were used to determine the unique contributions of the predictors and their subscales to violence.

The AUCs for the HCR-20 total score with violent crime, physical violence, and all violence were, respectively, .78, .73, and .73. The size of the AUCs for the HCR-20 were appreciable and compare well to AUCs published from other research (see Mossman, 1994). The AUCs for the PCL:SV with violent crime, physical violence, and all violence were .77, .69, and .66. The H and C scales produced AUCs with violent crime of .73, and an AUC for the R scale of .85 was achieved. Regression analyses indicated that between the HCR-20 and the PCL:SV the HCR-20 was the sole significant predictor of the rates of each of these violence indexes. Using all subscales of the HCR-20 and the PCL:SV as predictors of the rates of violence in regression analyses showed that the H scale was the most consistent predictor of the rates of violence—H scale was the sole predictor of violent crime and physical violence—and that the R scale was the only other subscale to enter regression equations.

Another study of civil psychiatric patients by Klassen (1996) examined the predictive power of the 10 H variables from the HCR-20 and the 12 items of the PCL:SV against on-ward violence as measured by the Overt Aggression Scale (Yudofsky, Silver, Jackson, Endicott, & Williams, 1986). The study showed that women were as likely as men to engage in violence on the ward, although their violence was typically less severe. Depending upon the outcome measure selected, the PCL:SV correlated significantly with aggression on the ward (.26). Part 2 of the PCL:SV, which taps historical antisocial behavior rather than interpersonal and affective symptoms (Part 1), correlated a little more highly (.33). The HCR-20 correlated at about the same level (.30), but only after one particular variable was eliminated (item H9 "Personality disorder"). This item correlated negatively (−.34) with outcome. It is possible that this unexpected finding had something to do with the composition of the study sample. The patients were all seriously disturbed on admission; emphasis during initial assessment, at the time of completion of the

HCR-20, would have been on the obvious, florid psychotic symptoms rather than the seemingly subtle personality considerations. It may indeed be difficult to assess such patients for personality disorders at time of admission. However this may be, further work will be required on this item if this preliminary finding should be substantiated. The Klassen (1996) project showed the expected separations between high- and low-scoring individuals. Those with high H scores exhibited violence earlier than those with low scores, and these differences were maintained. The data suggest that the H variables may have a role in predicting on-ward violence.

Wintrup (1996) recently coded the HCR-20 retrospectively for 80 patients assessed in a secure forensic hospital in 1986. An attractive feature of this undertaking was that, at the time of assessment, all patients were interviewed for psychopathy according to the PCL format. The remaining nine H items were coded from the files, as were the five C and five R items. Records were obtained from police and hospital sources after an interval of 6 years. In line with other recently published reports (e.g., Lidz et al., 1993; Menzies et al., 1994), level of violence was high at follow-up, with 70% of the sample acting violently in the community and 20% in institutions. Numbers of psychiatric readmissions were also high, at 42%. The study employed several outcome measures. H scores from the HCR-20 and Factor 2 (reflecting social deviance) scores from the PCL-R both correlated about .27 across various violent outcome measures. Survival analyses were clear in showing that those with medium (21–30) or high (31–40) total HCR-20 scores reoffended violently earlier than those with low scores (0–20). Although the C variables were not without a little predictive power across four outcome variables (.13), the five R variables contributed little to predictive efficiency. This relatively poor performance of the R variables may have been attributable in part to paucity of information in the files. The HCR-20 scores predicted quite well whether persons were rehospitalized to hospital or not during the follow-up period (.38). This was somewhat superior to the PCL-R Factor 2 scores (.25). As with outcome measures of violence, it was the H scores that provided the bulk of the power to predict rehospitalization (.36 by themselves). Scores from the HCR-20 predicted number of psychiatric admissions (.45 for either total scores or H scores alone). The PCL-R Factor 2 scores also yielded an appreciable correlation for the same correspondence (.36). Although the size of these correlations are unremarkable by conventional standards (though they are no smaller than the majority of effect sizes in this area), they are higher than many we have obtained in previous studies where we have had opportunity to work prospectively (e.g., Menzies et al., 1994). And, in accord with Harris et al. (1993) and Menzies and Webster (1995), the results of Wintrup (1996) give some encouragement as to what can be accomplished through the use of simple-to-gather additional information.

Douglas, Webster, and Wintrup (1996) investigated the interrater reliability and concurrent validity of the H and C scales of the HCR-20 in a sample of 72 inmates incarcerated in Canadian federal prisons. All data were coded retrospectively from files, except for psychopathy ratings, which had been earlier determined by other researchers with the assistance of an interview. The R items could not be coded because the majority of the sample had not yet been released from prison. Concerning interrater reliability, the Pearson correlation for the total scores (ranging from 0 to 30) was .80 between two raters. Scores on the HCR-20 were correlated with scores on the VRAG (Harris et al., 1993) and the PCL-R (Hare, 1991), as well as with the number of previous charges for violent offenses. For correlations with the PCL-R, the "Psychopathy" item of the HCR-20 (item H7) was removed from analyses to prevent inflation of the coefficient. For correlations with the number of previous charges, the "Previous violence" item (item H1) was removed from the HCR-20 for the same reason. The Pearson correlations between the HCR-20 total scores and the VRAG, PCL-R, and previous violent charges, were, respectively, .54, .64, and .44. The H scale correlated with these measures at .61, .54, and .52. Finally, the C scale's correlations were .28, .47, and .31. The VRAG correlated at .44, and the PCL-R at .34, with past violence.

As in Douglas's (1996) and Klassen's (1996) studies, the H scale related most strongly to violence. Nonetheless, the total scores were quite strongly related to violence (.44). The C scale may have performed less well because it was not possible to couple file reviews with interviews for these items, and file information was not necessarily collected to accord with the HCR-20 C items. Or perhaps most of these offenders were without psychiatric ailments, which would explain the lower correlation with past violence. Of course, the C items may simply bear less relation to violence than do the H items. Future research will help resolve these issues.

The various correlations with the PCL-R and VRAG, both of which have been demonstrated to relate to violence, suggest that the HCR-20 taps similar though somewhat different constructs, as it was designed to do. Based on Cohen's (1992) definitions of medium and large effect sizes for correlational data as .30 and .50, respectively, the HCR-20 H, C, and combined scores bear relationships of medium to large sizes with previous violence, psychopathy, and the VRAG.

THE FUTURE

Earlier in the chapter, we have noted that the HCR-20 was evolved for assessing individuals with mental and personality disorders. It seems to us that, since the H and R variables are likely to be crucial as factors in predicting violence, even in the absence of appreciable psychiatric disorder, there may now be value in substituting for clinical variables a set of

Impulsivity variables (e.g., through incorporating some version of the ICL sketched in Chapter 1 to yield an "HIR-20"). Such an HIR-20 could be of some possible use in probation or parole supervision, for example, where Axis I mental disorders and personality disorders are not features of the evaluation task which spring immediately to mind. Impulsivity could be assessed in experimental studies through the kinds of measures reviewed by Parker and Bagby (Chapter 8), BIS-11 version of the Barratt Impulsiveness Scale (Barratt, 1994), or, as noted already, the ICL (Chapter 1). A second line of research that will warrant attention concerns the use of specific-to-purpose instruments. We need to find out the extent to which predictive accuracy can be enhanced (if at all) by coupling scores from instruments like the VRAG and HCR-20 to the kinds of measures outlined in the chapters remaining in this section of the volume.

ACKNOWLEDGMENT

Preparation of this chapter was supported in part by a grant from the British Columbia Health Research Foundation. The views expressed herein are our own and do not necessarily reflect that of the funding agency.

Copies of the HCR-20 (both the original version and version 2) may be obtained by contacting the Mental Health, Law, and Policy Institute, Simon Fraser University, Burnaby, British Columbia V5A 1S6, Canada. Orders can be placed by e-mail (mhlpi@sfu.ca) or the World Wide Web (www.sfu.ca/psychology/groups/mhlpi/hcr-20.htm).

REFERENCES

Amador, X. F., Strauss, D. H., Yale, S. A., Flaum, M. M., Endicott, J., & Gorman, J. M. (1993). Assessment of insight in psychosis. *American Journal of Psychiatry, 150,* 873–879.

American Psychiatric Association. (1994). *Diagnostic and statistical manual of mental disorders* (4th ed.). Washington, DC: Author.

Andrews, D. A., Kiessling, J. J., Robinson, D., & Mickus, S. (1986). The risk principle of case classification: An outcome evaluation with young adult probationers. *Canadian Journal of Criminology, 28,* 377–384.

Andrews, D. A., Zinger, I., Hoge, R. D., Bonta, J., Gendreau, P., & Cullen, F. T. (1990). Does correctional treatment work: A clinically relevant and psychologically informed meta-analysis. *Criminology, 28,* 369–404.

Asnis, G. M., Kaplan, M. L., van Praag, H. M., & Sanderson, W. C. (1994). Homicidal behaviors among psychiatric outpatients. *Hospital and Community Psychiatry, 45,* 127–132.

Baker, E. (1993). Dangerousness, rights, and criminal justice. *Modern Law Review, 56,* 528–547.

Barratt, E. S. (1994). Impulsiveness and aggression. In J. Monahan & H. J. Steadman (Eds.), *Violence and mental disorder: Developments in risk assessment* (pp. 61–79). Chicago: University of Chicago Press.

Bartels, S. J., Drake, R. E., Wallach, M. A., & Freeman, D. H. (1991). Characteristic hostility in schizophrenic outpatients. *Schizophrenia Bulletin, 17,* 163–171.

Baxstrom v. Herald, 383 U.S. 107 (1966).

Bland, R., & Orn, H. (1986). Family violence and psychiatric disorder. *Canadian Journal of Psychiatry, 31,* 127–137.

Borum, R. (1996). Improving the clinical practice of violence risk assessment: Technology, guidelines, and training. *American Psychologist, 51,* 945–956.

Borum, R., Otto, R., & Golding, S. (1993). Improving clinical judgment and decision making in forensic evaluation. *Journal of Psychiatry and Law, Spring,* 35–76.

Cleckley, H. (1941). *The mask of sanity.* St. Louis, MO: Mosby.

Cohen, J. (1992). A power primer. *Psychological Bulletin, 112,* 155–159.

Convit, A., Jaeger, J., Lin, S. P., Meisner, M. & Volavka, J. (1988). Predicting assaultiveness in psychiatric inpatients: A pilot study. *Hospital and Community Psychiatry, 39,* 429–434.

Cooper, R. P., & Werner, P. D. (1990). Predicting violence in newly admitted inmates: A lens model analysis of staff decision making. *Criminal Justice and Behavior, 17,* 431–447.

Cote, G., & Hodgins, S. (1992). The prevalence of major mental disorders among homicide offenders. *International Journal of Law and Psychiatry, 15,* 89–99.

Criminal Code of Canada, (1985). R. S. C. ch. C-47.

Dixon v. Attorney General of Pennsylvania, 325 F. Supp. 966 (1971).

Dodge, K. A., Price, J. M., Bachorowski, J., & Newman, J. P. (1990). Hostile attributional biases in severely aggressive adolescents. *Journal of Abnormal Psychology, 99,* 385–392.

Douglas, K. S. (1996). *Assessing the risk of violence in civil psychiatric outpatients: The predictive validity of the HCR-20 risk assessment scheme.* Unpublished master's thesis, Simon Fraser University, Burnaby, British Columbia.

Douglas, K. S., & Hart, S. D. (1996, February–March). *Major mental disorder and violent behavior: A meta-analysis of study characteristics and substantive factors influencing effect size.* Poster presented at the biennial meeting of the American Psychology–Law Society, Hilton Head, SC.

Douglas, K. S., & Webster, C. D. (in press). Predicting violence in mentally and personality disordered individuals. In R. Roesch & S. D. Hart (Eds.), *Psychology and law: The state of the discipline.* New York: Plenum Press.

Douglas, K. S., Webster, C. D., & Wintrup, A. (1996, August). *The HCR-20 risk assessment scheme: Psychometric properties in two samples.* Poster presented at the annual conference of the American Psychological Association, Toronto.

Estroff, S. E., & Zimmer, C. (1994). Social networks, social support, and violence among persons with severe, persistent mental illness. In J. Monahan & H. J. Steadman (Eds.), *Violence and mental disorder: Developments in risk assessment* (pp. 259–295). Chicago: University of Chicago Press.

Farrington, D. P. (1995). The psychology of crime: Influences and constraints on offending. In R. Bull & D. Carson (Eds.), *Handbook of psychology in legal contexts* (pp. 291–314). Chichester, England: Wiley.

Feder, L. (1991). A comparison of the community adjustment of mentally ill offenders with those from the general prison population. *Law and Human Behavior,* 15, 477–493.

Felson, R. B. (1992). "Kick 'em when they're down": Explanations of the relationship between stress and interpersonal aggression and violence. *Sociological Quarterly,* 33, 1–16.

Forth, A. E., Hart, S. D., & Hare, R. D. (1990). Assessment of psychopathy in male young offenders. *Psychological Assessment: A Journal of Consulting and Clinical Psychology,* 2, 342–344.

Guerra, N. G., Huesmann, L. R., Tolan, P. H., Van Acker, R., & Eron, L. D. (1995). Stressful events and individual beliefs as correlates of economic disadvantage and aggression among urban children. *Journal of Consulting and Clinical Psychology,* 63, 518–528.

Hare, R. D. (1991). *Manual for the Hare Psychopathy Checklist—Revised.* Toronto: Multi-Health Systems.

Hare, R. D. (1993). *Without conscience: The disturbing world of the psychopaths among us.* New York: Simon & Schuster.

Hare, R. D. (1996). Psychopathy: A clinical construct whose time has come. *Criminal Justice and Behavior,* 23, 25–54.

Harris, G. T., Rice, M. E., & Cormier, C. A. (1991). Psychopathy and violent recidivism. *Law and Human Behavior,* 15, 625–637.

Harris, G. T., Rice, M. E., & Quinsey, V. L. (1993). Violent recidivism of mentally disordered offenders: The development of a statistical prediction instrument. *Criminal Justice and Behavior,* 20, 315–335.

Hart, S. D., Cox, D. N., & Hare, R. D. (1995). *The Hare Psychopathy Checklist—Revised: Screening Version (PCL:SV).* Toronto: Multi-Health Systems.

Hart, S. D., Hare, R. D. & Forth, A. E. (1994). Psychopathy as a risk marker for violence: Development and validation of a screening version of the Revised Psychopathy Checklist. In J. Monahan & H. J. Steadman (Eds.), *Violence and mental disorder: Developments in risk assessment* (pp. 81–97). Chicago: University of Chicago Press.

Haywood, T. W., Kravitz, H. M., Grossman, L. S., Cavanaugh, J. L., Davis, J. M., & Lewis, D. A. (1995). Predicting the "revolving door" phenomenon among patients with schizophrenic, schizoaffective, and affective disorders. *American Journal of Psychiatry,* 152, 856–861.

Hellman, D., & Blackman, J. (1966). Enuresis, firesetting, and cruelty to animals: A triad predictive of adult crime. *American Journal of Psychiatry,* 122, 1431–1436.

Hill, C. D., Rogers, R., & Bickford, M. E. (1996). Predicting aggressive and socially disruptive behavior in a maximum security forensic hospital. *Journal of Forensic Sciences,* 41, 56–59.

Hillbrand, M. (1995). Aggression against self and aggression against others in violent psychiatric patients. *Journal of Consulting and Clinical Psychology,* 63, 668–671.

Hodgins, S. (1990). Prevalence of mental disorders among penitentiary inmates in Quebec. *Canada's Mental Health,* 38, 1–4.

Hodgins, S., & Cote, G. (1993). The criminality of mentally disordered offenders. *Criminal Justice and Behavior,* 20, 115–129.

Hoffman, P. B., & Beck, J. L. (1985). Recidivism among released federal prisoners: Salient factor score and five-year follow-up. *Criminal Justice and Behavior, 12,* 501–507.

Jakimiec, J., Porporino, F., Addario, S., & Webster, C. D. (1986). Dangerous offenders in Canada, 1977–1985. *International Journal of Law and Psychiatry, 9,* 135–146.

Kay, S. R., Wolkenfeld, F., & Murrill, L. M. (1988). Profiles of aggression among psychiatric patients: II. Covariates and predictors. *Journal of Nervous and Mental Disease, 176,* 547–557.

Klassen, C. (1996). *Predicting aggression in psychiatric inpatients using 10 historical risk factors: Validating the "H" of the HCR-20.* Unpublished B.A. honours thesis, Simon Fraser University, Burnaby, British Columbia.

Klassen, D., & O'Connor, W. A. (1988a). Crime, inpatient admissions, and violence among male mental patients. *International Journal of Law and Psychiatry, 11,* 305–312.

Klassen, D., & O'Connor, W. A. (1988b). Predicting violence in schizophrenic and non-schizophrenic patients: A prospective study. *Journal of Community Psychology, 16,* 217–227.

Klassen, D., & O'Connor, W. A. (1989). Assessing the risk of violence in released mental patients: A cross-validation study. *Psychological Assessment: A Journal of Consulting and Clinical Psychology, 1,* 75–81.

Klassen, D., & O'Connor, W. A. (1994). Demographic and case history variables in risk assessment. In J. Monahan & H. J. Steadman (Eds.), *Violence and mental disorder: Developments in risk assessment* (pp. 229–258). Chicago: University of Chicago Press.

Kozol, H. L., Boucher, R. J., & Garofalo, R. F. (1972). The diagnosis and treatment of dangerousness. *Crime and Delinquency, 18,* 371–392.

Krakowski, M., Volavka, J., & Brizer, D. (1986). Psychopathology and violence: A review of the literature. *Comprehensive Psychiatry, 27,* 131–148.

Lattimore, P. K., Visher, C. A., & Linster, R. L. (1995). Predicting rearrest for violence among serious youthful offenders. *Journal of Research in Crime and Delinquency, 32,* 54–83.

Lewis, G., & Appleby, L. (1988). Personality disorder: The patients psychiatrists dislike. *British Journal of Psychiatry, 153,* 44–49.

Lidz, C. W., Mulvey, E. P., & Gardner, W. (1993). The accuracy of predictions of violence to others. *Journal of the American Medical Association, 269,* 1007–1111.

Link, B. G., Andrews, H., & Cullen, F. T. (1992). The violent and illegal behavior of mental patients reconsidered. *American Sociological Review, 57,* 275–292.

Link, B. G., & Stueve, A. (1994). Psychotic symptoms and the violent/illegal behavior of mental patients compared to community controls. In J. Monahan & H. J. Steadman (Eds.), *Violence and mental disorder: Developments in risk assessment* (pp. 137–159). Chicago: University of Chicago Press.

MacCulloch, M. J., Snowden, P. R., Wood, P. J. W., & Mills, H. E. (1983). Sadistic fantasy, sadistic behavior, and offending. *British Journal of Psychiatry, 143,* 20–29.

McNiel, D. E. (1994). Hallucinations and violence. In J. Monahan & H. J. Steadman (Eds.), *Violence and mental disorder: Developments in risk assessment* (pp. 183–202). Chicago: University of Chicago Press

McNiel, D. E., & Binder, R. L. (1994a). The relationship between acute psychiatric symptoms, diagnosis, and short-term risk of violence. *Hospital and Community Psychiatry, 45,* 133–137.

McNiel, D. E., & Binder, R. L. (1994b). Screening for risk of inpatient violence: Validation of an actuarial tool. *Law and Human Behavior, 18,* 579–586.

Megargee, E. I. (1976). The prediction of dangerous behavior. *Criminal Justice and Behavior, 3,* 3–22.

Menzies, R. J. (1989). *Survival of the sanest: Order and disorder in a pretrial psychiatric clinic.* Toronto: University of Toronto Press.

Menzies, R. J., & Webster, C. D. (1995). Construction and validation of risk assessments in a six-year follow-up of forensic patients: A tridimensional analysis. *Journal of Consulting and Clinical Psychology, 63,* 766–778.

Menzies, R. J., Webster, C. D., McMain, S., Staley, S., & Scaglione, R. (1994). The dimensions of dangerousness revisited: Assessing forensic predictions about violence. *Law and Human Behavior, 18,* 1–28.

Menzies, R. J., Webster, C. D., & Sepejak, D. S. (1985a). The dimensions of dangerousness: Evaluating the accuracy of psychometric predictions of violence among forensic patients. *Law and Human Behavior, 9,* 35–56.

Menzies, R. J., Webster, C. D., & Sepejak, D. S. (1985b). Hitting the forensic sound barrier: Predictions of dangerousness in a pre-trial psychiatric clinic. In C. D. Webster, M. H. Ben-Aron, & S. J. Hucker (Eds.), *Dangerousness: Probability and prediction, psychiatry and public policy* (pp. 115–143). New York: Cambridge University Press.

Monahan, J. (1981). *Predicting violent behavior: An assessment of clinical techniques.* Beverly Hills, CA: Sage.

Monahan, J. (1984). The prediction of violent behavior: Toward a second generation of theory and policy. *American Journal of Psychiatry, 141,* 10–15.

Monahan, J. (1988). Risk assessment of violence among the mentally disordered: Generating useful knowledge. *International Journal of Law and Psychiatry, 11,* 249–257.

Monahan, J. (1992). Mental disorder and violent behavior. *American Psychologist, 47,* 511–521.

Monahan, J., & Steadman, H. J. (Eds.). (1994). *Violence and mental disorder: Developments in risk assessment.* Chicago: University of Chicago Press.

Monahan, J., & Steadman, H. J. (1996). Violent storms and violent people: How meteorology can inform risk communication in mental health law. *American Psychologist, 51,* 931–938.

Moore, M. H., Estrich, S. R., McGillis, D., & Spelman, W. (1984). *Dangerous offenders: The elusive target of justice.* Cambridge, MA: Harvard University Press.

Mossman, D. (1994). Assessing predictions of violence: Being accurate about accuracy. *Journal of Consulting and Clinical Psychology, 62,* 783–792.

Mulvey, E. P. (1994). Assessing the evidence of a link between mental illness and violence. *Hospital and Community Psychiatry, 45,* 663–668.

Novaco, R. W. (1994). Anger as a risk factor for violence among the mentally disordered. In J. Monahan & H. J. Steadman (Eds.), *Violence and mental disorder: Developments in risk assessment* (pp. 21–59). Chicago: University of Chicago Press.

Pfohl, S. J. (1978). *Predicting dangerousness: The social construction of psychiatric reality.* Lexington, MA: Lexington Books.

Prentky, R. A., Knight, R. A., Lee, A. F. S., & Cerce, D. D. (1995). Predictive validity of lifestyle impulsivity for rapists. *Criminal Justice and Behavior, 22,* 106–128.

Quinsey, V. L., Rice, M. E., & Harris, G. T. (1995). Actuarial prediction of sexual recidivism. *Journal of Interpersonal Violence, 10,* 85–105.

Rice, M. E., & Harris, G. T. (1995). Violent recidivism: Assessing predictive validity. *Journal of Consulting and Clinical Psychology, 63,* 737–748.

Robins, L. N., Tipp, J., & Przybeck, T. (1991). Antisocial personality. In L. N. Robins & D. Reiger (Eds.), *Psychiatric disorders in America* (pp. 258–290). New York: Free Press.

Roesch, R., Webster, C. D., & Eaves, D. (1984). The fitness interview test: A method for examining fitness to stand trial. Toronto: University of Toronto, Centre of Criminology.

Selby, M. J. (1984). Assessment of violence potential using measures of anger, hostility, and social desirability. *Journal of Personality Assessment, 48,* 531–543.

Serin, R. C. (1991). Psychopathy and violence in criminals. *Journal of Interpersonal Violence, 6,* 423–431.

Serin, R. C., & Amos, N. L. (1995). The role of psychopathy in the assessment of dangerousness. *International Journal of Law and Psychiatry, 18,* 231–238.

Smith, C., & Thornberry, T. P. (1995). The relationship between childhood maltreatment and adolescent involvement in delinquency. *Criminology, 33,* 451–481.

Snyder, S., Pitts, W. M., & Pokorny, A. D. (1986). Selected behavioral features of patients with borderline personality traits. *Suicide and Life-Threatening Behavior, 16,* 28–39.

Steadman, H. J., & Cocozza, J. J. (1974). *Careers of the criminally insane: Excessive social control of deviance.* Lexington, MA: Lexington Books.

Steadman, H. J., Monahan, J., Appelbaum, P. S., Grisso, T., Mulvey, E. P., Roth, L. H., Robbins, P. C., & Klassen, D. (1994). Designing a new generation of risk assessment research. In J. Monahan & H. J. Steadman (Eds.), *Violence and mental disorder: Developments in risk assessment* (pp. 297–318). Chicago: University of Chicago Press

Swanson, J. W. (1994). Mental disorder, substance abuse, and community violence: An epidemiological approach. In J. Monahan & H. J. Steadman (Eds.), *Violence and mental disorder: Developments in risk assessment* (pp. 101–136). Chicago: University of Chicago Press.

Swanson, J. W., Borum, R., Swartz, M. S., & Monahan, J. (1996). Psychotic symptoms and disorders and the risk of violent behavior in the community. *Criminal Behaviour and Mental Health, 6,* 309–329.

Taylor, P. J. (1986). Psychiatric disorder in London's life-sentenced offenders. *British Journal of Criminology, 26,* 63–78.

Teplin, L. A. (1990). The prevalence of severe mental disorder among male urban jail detainees: Comparison with the Epidemiologic Catchment Area program. *American Journal of Public Health, 80,* 663–669.

Thornberry, T. P., & Jacoby, J. E. (1979). *The criminally insane: A community follow-up of mentally ill offenders.* Chicago: University of Chicago Press.

Torrey, E. F. (1994). Violent behavior by individuals with serious mental illness. *Hospital and Community Psychiatry, 45,* 653–662.

Webster, C. D. (1984). How much of the clinical predictability of dangerousness issue is due to language and communication difficulties?: Some sample courtroom questions and some inspired but heady answers. *International Journal of Offender Therapy and Comparative Criminology, 28,* 159–167.

Webster, C. D. (1985). Defending dangerous offenders. *Criminal Lawyer's Association Newsletter, 6,* 6–10.

Webster, C. D., Dickens, B. M., & Addario, S. M. (1985). *Constructing dangerousness: Scientific, legal and policy implications.* Toronto: University of Toronto, Centre of Criminology.

Webster, C. D., Douglas, K. S., Eaves, D., & Hart, S. D. (1997). *HCR-20: Assessing risk for violence (version 2).* Vancouver: Mental Health, Law, & Policy Institute, Simon Fraser University.

Webster, C. D., Eaves, D., Douglas, K. S., & Wintrup, A. (1995). *The HCR-20 scheme: The assessment of dangerousness and risk.* Vancouver: Simon Fraser University and Forensic Psychiatric Services Commission of British Columbia.

Webster, C. D., Harris, G. T., Rice, M. E., Cormier, C., & Quinsey, V. L. (1994). *The Violence Prediction Scheme: Assessing dangerousness in high risk men.* Toronto: University of Toronto, Centre of Criminology.

Webster, C. D., & Menzies, R. (1993). Supervision in the deinstitutionalized community. In S. Hodgins (Ed.), *Crime and mental disorder* (pp. 22–38). Newbury Park, CA: Sage.

Webster, C. D., & Polvi, N. H. (1995). Challenging assessments of dangerousness and risk. In J. Ziskin (Ed.), *Coping with psychiatric and psychological testimony* (5th ed., pp. 1372–1399). Los Angeles: Law and Psychology Press.

Welsh, W. N., & Gordon, A. (1991). Cognitive mediators of aggression: Test of a causal model. *Criminal Justice and Behavior, 18,* 125–145.

Wessely, S. (1993). Violence and psychosis. In C. Thompson & P. Cohen (Eds.), *Violence: Basic and clinical science* (pp. 119–134). Oxford: Butterworth–Heinemann.

Williamson, S., Hare, R. D., & Wong, S. (1987). Violence: Criminal psychopaths and their victims. *Canadian Journal of Behavioural Science, 19,* 454–462.

Wintrup, A. (1996). *Assessing risk of violence in mentally disordered offenders with the HCR-20.* Unpublished master's thesis, Simon Fraser University, Burnaby, British Columbia.

Woodcock, J. H. (1986). A neuropsychiatric approach to impulse disorders. *Psychiatric Clinics of North America, 9,* 341–352.

Yarvis, R. M. (1990). Axis I and Axis II diagnostic parameters of homicide. *Bulletin of the American Academy of Psychiatry and the Law, 18,* 249–269.

Yudofsky, S. C., Silver, J. M., Jackson, W., Endicott, J., & Williams, D. (1986). The Overt Aggression Scale for the objective rating of verbal and physical aggression. *American Journal of Psychiatry, 143,* 35–39.

Scoring Sheet for the 20-Item Historical/Clinical/ Risk Management (HCR-20) Scheme, Version 2

Participant's Name _____   Date _____

Assessor's Name _____   Participant's Gender _____

Participant's Current Age _____

Historical Items	Omit	0	1	2	Total
H1 Previous violence					
H2 Young age at first violent incident					
H3 Relationship instability					
H4 Employment problems					
H5 Substance use problems					
H6 Major mental illness					
H7 Psychopathy					
H8 Early maladjustment					
H9 Personality disorder					
H10 Prior supervision failure					
Historical Item Total					**/20**

Clinical Items

C1 Lack of insight					
C2 Negative attitudes					
C3 Active symptoms of major mental illness					
C4 Impulsivity					
C5 Unresponsive to treatment					
Clinical Item Total					**/10**

Risk Management Items   Out [   ]   In [   ]

Risk Management Items

R1 Plans lack feasibility					
R2 Exposure to destabilizers					
R3 Lack of personal support					
R4 Noncompliance with remediation attempts					
R5 Stress					
Risk Management Item Total					**/10**

Overall Total Score					**/40**

15

Assessing Risk of Suicide in Correctional Settings

NATALIE H. POLVI

Although impulsivity is often connected with acting violently toward others, it can also be a factor in acting against the self as in the case of attempted or completed suicide. Both psychological and pharmacological research have provided evidence for a link between impulsivity and suicidal behavior. For example, psychometric measures of impulsivity have distinguished between suicidal and nonsuicidal psychiatric inpatients (Apter, Plutchik, & van Praag, 1993; Kotler et al., 1993), and an examination of 350 suicide attempters revealed that 40% exhibited less than 5 minutes' premeditation in contemplating their act (Williams, Davidson, & Montgomery, 1980). Research evidence for a biological basis to any relationship between impulsivity and suicide has involved demonstrating that abnormalities in the serotonergic system play a role in suicidal behavior (Bourgeois, 1991; Golden et al., 1991; Stanley, Winchel, Molcho, Simeon, & Stanley, 1992). Given this evidence of a link between impulsivity and suicidal behavior, it is the purpose of this chapter to explore the issue of assessment and prediction of suicide, with emphasis on the correctional context.

The assessment and estimation of suicidal risk constitute a serious and difficult task for any mental health professional. Add to this the challenges that may be presented by a specific population (e.g., youths, native peoples, the severely drug-addicted), and the task may appear even more complicated. This chapter not only outlines the factors relevant to assessing suicidal risk in incarcerated sentenced clients, but provides a checklist—Estimate of Suicide Risk (ESR)—that quantifies the assessed level of suicide risk by consolidating these factors. The preliminary form of the ESR presented here is based on (1) the research literature examining suicide prediction in general and in the prison population in particular, and (2) my own clinical experience in a Canadian medium-security federal penitentiary, Warkworth Institution.

The ESR is not intended for long-term prediction, but rather for short-term assessment of suicide risk in a clinical forensic setting. In addition, the scale is primarily targeted toward sentenced prisoners as opposed to remand or jail inmates. This differentiation is necessary, given the body of research addressing jail suicides, which demonstrates that jail suicides have some distinct characteristics (Bonner, 1992; Haycock, 1991; Hayes, 1995a; Lloyd, 1990). Although the ESR has been based on relevant research literature as much as possible, neither its psychometric properties nor its predictive power has yet been demonstrated. However, even in the absence of an empirically based assessment tool, one can argue that simply constructing a model for decision making may improve accuracy (Dawes, Faust, & Meehl, 1989). Currently there exist several suicide risk scales for the general population that have demonstrated psychometric properties (for a review, see Rothberg & Geer-Williams, 1992); one of these instruments is an empirically derived scale based on a large prospective study (Motto, 1985; Motto, Heilbron, & Juster, 1985). Some suicide screening instruments have also been designed for jail populations (Arboleda-Florez & Holley, 1988; Sherman & Morschauser, 1989). At present, however, there appears to be no scale specifically addressing the estimation of suicidal risk in sentenced prison populations.

Sherman and Morschauser's (1989) screening guidelines for jail detainees and Kropp, Hart, Webster, and Eaves's (1994) manual for the Spousal Assault and Risk Assessment Guide (SARA), were used as guides for structuring the ESR checklist. Also taken into account were reviews of suicide predictors in the general population (Clark & Fawcett, 1992; Maris, 1992a). The risk factors that make up the ESR include 9 historical and actuarial factors and 11 clinical factors. Research demonstrating each factor's relevance to suicidal risk is summarized, and literature relevant to both the general population and incarcerated populations is reviewed whenever such literature exists. In what follows, the ESR items are considered in their order of appearance on the preliminary score sheet presented in the Appendix. Readers who wish more information on a proposed scoring procedure may receive it by writing to me (see the Acknowledgments).

HISTORICAL RISK FACTORS

Psychiatric History

Having a psychiatric history is associated with an elevated risk for suicidal behavior in both the general population (Clark & Fawcett, 1992;

Roy & Draper, 1995; Tanney, 1992; Westermeyer, Harrow, & Marengo, 1991) and the prison population (Anno, 1985; Bonner, 1992; Burtch & Ericson, 1979; Dooley, 1990; Green, Kendall, Andre, Looman, & Polvi, 1993; Levey, 1990; Topp, 1979). It is difficult to identify the precise degree of increased suicide risk presented by specific psychiatric diagnoses, since studies vary in the populations examined (e.g., inpatient, outpatient, or both), the length of follow-up, and the disorders (or combination of disorders) targeted for study (Appleby, 1992).

Clark and Fawcett (1992) made an admirable effort to provide some general conclusions about the risk presented by certain psychiatric disorders. They reviewed six studies, each of which investigated the psychological autopsies of 100 or more community-based suicides. Clark and Fawcett concluded that these studies, representing four different countries, "converge on the conclusion that a recent major psychiatric disorder is implicated in no less than 93% of cases of adult suicide" (p. 18). Regarding the prevalence of specific psychiatric disorders among suicides, they concluded that 40–60% of the cases displayed major depression, 20% chronic alcoholism, and 10% schizophrenia. Combining depression and alcoholism accounted for 57–86% of all suicides. Related to the specific risk experienced by schizophrenics, both Tanney (1992) and Clark and Fawcett (1992) reviewed recent research suggesting that individuals with "atypical psychoses (i.e., schizoaffective disorder, schizophreniform disorder, and other atypical psychoses)" (Clark & Fawcett, 1992, pp. 39–40) have an increased risk of suicide. In particular, these researchers, as well as Westermeyer et al. (1991), have concluded that young male schizophrenics are at particularly high risk for suicide.

In research predominantly examining sentenced prisoners, this factor of psychiatric history is usually broadly defined. Typically, it refers to previous psychiatric contact, admissions, unspecified diagnosis, or unspecified treatment. Estimated proportions of prison suicide samples with a psychiatric history range from 33% as calculated by Dooley (1990) to 78% as reported by Burtch and Ericson (1979). Studies of prisoner suicide make little differentiation among types of psychiatric diagnoses, very possibly because of deficits in the completeness or availability of prisoner records. Several studies have specifically identified the prevalence of depressive disorders or diagnoses among the respective suicide sample. Backett (1987) found that 6% of 33 prisoner suicides in Scottish prisons had a depressive disorder; Burtch and Ericson (1979) reported that 30% of 96 suicides in Canadian maximum-security penitentiaries had a history of depression; Schimmel, Sullivan, and Mrad (1989) found that 9% of 43 U.S. federal prisoner suicides had been treated for depression; and Dooley (1990) reported that 7% of 295 prisoner suicides in England and Wales had a history of depressive illness. Finally, Topp (1979) found that 10% of 186 suicides in English prisons had a history of definite depressive episodes, whereas an additional 42% "had shown some tendency to depression in the past" (p. 25). In a study examining the prevalence of mental disorders and suicide attempts in sentenced prisoners (Bland, Newman, Dyck, & Orn, 1990), suicide attempters exhibited a higher prevalence of antisocial personality disorder (1.5 times that of nonattempters), major depressive episode (2.3 times), and anxiety and somatoform disorders (4.5 times).

History of Alcohol or Drug Abuse

In a review of the literature on the relationship between substance abuse and the risk of suicide, Lester (1992) concluded that substance abuse increases this risk. Research subsequent to Lester's review has supported this conclusion (Klatsky & Armstrong, 1993; Suokas & Lonnqvist, 1995; Wasserman, Varnik, & Eklund, 1994). A meta-analysis of published studies examining the lifetime risk of suicide in alcoholics indicated that they have a risk 60 to 120 times that of the general population (Murphy & Wetzel, 1990). In addition, there is evidence that the combination of alcoholism and depression further increases the risk of suicidal behavior (Bulik, Carpenter, Kupfer, & Frank, 1990; Fawcett, Clark, & Busch, 1993; Fowler, Liskow, & Tanna, 1980; Murphy & Wetzel, 1990).

Research on prison suicides suggests that a history of substance abuse may be particularly prevalent among this population. For example, Green et al. (1993) found that 65% of 133 Canadian prison suicides had a history of alcohol abuse, and that 54% of this sample had a history of drug abuse. Similarly, the New York State Commission of Corrections reported that 62% of suicides had documented histories of alcohol or other substance abuse (as cited in Sherman & Morschauser, 1989). Dooley (1990) discovered that 29% of 295 suicides had a history of alcohol abuse and 23% had a history of drug abuse. Bland et al. (1990) found that prisoners with a history of suicide attempt(s) had a prevalence rate of alcohol abuse or dependence 1.2 times greater, and a prevalence rate for drug abuse or dependence 1.4 times greater, than the rates for nonattempters. Finally, a prospective 6-year follow-up study on pretrial forensic patients revealed that both drug abuse and alcohol abuse were significant (and separate) predictors of later suicidal behavior (in the form of thoughts, threats, attempts, and completed suicides) (Daley, 1987).

Prior Suicide Attempt(s)

Research on suicide in both the general population (Maris, 1992b; Moller, 1990; Steer, Beck, Garrison, & Lester, 1988) and psychiatric populations (Allebeck, Varla, Kristjansson, & Wistedt, 1987; Roy & Draper, 1995) indicates that one or more prior suicide attempts increase the risk of a later completed suicide. Although a number of factors affect the relative risk of an attempter's eventually completing a suicide (e.g., gender, marital status, age, psychosocial factors), studies indicate that the proportion of suicide completers with previous nonfatal suicide attempts ranges from 1% to 11% (Maris, 1992b). From examining a different set of studies—those based on psychological autopsies of community-based (rather than institutional) suicides—Clark and Fawcett (1992) concluded that 18–38% of suicide completers had attempted suicide on a previous occasion. Finally, recent research (Rudd, Joiner, & Rajab, 1996) indicates that people with multiple prior attempts present with more severe clinical symptoms (e.g., severity of suicidal ideation, more hopelessness, more depressive symptomatology) than do people with a history of either one attempt or just suicidal ideation.

This variable has been examined quite consistently in prisoner suicide research (Anno, 1985; Bonner, 1992; Burtch & Ericson, 1979; Dooley, 1990; Green et al., 1993; Lloyd, 1990; Topp, 1979), and these studies have found that from 40% to 55% of the suicide samples had a suicidal history. There is some indication that these percentages represent a disproportionately high level of suicide attempts in the suicide samples as compared to the general prison population. Bland et al. (1990) compared a sample of 180 randomly selected male prisoners with 1,006 matched community male residents, and reported a 23% lifetime prevalence of suicide attempts among sentenced prisoners. Thus, the estimated prior-attempt rate of 40–55% among prisoner suicides is approximately twice the rate found in Bland et al.'s sample. Of particular note is a finding (Green et al., 1993) that 94% of prisoner suicides had made a prior attempt within a year of the actual completed suicide. This finding is consistent with a generalization made by Maris (1992b), based on his examination of the relationship between nonfatal suicide attempts and completed suicide: "The probability of completing suicide is especially high in the first year or two after the initial nonfatal suicide attempt" (p. 374).

History of Impulsive Behavior

As mentioned earlier, some psychological and pharmacological research has indicated that impulsivity is positively related to an elevated risk for attempting or committing suicide. The precise role that impulsivity plays in elevating suicidal risk continues to be the subject of research. However, the relationship between impulsivity and suicidal behavior is often examined in relation to violent behavior (e.g., Apter et al., 1993; Brown, Linnoila, & Goodwin, 1992; Kotler et al., 1993). Indeed, Plutchik and van Praag (1990) reviewed two different bodies of research and concluded that there is a definite relationship between suicide and violence. Based on this conclusion and their subsequent study of psychiatric inpatients, Plutchik and van Praag proposed a two-stage model of suicide and violence. They suggested that certain classes of events (e.g., challenges, threats, losses) trigger aggressive impulses, and that the likelihood of violent behavior depends on a large number of factors that may serve to increase or decrease the aggressive impulse (e.g., weapons availability, history of assaultive behavior, personality style, interpersonal style). However, "a separate set of variables determines whether the goal of aggressive actions will be other people or oneself" (1990, p. 60). Their interviews of 100 psychiatric inpatients suggested which variables might be related to suicide but not violence, or vice versa. Specifically, impulsivity was found to be a correlate of violence only. Plutchik and van Praag (1990) suggested that the presence and interaction of these two sets of variables (with one variable being impulsivity) is what ultimately determines the strength and target (i.e., others or self) of aggressive behavior.

In a further examination of this issue, Plutchik and van Praag (1995) reviewed research on the relationship among impulsivity, suicidal behavior, and violent behavior. Upon examining four studies that used a psychometric measure of impulsivity, they concluded that both suicidal and violent patients exhibited significantly higher levels of impulsivity. In one study, when the relationship between impulsivity and violence was partialed out, the correlation between impulsivity and suicide risk was .22. Some additional support for a relationship among impulsivity, suicidal behavior, and violence is offered by Swedish researchers. Bergman and Brismar (1994) investigated the hormonal levels and personality characteristics of 49 male alcoholics as these factors related to the patients' violence and suicidal history. They found a significant positive correlation between the number of prior violent episodes and the number of suicide attempts. Psychometric measures of impulsivity and muscle tension significantly differentiated patients with or without prior suicide attempt(s). Bergman and Brismar concluded: "Our results confirm that there is a positive correlation between suicidal and abusive behavior. As the correlation coefficient was 0.33, ~10% of the variation in suicide attempts in this material can be explained by the abusive behavior" (1994, p. 313).

Overall, though the relationship appears complex, the empirical research suggests that impulsivity is associated with an increased risk of suicidal behavior. Even if this relationship is mediated or determined by proneness to violence, this is reason enough to consider it in a correctional population, since such a population will probably contain a high proportion of individuals who have demonstrated histories of violent behavior.

Family History of Suicide

Research has demonstrated that suicide tends to run in families, and that a genetic factor is implicated in familial histories of suicide (Kety, 1986; Mitterauer, 1990; Roy, 1992; Tsuang, 1983). Generally, first-degree relatives (i.e., offspring and siblings) of people who have committed suicide are at greater risk of suicide. In addition, studies on psychiatric patient populations indicate that relatives of people with mood disorders (i.e., bipolar disorders, depression) who committed suicide are at an even greater risk of suicide (Mitterauer, 1990; Roy, 1994; Tsuang, 1983). Roy (1992), reviewing Danish adoption studies that investigated the genetic factors in suicide, concluded: "the Copenhagen adoption studies strongly suggest that there may be a genetic factor for suicide that is independent of, or additive to, the genetic transmission of affective disorder" (p. 579). Kety (1986) reached a similar conclusion in an earlier review of research examining genetic aspects of suicide. Recent research provides additional support for such a conclusion. Brent, Bridge, Johnson, and Connolly (1996) studied the first- and second-degree relatives of 58 adolescent suicides and 55 matched control subjects. They compared the two groups of relatives in terms of suicidal behavior, Axis I and II psychiatric disorders, and lifetime history of aggressive behavior. Brent et al. found that the relatives of adolescent suicides had a higher rate of suicidal behavior (i.e., attempts or completions) even after controlling for the prevalence of Axis I and II disorders. Kety (1986) hypothesized that impulsive behavior may be the mediating genetic factor in suicide. He suggested:

> It is an interesting possibility that the genetic predisposition to suicide may represent a tendency to impulsive behavior of which suicide is a prime example. . . . We cannot dismiss the possibility that the genetic factor in suicide is an inability to control impulsive behavior, while depression and other mental illness as well as overwhelming environmental stress serve as potentiating mechanisms which foster or trigger the impulsive behavior, directing it toward a suicidal outcome. (1986, p. 44)

ACTUARIAL RISK FACTORS

Several actuarial factors related to the risk of prisoner suicide are consistently mentioned in the research literature. Unfortunately, these factors alone tend to provide low predictive ability, because they are common to a large proportion of the prisoner population and are not limited to prisoners prone to suicide. In addition, because of methodological weaknesses such as the lack of comparison groups in many studies (Bonner, 1992; Haycock, 1991; Liebling, 1992; Lloyd, 1990), the research results are difficult to interpret. However, given the consistency of the literature in relating these factors to prisoner suicide, it appeared important to include them in the ESR. The following is a summary of these actuarial factors.

Age

In contrast to studies of suicide in the general population, which demonstrate that suicide occurs disproportionately in older age groups (i.e., those aged 45 and over; Clark & Fawcett, 1992; Garrison, 1992; Maris, 1992a), research on prisoner suicide (Bonner, 1992; Hatty & Walker, 1986; Lloyd,

1990; Salive, Smith, & Brewer, 1989) indicates that prisoners committing suicide tend to represent the younger age groups. Although no clear age cutoff emerges from the research, Liebling (1992) concluded from her review that the ages of prisoners who completed suicide were below the mean prisoner age in many studies. Salive et al. (1989) reported that the highest rate of prisoner suicide occurred in the 25-to-34 age group, whereas Schimmel et al. (1989) found that the highest proportion of prisoner suicides took place among those aged 30 to 39. Hatty and Walker (1986) reported that, compared to the general prison population, the highest proportion of Australian prison suicides occurred in the 20-to-29 age group, and the second highest in the 30-to-39 age group. Burtch and Ericson (1979) also found a bimodal distribution, in which younger inmates (aged 15 to 24) and older inmates (aged 50 and above) were more prone to commit suicide.

Marital Status

As in the general population, where unmarried males (Maris, 1992b) are more prone to suicide, single prisoners appear to be at greater risk of suicide (Backett, 1987; Burtch & Ericson, 1979; Dooley, 1990; Topp, 1979). Although most of the studies reviewed by Liebling (1992) suggested that the majority of prisoners committing suicide are single, she pointed out that comparison groups were rarely used in these studies. Lloyd (1990) stated that U.S. and British studies agreed that between 70% and 80% of prisoner suicides were not married. He noted the lack of control groups in the relevant research, but stated that in studies where control groups were used, the results demonstrated that comparatively more prisoner suicides were single. Lloyd also pointed out a confounding factor: The research generally does not account for cohabitation of unmarried prisoners.

Sentence Length

Most reviewers have concluded that prisoners with longer sentences are disproportionately represented among suicides (Bonner, 1992; Haycock, 1991; Hayes, 1995a; Liebling, 1992; Lloyd, 1990). Indeed, some have suggested that those serving life sentences constitute a distinct subgroup in terms of presenting elevated risk for suicide (Haycock, 1991; Liebling, 1992; Lloyd, 1990). Some researchers have found no relationship between sentence length and prisoner suicide (Anno, 1985; Green et al., 1993), but others have done so. Dooley (1990) found the highest suicide rate among prisoners serving sentences 4 years or longer, whereas Topp (1979) found the highest rate among prisoners serving more than 18 months. Burtch and Ericson (1979) reported that two groups were overrepresented among suicides: (1) prisoners serving 2 to 4 years, and (2) those serving life sentences. Hatty and Walker (1986) concluded that prisoners serving indefinite sentences are disproportionately represented among prisoner suicides. One difficulty in interpreting research findings relating sentence length to suicide is that sentence length is confounded with seriousness of crime, given that more serious and/or violent crimes tend to result in longer sentences (Haycock, 1991; Lloyd, 1990).

Time Served in Sentence

Generally, prisoners who commit suicide tend to do so early in their sentences (Burtch & Ericson, 1979; Dooley, 1990; Green et al., 1993). However, as Lloyd (1990) pointed out in his review, it is difficult to assess the available research on this variable, since researchers typically have not clearly differentiated between sentenced and unsentenced prisoners in their samples. Studies on suicide in temporary detention facilities (e.g., police lockups, remand facilities, jails) indicate that a disproportionate number of offenders commit suicide within 24 hours of lockup (Hayes, 1989). Lloyd's (1990) overall conclusion regarding this population was that there is a high rate of suicides within the first 2 weeks of remand custody. Studies using samples of either exclusively sentenced prisoners or a combination of remand and sentenced prisoners suggest very broadly that 3 months and 2 years may be important milestones. Upon examining a Canadian sample of 133 federally sentenced prisoners, we (Green et al., 1993) found that 25% of those committing suicide did so within 90 days of sentence commencement, and that a total of 51.5% of that group committed suicide within 1 year of beginning their sentences. In an earlier sample of federally sentenced prisoners, Burtch and Ericson (1979) calculated that 60.2% of 96 inmate suicides occurred within the first year of sentence, whereas an additional 21.9% of suicides occurred within 13–24 months of sentence commencement. Hayes (1995a) cited a study completed by the New York State Department of Correctional Services, in which 64% of 53 prisoner suicides were found to have committed suicide within the first 2 years of sentence. In a sample of 186 English prisoners (of whom 37% were remand or unsentenced) who committed suicide, Topp (1979) found that 61% committed suicide within 3 months of entering custody (the cumulative percentages at the 1-, 2-, and 3-month marks were 41.5%, 53%, and 61%, respectively).

CLINICAL RISK FACTORS

Suicidal Ideation and Suicidal Intent

Traditionally, assessment of suicidal risk has involved determining the presence of ideation, intention, and planning with respect to suicide (Fremouw, de Perczel, & Ellis, 1990; Sommers-Flanagan & Sommers-Flanagan, 1995). Beck and his colleagues have developed scales for assessing some of these classic clinical factors (for a review of these scales, see

Eyman & Eyman, 1992, and Weishaar & Beck, 1992). Indeed, by opera-
tionalizing suicidal ideation, suicidal intent, depression, and hopelessness, Beck and his colleagues have been able to demonstrate empirically
that these clinical factors are associated with an elevated risk for suicidal
behavior. Such scales assist both in the clinical assessment of individuals
and in research on suicide. Although Eyman and Eyman (1992) believe it
is likely that information about current suicidal risk is most effectively
obtained via interview, they have opined that using some suicide scales
can provide useful information about an individual's vulnerability to
suicidal behavior.

Suicidal Plan

Assessing a client's suicidal plan involves examining several factors: the
specificity of the plan, the lethality of the intended method, the availability of means, and the proximity of help or rescue (Bednar, Bednar,
Lamber, & Waite, 1991; Sommers-Flanagan & Sommers-Flanagan, 1995).
Particularly relevant are the chosen suicide method and its inherent
lethality. In a review of the literature on suicide methods, McIntosh (1992)
defined "lethality" as the probability of death as presented by a particular
method. He explained that lethality consists of two components. The first
component is the elapsed time between initiating the suicidal act and
death, with shorter time period being associated with greater lethality.
The second component is the potential for, and availability of, medical
intervention after the method has been used. Using official U.S. mortality
statistics for the years 1985 to 1987, McIntosh determined the percentages
of deaths attributable to various method types across three demographic
variables (sex, age, and ethnicity), and compared these data to those from
previous research to determine the trend over time. He found that the use
of firearms was consistently the most common method of suicide across
sex and age groups, and all but two ethnicity categories. Also, the use of
firearms has increased over time. Hanging was the second most common
method among males, whereas the use of solid or liquid poison was the
second most common method among females. Given that research reveals
hanging to be the predominant method of suicide in prison (Anno, 1985;
Bonner, 1992; Burtch & Ericson, 1979; Dooley, 1990; Green et al., 1993;
Hardyman, 1983; Lloyd, 1990; Salive et al., 1989; Schimmel et al., 1989;
Topp, 1979), the forensic clinician may wish to inquire of the prisoner
about this method specifically. In this respect, it is especially important
for the examiner to have precise knowledge of the potential means within
the prisoner's living space.

Hopelessness

Theory and research related to cognitive therapy as pioneered by Beck
and his colleagues have indicated that hopelessness is one of the key

factors related to suicidal behavior (Weishaar & Beck, 1992). Defining "hopelessness" as "a state of negative expectancies" (p. 471), Weishaar and Beck (1992) reviewed the research demonstrating the relationship between hopelessness and facets of suicidal behavior. Their statement that hopelessness is more strongly associated with suicidal intent and ideation than is depression was supported by subsequent research, which demonstrated that hopelessness in mood-disordered patients was 1.3 times more important than depression in predicting suicidal ideation (Beck, Steer, Beck, & Newman, 1993). Overall, after examining both prospective and longitudinal research, Weishaar and Beck (1992) concluded that the construct of hopelessness has predictive utility in regard to suicidality.

Consistent with such a conclusion, two studies have supported hopelessness as a significant predictor of suicidal behavior in sentenced prisoners (Holden, Mendonca, & Serin, 1989; Ivanoff & Jang, 1991). In addition, these studies have demonstrated that social desirability interacts with hopelessness in the prediction of suicidality. However, the respective researchers have offered differing interpretations of this interaction, which may well be a result of their using two different social desirability measures. In discussing their research, Holden et al. (1989) suggested that higher levels of perceived self-efficacy moderate the relationship between hopelessness and suicidality. In their paper, Ivanoff and Jang (1991) stated that the interaction involves an inverse relationship between hopelessness and social desirability, whereby the predictive ability of hopelessness decreases as social desirability increases.

Sudden Change in Psychological Functioning

Traditionally, in the clinical assessment and treatment of suicidality, a sudden, unexplained change in a client's mood and/or functioning has been associated with increased risk of suicide. Both Fremouw et al. (1990) and Maris (1992a) have discussed this clinical sign as it relates to depressive illness, and Drake, Gates, Whitaker and Cotton (1985) have concluded that it is a factor relevant to suicidal behavior in schizophrenics. Generally, it is thought that a slight improvement in a client's mental illness makes energy available for the client to act on suicidal intentions or plans. Having made the decision to commit suicide, the client may experience a reduction in tension or ambivalence and present a better mood than previously. It is not hard for correctional and clinical staff members to be beguiled by such superficially positive signs.

Stress, Vulnerability, and Coping

Reviewers of the research literature on the relationship between both recent and long-standing stressful life events and suicidality have concluded that such circumstances can play an important role in an individual's suicidal behavior (Heikkinen, Aro, & Lonnqvist, 1993; Yufit & Bongar, 1992). However, Yufit and Bongar (1992) cautioned that this is not a simple and direct relationship. Rather, they stated that stressful life events "must be contextualized within the larger overall picture of the individual's personality structure and lifelong characterological ability to cope with (or to be vulnerable to) stress, failure, and loss" (p. 557). Significantly, some research indicates that life stressors in general (Heikkinen et al., 1993) and interpersonal loss in particular (Murphy & Wetzel, 1990) may exacerbate the suicidal risk of alcoholics.

Bonner (1992) described the occurrence of prisoner suicide in a similar vein by referring to a "stress–vulnerability process" (p. 406). By drawing on the suicidology literature, which conceptualizes suicide as a process occurring over time, he hypothesized that "certain individuals are unprepared, ill equipped, and/or at a loss for resources to cope effectively with incarceration" (p. 415). Risk factors such as loneliness, alienation, and isolation break down the coping mechanisms of these individuals. Thus, they are left vulnerable to negative life events. Bonner concluded that the interaction of these risk factors and negative life events is what may lead to emotional breakdown over time, and, given certain conditions, to eventual suicide. Subsequent research (Bonner & Rich, 1992) has lent some support to this hypothesis by demonstrating a relationship between cognitive vulnerability and hopelessness in a sample of correctional inmates.

Levey (1990) also attributed a role to stress and stressors in prisoner suicide. In her review of suicide in U.K. correctional institutions, Levey linked suicide to the way stressors come together. She stated that "suicides in custody seem to be less the result of formal mental illness than a function of the clustering of stresses, together with a lack of adequate coping strategies to adjust to the stress of imprisonment" (p. 607).

Recent research by Liebling (1995) lends support to the proposed role of stress, vulnerability, and coping ability in the suicidal behavior of prisoners. Drawing subjects from four institutions for young offenders, three remand centers, and one prison, Liebling's research involved interviewing 100 prisoners who had attempted suicide and 112 randomly selected prisoners who had not attempted suicide. In comparing the two groups, she found significant differences in background variables and characteristics of their prison life. She used the term "vulnerable" to describe the attempters, and stated that "their vulnerability, characterized by a history of adverse life circumstances followed by persistent problems in 'coping', was exposed by many different aspects of the prison world, from activities and relationships to planning for the future" (p. 179). Liebling realized that a large proportion of the prison populations shared the characteristics of her suicide attempter group. Therefore, she examined completed suicides in England and Wales from 1987 to 1993 and identified three distinct groups, which differed in age, history of self-injury, motivation for suicide, and situational factors attributable to death. Not only did she demonstrate that one of the three groups closely resembled the vulnerable "poor copers" who constituted most of the attempters in her study; she also showed that this same group accounted for more completed suicides (30–45%) than the other two groups combined. Consistent with Liebling's research is a study based on the completion of self-report scales by prisoners who had attempted suicide or perpetrated intentional self-harm (Holden et al., 1989). The authors concluded that higher levels of capability or self-efficacy on the part of prisoners moderated the relationship between hopelessness and suicidality.

Depressive Symptomatology

The role of depression as a risk factor in suicide can be a subject of confusion. Tanney (1992) pointed out that some researchers have failed to distinguish between depression as a syndrome or symptom and depression as a mental disorder. This has resulted in difficulties in interpreting the results of some research. Despite this, Tanney acknowledged that one consistent finding of psychological autopsy studies is that mood disorders are the most important mental disorder diagnoses related to suicide. Upon reviewing the research literature on mental disorders and suicide, Tanney concluded that major depression (unipolar) and psychotic/melancholic depression are the depression subtypes most strongly related to suicidal behaviors.

In terms of depressive symptomatology, Smith (1986) found a significant correlation between dysphoric mood and suicidal ideation/attempts in young adults. These measures were also correlated with other measures of psychological distress, as well as with substance use. Beck et al. (1993) found a significant interaction between depression and hopelessness, such that "increasing levels of both self-reported depression and hopelessness were positively related to suicidal ideation" (p. 144). Other researchers have demonstrated a relationship between current depressive symptoms and suicidality (Cohen, Lavelle, Rich, & Bromet, 1994; DeMan & Leduc, 1995; Drake et al., 1985; Drake, Gates, & Cotton, 1986; Roy, 1982; Strakowski, McElroy, Keck, & West, 1996).

Given some empirical evidence of a causal relationship between depressive symptomatology and suicidal risk, as well as a link between depression and hopelessness (Beck et al., 1993; Sommers-Flanagan & Sommers-Flanagan, 1995; Weishaar & Beck, 1992), depressive symptomatology is included on the ESR. Certainly, given the conceptual relationship among depression, hopelessness, and suicidality, there is an argument for considering such active symptomatology in the assessment of suicidality. This conceptual connection consists of the "cognitive triad" in depressed patients, which is described as a "negative view of the self, the world, and the future" (Weishaar & Beck, 1992, p. 467), and the concomitant occurrence of hopelessness, which is described as being "associated with a pessimistic view of the future" (Weishaar & Beck, 1992, p. 467).

Current Use of Alcohol or Drugs

Although in theory prisons are not supposed to allow the consumption of alcohol or drugs on the premises, the fact is these substances tend to be present and obtainable by prisoners. Given these substances' disinhibiting effects on behavior, it is prudent to consider the possibility of a client's being under the influence of a substance. Research suggests that alcohol or drug dependence as a diagnosis is predictive of elevated risk for suicidal behavior (Klatsky & Armstrong, 1993; Maris, 1981; Sundry, 1972). In addition, according to some research, alcohol use can be both an epidemiological and a clinical risk factor (Hawton, Fagg, & McKeown, 1989; Murphy, Wetzel, Robins, & McEvoy, 1992; Suokas & Lonnqvist, 1995; Weishaar & Beck, 1992). For instance, Weishaar and Beck (1992) reviewed several relevant studies demonstrating a relationship between alcohol consumption and suicidal action. They concluded that a person need not be an alcoholic for this risk to be present, since "use of alcohol at the time of suicidal ideation may increase the possibility of poor judgment, lack of control, and mood changes" (p. 471). Weiss and Stephens (1992) suggested that a greater risk of suicide can result from increased aggressiveness, impaired judgment, greater impulsivity, and/or engagement in high-risk activities.

Psychotic Symptoms

Research investigating the connection between psychotic symptoms and suicidal risk can be difficult to interpret and consolidate because of semantic differences. Some researchers use the term "psychotic" to refer to a disorder, while others use the term to refer to a temporary state or discrete symptoms (e.g., delusions). As an example of the former, Tanney (1992) concluded that suicide occurs more frequently among people with psychotic versus neurotic disorders. As an example of the latter, Clark and Fawcett (1992) stated that in schizophrenics, suicide is less likely to occur during "exacerbations of florid psychosis" (p. 40) but more likely to occur with delusions of persecution (i.e., paranoia). In addition, they concluded that "the presence of 'command hallucinations,' or hallucinations instructing the patient to perform specific acts, particularly violent or destructive acts, does not appear to be associated with greater suicide risk" (p. 40). Furthermore, some researchers study psychotic patients whose diagnosis is depression (Miller & Chabrier, 1987); some study psychotic patients whose diagnosis is schizophrenia (Virkkunen, 1974);

and some study both populations (Westermeyer & Harrow, 1989). In their review, Weiden and Roy (1992) supported the conclusion that there is little empirical support for hallucinations as a risk factor for suicidal behavior. However, they also pointed out that methodological difficulties in this research may mask the true effects of psychotic symptoms on suicidality. For instance, clinicians tend to hospitalize schizophrenics with psychotic symptoms more often than they do those with depressive symptoms. As a result, psychotic schizophrenics are protected from suicide, and the potential influence of psychotic symptoms on their behavior is affected by clinical intervention.

Overall, the literature appears to suggest that some psychotic symptoms represent an elevated risk for suicide in people diagnosed with primarily affective disorders (e.g., depression) (e.g., Cohen et al., 1994; Fawcett et al., 1987; Miller & Chabrier, 1987; Roose, Glassman, Walsh, Woodring, & Vital-Herne, 1983). Although Fremouw et al. (1990) drew the general conclusion that "psychosis, whether secondary to affective disorder or schizophrenia, presents a major risk for suicide" (p. 110), they based their conclusion on a limited amount of research. Fremouw et al. suggested that the symptoms most likely to be associated with suicidal risk are delusions or command hallucinations in which there is a compulsion to die. Research by Robins (1986) may lend some support to Fremouw et al.'s conclusion. Robins retrospectively diagnosed psychoses (defined as delusions; hallucinations; bizarre behaviors; formal thought disorder; or experiencing confusion, disorientation, or memory loss) in 25 of 134 suicides occurring in St. Louis in a 1-year period. Active psychoses occurred not solely in those with affective disorders, but also in those with diagnoses of alcohol dependence, organic brain syndrome, and schizophrenia.

Physical Isolation

There are two types of isolation that appear relevant as risk factors in the suicidal prisoner. The first is physical isolation. Research on prison and jail suicide has revealed that a disproportionate percentage (60–79%) of suicides occur while the prisoners are confined to locations that are remote from the general prison population (Bonner, 1992; Burtch & Ericson, 1979; Hayes, 1989; Liebling, 1992; Lloyd, 1990; Schimmel et al., 1989). Typically these locations are isolation cells in a segregated area of the prison/jail, but they may also include single cells in observation units or psychiatric/medical units of a prison.

Psychosocial Isolation

The second type of isolation is psychosocial, in which the prisoner is isolated from emotional and social sources of support (Sherman & Morschauser, 1989). A lack of social support has been identified as a risk factor for suicidality in a number of populations (Drake et al., 1986; Heikkinen et al., 1993; Kotler et al., 1993; Roy, 1982; Veiel, Brill, Hafner, & Welz, 1988). In regard to incarceration, Bonner (1992) outlined the potential mechanisms by which physical and psychosocial isolation interact and contribute to enhanced suicidal risk. He suggested that those in prison experience psychosocial isolation, and that some individuals are more vulnerable to both isolation and life stressors than are other prisoners. These vulnerable persons, who are already apt to be at heightened risk for suicidal behavior, tend to be at even greater risk with the addition of physical isolation.

CONCLUSION

In a book devoted to examining impulsive behavior, it is fitting to consider suicidal behavior. Attempted or completed suicide appears linked to impulsivity, according to psychometric, biological, and genetic research that has examined the relationship between impulsiveness and suicidal behavior. However, the assessment and prediction of suicidal risk require consideration of multiple factors. To this end, the present chapter has endeavored to summarize and consolidate the factors most relevant to assessing suicidality in incarcerated populations. The ESR checklist is presented primarily as a guide to the forensic clinician in assessing the level of a prisoner's suicidal risk. Although its predictive validity and psychometric integrity have not yet been demonstrated, the ESR is expected to be directly relevant to estimating suicide risk in sentenced prisoners, given that it has been thoroughly grounded in the relevant literature.

It should be noted that the majority of prisoner suicide research focuses on the suicidal risk factors related to the male prisoner; therefore, the ESR is heavily weighted toward assessing risk of suicide in male prisoners. However, the risk factors outlined in the present chapter may provide some assistance to clinicians assessing suicidality in female offenders as well. Liebling (1994) has outlined the commonalities and differences in suicide risk factors between male and female prisoners. The common factors include being at an early stage of custody, being mentally disordered, being charged or convicted of murder, having a history of drug or alcohol abuse, making previous suicide attempts, and being physically isolated in the prison. The risk factors specific to female prisoners include having a history of arson or violence, having major alcohol problems, and having many self-inflicted injuries.

Other conditions limiting the predictive power of the ESR include the inherent difficulties in the prediction of suicide and the methodological weaknesses in prisoner suicide research (Cohen, 1986; Robins & Kulbok, 1986). One major difficulty resides in the fact that suicide is a relatively infrequent event, and thus is automatically difficult to predict. In addition, a number of factors in the ESR (e.g., history of substance abuse, age, marital status) are characteristic of a large proportion of the prisoner population, and thus have only limited power in the prediction of suicide. Furthermore, several methodological weaknesses in the prisoner suicide research (Bonner, 1992; Haycock, 1991; Liebling, 1992; Lloyd, 1990) restrict the degree to which solid conclusions can be drawn from many studies. The descriptive and retrospective nature of most suicide research makes it difficult to establish the causal role of some factors. The general lack of control and comparison groups, particularly in research examining historical and actuarial factors, limits definitive conclusions about differences between offenders who do and do not commit suicide. In addition, although dynamic clinical factors were incorporated into the ESR, suicide research generally focuses on static risk factors and a concomitant conceptualization of suicide as a distinct occurrence. This limits the extent to which the process of *becoming* suicidal can be considered when prisoner suicides are examined (Bonner, 1992).

Finally, it is recognized that assessing an individual's risk of suicide is only one element in the management and treatment of suicidal behavior. However, it has not been my intention here to discuss the separate issue of management of the suicidal client. There are several good sources to consult in this regard. A portion of Bongar's (1992) edited book is devoted to the management and treatment of suicidal clients. Bednar et al. (1991) provide two excellent chapters in which they discuss clinical interviews, case management, and the mental health professional's legal duties with respect to suicidal clients. It is also recommended that the reader consult articles on standards of care, despite the fact that they are not tailored to prisoner suicide (Bongar, Maris, Berman, Litman, & Silverman, 1993; Silverman, Berman, Bongar, Litman, & Maris, 1994). With particular reference to the correctional population, several sources can be consulted regarding the management of suicidal prisoners (Lester & Danto, 1993; Rakis & Monroe, 1989; Rosine, 1995) and suicide prevention in prison settings (Hayes, 1995a, 1995b; Liebling, 1992).

ACKNOWLEDGMENTS

The Estimate of Suicide Risk (ESR) checklist was conceptualized, and this chapter was written, while I was on education leave from my position as institutional psychologist at Warkworth Institution, Campbellford, Ontario. I gratefully acknowledge the sponsorship and support of this education leave by both Warkworth Institution and the Ontario Region of the Correctional Service of Canada. The opinions expressed in this chapter do not necessarily reflect those of the Correctional Service of Canada.

For a copy of the ESR, contact me at the Department of Psychology, Regional Reception and Assessment Centre, c/o Matsqui Institution, Correctional Service of Canada, Pacific Region, Box 2500, Abbotsford, British Columbia V2S 4P3, Canada.

REFERENCES

Allebeck, P., Varla, A., Kristjansson, E., & Wistedt, B. (1987). Risk factors for suicide among patients with schizophrenia. *Acta Psychiatrica Scandinavica, 76,* 414–419.

Anno, B. J. (1985). Patterns of suicide in Texas Department of Corrections, 1980–1985. *Journal of Prisons and Jail Health, 5,* 82–93.

Appleby, L. (1992). Suicide in psychiatric patients: Risk and prevention. *British Journal of Psychiatry, 161,* 749–758.

Apter, A. & Plutchik, R., & van Praag, H. M. (1993). Anxiety, impulsivity and depressed mood in relation to suicidal and violent behavior. *Acta Psychiatrica Scandinavica, 87,* 1–5.

Arboleda-Florez, J., & Holley, H. L. (1988). Development of a suicide screening instrument for use in a remand centre setting. *Canadian Journal of Psychiatry, 33,* 595–598.

Backett, S. A. (1987). Suicide in Scottish prisons. *British Journal of Psychiatry, 151,* 210–221.

Beck, A. T., Steer, R. A., Beck, J. S., & Newman, C. F. (1993). Hopelessness, depression, suicidal ideation, and clinical diagnosis of depression. *Suicide and Life-Threatening Behavior, 23,* 139–145.

Bednar, R. L., Bednar, S. C. Lamber, M. J., & Waite, D. R. (1991). *Psychotherapy with high-risk clients: Legal and professional standards.* Pacific Grove, CA: Brooks/Cole.

Bergman, B., & Brismar, B. (1994). Hormone levels and personality characteristics in abusive and suicidal male alcoholics. *Alcoholism: Clinical and Experimental Research, 18,* 311–316.

Bland, R. C., Newman, S. C., Dyck, R. J., & Orn, H. (1990). Prevalence of psychiatric disorders and suicide attempts in a prison population. *Canadian Journal of Psychiatry, 35,* 407–413.

Bongar, B. (Ed.). (1992). *Suicide: Guidelines for assessment, management, and treatment.* New York: Oxford University Press.

Bongar, B., Maris, R. W., Berman, A. L., Litman, R. E., & Silverman, M. M. (1993). Inpatient standards of care and the suicidal patient: Part I. General clinical formulations and legal considerations. *Suicide and Life-Threatening Behavior, 23,* 245–256.

Bonner, R. L. (1992). Isolation, seclusion, and psychosocial vulnerability as risk factors for suicide behind bars. In R. W. Maris, A. L. Berman, J. T. Maltsberger, & R. I. Yufit (Eds.), *Assessment and prediction of suicide* (pp. 398–419). New York: Guilford Press.

Bonner, R. L., & Rich, A. R. (1992). Cognitive vulnerability and hopelessness among correctional inmates: A state of mind model. *Journal of Offender Rehabilitation, 17,* 113–122.

Bourgeois, M. (1991). Serotonin, impulsivity and suicide. *Human Psychopharmacology, 6,* 31–36.

Brent, D. A., Bridge, J., Johnson, B. A., & Connolly, J. (1996). Suicidal behavior runs in families: A controlled family study of adolescent suicide victims. *Archives of General Psychiatry, 53,* 1145–1152.

Brown, G. L., Linnoila, M. K., & Goodwin, F. K. (1992). Impulsivity, aggression, and associated affects: Relationship to self-destructive behavior and suicide. In R. W. Maris, A. L. Berman, J. T. Maltsberger, & R. I. Yufit (Eds.), *Assessment and prediction of suicide* (pp. 589–606). New York: Guilford Press.

Bulik, C., Carpenter, L., Kupfer, D., & Frank, E. (1990). Features associated with suicide attempts in recurrent major depression. *Journal of Affective Disorders, 18,* 29–37.

Burtch, B. E., & Ericson, R. B. (1979). *The silent system: An inquiry into prisoners who suicide.* Toronto: University of Toronto, Centre of Criminology.

Clark, D. C., & Fawcett, J. (1992). Review of empirical risk factors for evaluation of the suicidal patient. In B. Bongar (Ed.), *Suicide: Guidelines for assessment, management, and treatment* (pp. 16–48). New York: Oxford University Press.

Cohen, J. (1986). Statistical approaches to suicide risk factor analysis. *Annals of the New York Academy of Sciences, 487,* 34–41.

Cohen, S., Lavelle, J., Rich, C. L., & Bromet, E. (1994). Rates and correlates of suicide attempts in first-admission psychotic patients. *Acta Psychiatrica Scandinavica, 90,* 167–171.

Daley, M. (1987). *The clinical prediction of dangerousness to self: A six-year follow-up of 283 forensic cases.* Unpublished master's thesis, University of Toronto.

Dawes, R. M., Faust, D., & Meehl, P. E. (1989). Clinical versus actuarial judgment. *Science, 243,* 1668–1674.

DeMan, A. F., & Leduc, C. P. (1995). Suicidal ideation in high school students: Depression and other correlates. *Journal of Clinical Psychology, 51,* 173–181.

Dooley, E. (1990). Prison suicide in England and Wales, 1972–87. *British Journal of Psychiatry, 156,* 40–45.

Drake, R., Gates, C., & Cotton, P. G. (1986). Suicide among schizophrenics: A comparison of attempters and completed suicides. *British Journal of Psychiatry, 149,* 784–787.

Drake, R., Gates, C., Whitaker, A., & Cotton, P. G. (1985). Suicide among schizophrenics: A review. *Comprehensive Psychiatry, 26,* 90–100.

Eyman, J. R., & Eyman, S. K. (1992). Psychological testing for potentially suicidal individuals. In B. Bongar (Ed.), *Suicide: Guidelines for assessment, management, and treatment* (pp. 127–143). New York: Oxford University Press.

Fawcett, J., Clark, D. C., & Busch, K. A. (1993). Assessing and treating the patient at risk for suicide. *Psychiatric Annals, 23,* 244–255.

Fawcett, J., Scheftner, W., Clark, D., Hedeker, D., Gibbons, R., & Coryell, W. (1987). Clinical predictors of suicide in patients with major affective disorders: A controlled prospective study. *American Journal of Psychiatry, 144,* 35–40.

Fowler, R. C., Liskow, B. I., & Tanna, V. L. (1980). Alcoholism, depression, and life events. *Journal of Affective Disorders, 2,* 127–135.

Fremouw, W. J., de Perczel, M., & Ellis, T. E. (1990). *Suicide risk: Assessment and response guidelines.* Elmsford, NY: Pergamon Press.

Garrison, C. Z. (1992). Demographic predictors of suicide. In R. W. Maris, A. L. Berman, J. T. Maltsberger, & R. I. Yufit (Eds.), *Assessment and prediction of suicide* (pp. 484–498). New York: Guilford Press.

Golden, R. N., Gilmore, J. H., Corrigan, M. H. N., Ekstrom, R. D., Knight, B. T., & Garbutt, J. C. (1991). Serotonin, suicide, and aggression: Clinical studies. *Journal of Clinical Psychiatry, 52,* 61–29.

Green, C., Kendall, K., Andre, G., Looman, T., & Polvi, N. (1993). A study of 133 suicides among Canadian federal prisoners. *Medicine, Science and the Law, 33,* 121–127.

Hardyman, P. L. (1983). *The ultimate escape: Suicide in Ohio's jails and temporary detention facilities: 1980–1981.* Columbus: Ohio Bureau of Adult Detention Facilities and Services.

Hatty, S. E., & Walker, J. R. (1986). *A national study of deaths in Australian prisons.* Canberra: Australian Institute of Criminology.

Hawton, K., Fagg, J., & McKeown, S. P. (1989). Alcoholism, alcohol and attempted suicide. *Alcohol and Alcoholism, 24,* 3–9.

Haycock, J. (1991). Crimes and misdemeanors: A review of recent research on suicides in prison. *Omega: Journal of Death and Dying, 23,* 81–94.

Hayes, L. M. (1989). National study of jail suicides: Seven years later. *Psychiatric Quarterly, 60,* 7–29.

Hayes, L. M. (1995a). Prison suicide: An overview and a guide to prevention. *The Prison Journal, 75,* 431–456.

Hayes, L. M. (1995b). *Prisoner suicide: An overview and guide to prevention.* Washington, DC: U.S. Department of Justice, National Institute of Corrections.

Heikkinen, M., Aro, H., & Lonnqvist, J. (1993). Life events and social support in suicide. *Suicide and Life-Threatening Behavior, 23,* 343–358.

Holden, R. R., Mendonca, J. D., & Serin, R. C. (1989). Suicide, hopelessness, and social desirability: A test of an interactive model. *Journal of Consulting and Clinical Psychology, 57,* 500–504.

Ivanoff, A., & Jang, S. J. (1991). The role of hopelessness and social desirability in predicting suicidal behavior: A study of prison inmates. *Journal of Consulting and Clinical Psychology, 59,* 394–399.

Kety, S. (1986). Genetic factors in suicide. In A. Roy (Ed.), *Suicide* (pp. 41–45). Baltimore: Williams & Wilkins.

Klatsky, A. L., & Armstrong, M. A. (1993). Alcohol use, other traits, and risk of unnatural death: A prospective study. *Alcoholism: Clinical and Experimental Research, 17,* 1156–1162.

Kotler, M., Finkelstein, G., Molcho, A., Botsis, A. J., Plutchik, R., Brown, S. L., & van Praag, H. M. (1993). Correlates of suicide and violence risk in an inpatient population: Coping styles and social support. *Psychiatry Research, 47,* 281–290.

Kropp, R. P., Hart, S. D., Webster, C. D., & Eaves, D. (1994). *Manual for the Spousal Assault Risk Assessment Guide.* Vancouver: British Columbia Institute on Family Violence.

Lester, D. L. (1992). Alcoholism and drug abuse. In R. W. Maris, A. L. Berman, J. T. Maltsberger, & R. I. Yufit (Eds.), *Assessment and prediction of suicide* (pp. 321–336). New York: Guilford Press.

Lester, D. L., & Danto, B. L. (1993). *Suicide behind bars: Prediction and prevention.* Philadelphia: Charles Press.

Levey, S. (1990). Suicide. In R. Bluglass & P. Bowden (Eds.), *Principles and practice of forensic psychiatry* (pp. 597-610). New York: Churchill Livingstone.

Liebling, A. (1992). *Suicides in prisons.* London: Routledge.

Liebling, A. (1994). Suicide amongst women prisoners. *Howard Journal of Criminal Justice, 33,* 1–9.

Liebling, A. (1995). Vulnerability and prison suicide. *British Journal of Criminology, 35,* 173–187.

Lloyd, C. (1990). *Suicide and self-injury in prison: A literature review* (Home Office Research Study No. 115). London: Her Majesty's Stationery Office.

Maris, R. W. (1992a). Overview of the study of suicide assessment and prediction. In R. W. Maris, A. L. Berman, J. T. Maltsberger, & R. I. Yufit (Eds.), *Assessment and prediction of suicide* (pp. 3–22). New York: Guilford Press.

Maris, R. W. (1992b). The relation of nonfatal suicide attempts to completed suicides. In R. W. Maris, A. L. Berman, J. T. Maltsberger, & R. I. Yufit (Eds.), *Assessment and prediction of suicide* (pp. 362–380). New York: Guilford Press.

Maris, R. W. (1981). *Pathways to suicide: A survey of self-destructive behaviors.* Baltimore: Johns Hopkins University Press.

McIntosh, J. L. (1992). Methods of suicide. In R. W. Maris, A. L. Berman, J. T. Maltsberger, & R. I. Yufit (Eds.), *Assessment and prediction of suicide* (pp. 381–397). New York: Guilford Press.

Miller, F., & Chabrier, L. A. (1987). The relation of delusional content in psychotic depression to life-threatening behavior. *Suicide and Life-Threatening Behavior, 17,* 13–17.

Mitterauer, B. (1990). A contribution to the discussion of the role of the genetic factor in suicide, based on five studies in an epidemiologically defined area (Province of Salzburg, Austria). *Comprehensive Psychiatry, 31,* 557–565.

Moller, H. J. (1990). Suicide risk and treatment problems in patients who have attempted suicide. In D. Lester (Ed.), *Current concepts in suicide* (pp. 168–181). Philadelphia: Charles Press.

Motto, J. A. (1985). Preliminary field testing of a risk estimator for suicide. *Suicide and Life-Threatening Behavior, 15,* 139–150.

Motto, J. A., Heilbron, D. C., & Juster, R. P. (1985). Development of a clinical instrument to estimate suicide risk. *American Journal of Psychiatry, 141,* 680–686.

Murphy, G. E., & Wetzel, R. D. (1990). The lifetime risk of suicide in alcoholism. *Archives of General Psychiatry, 47,* 383–392.

Murphy, G. E., Wetzel, R. D., Robins, E., & McEvoy, L. (1992). Multiple risk factors predict suicide in alcoholism. *Archives of General Psychiatry, 49,* 459–463.

Plutchik, R., & van Praag, H. M. (1990). Psychosocial correlates of suicide and violence risk. In H. M. van Praag, R. Plutchik, & A. Apter (Eds.), *Violence and suicidality: Perspectives in clinical and psychobiological research* (pp. 37–62). New York: Brunner/Mazel.

Plutchik, R., & van Praag, H. M. (1995). The nature of impulsivity: Definitions, ontology, genetics and relations to aggression. In E. Hollander & D. J. Stein (Eds.), *Impulsivity and aggression* (pp. 7–24). Chichester, England: Wiley.

Rakis, J., & Monroe, J. (1989). Monitoring and managing the suicidal prisoner. *Psychiatric Quarterly, 60,* 151–160.

Robins, E. (1986). Psychosis and suicide. *Biological Psychiatry, 21,* 665–672.

Robins, L. N., & Kulbok, P. A. (1986). Methodological strategies in suicide. *Annals of the New York Academy of Sciences, 487,* 1–15.

Roose, S. P., Glassman, A. H., Walsh, B. T., Woodring, S., & Vital-Herne, J. (1983). Depression, delusions, and suicide. *American Journal of Psychiatry, 140,* 1159–1162.

Rosine, L. (1995). Assessment of suicides in incarcerated populations. In T. A. Lies, L. Motiuk, & J. R. P. Ogloff (Eds.), *Forensic psychology: Policy and practice in corrections*. Ottawa: Correctional Service of Canada.

Rothberg, J. M., & Geer-Williams, C. (1992). A comparison and review of suicide prediction scales. In R. W. Maris, A. L. Berman, J. T. Maltsberger, & R. I. Yufit (Eds.), *Assessment and prediction of suicide* (pp. 202–217). New York: Guilford Press.

Roy, A. (1982). Risk factors for suicide in psychiatric patients. *Archives of General Psychiatry, 39,* 1089–1095.

Roy, A. (1992). Genetics, biology, and suicide in the family. In R. W. Maris, A. L. Berman, J. T. Maltsberger, & R. I. Yufit (Eds.), *Assessment and prediction of suicide* (pp. 574–588). New York: Guilford Press.

Roy, A. (1994). Affective disorders. In M. Hersen, R. T. Ammerman, & L. Sisson (Eds.), *Handbook of aggressive and destructive behavior in psychiatric patients* (pp. 221–236). New York: Plenum Press.

Roy, A., & Draper, R. (1995). Suicide among psychiatric hospital inpatients. *Psychological Medicine, 25,* 199–202.

Rudd, M. D., Joiner, T., & Rajab, M. H. (1996). Relationships among suicide ideators, attempters, and multiple attempters in a young-adult sample. *Journal of Abnormal Psychology, 105,* 541–550.

Salive, M. E., Smith, G. S., & Brewer, T. F. (1989). Suicide mortality in the Maryland state prison system, 1979 through 1987. *Journal of the American Medical Association, 262,* 365–369.

Schimmel, D., Sullivan, J., & Mrad, D. (1989). Suicide prevention: Is it working in the federal prison system? *Federal Prisons Journal, 1,* 20–24.

Sherman, L. G., & Morschauser, P. C. (1989). Screening for suicide risk in inmates. *Psychiatric Quarterly, 60,* 119–138.

Silverman, M. M., Berman, A. L., Bongar, B., Litman, R. E., & Maris, R. W. (1994). Inpatient standards of care and the suicidal patient: Part II. An integration with clinical risk management. *Suicide and Life-Threatening Behavior, 24,* 152–169.

Smith, G. (1986). Interrelations among measures of depressive symptomatology, other measures of psychological distress and young adult substance abuse. In G. L. Klerman (Ed.) *Suicide and depression among adolescents and young adults* (pp. 299–315). Washington, DC: American Psychiatric Press.

Sommers-Flanagan, J., & Sommers-Flanagan, R. (1995). Intake interviewing with suicidal patients: A systematic approach. *Professional Psychology: Research and Practice, 26,* 41–47.

Stanley, B., Winchel, R., Molcho, A., Simeon, D., & Stanley, M. (1992). Suicide and the self-harm continuum: Phenomenological and biochemical evidence. *International Review of Psychiatry, 4,* 149–155.

Steer, R. A., Beck, A. T., Garrison, B., & Lester, D. (1988). Eventual suicide in interrupted and uninterrupted attempters: A challenge to the cry-for-help hypothesis. *Suicide and Life-Threatening Behavior, 18,* 119–128.

Strakowski, S. M., McElroy, S. C., Keck, P. E., & West, S. A. (1996). Suicidality among patients with mixed and manic bipolar disorder. *American Journal of Psychiatry, 153,* 674–676.

Sundry, P. (1972). Socio-cultural studies in specific situations: Drug addicts and alcoholics. In J. Waldenstrom, T. Larsson, & N. Ljunstedt (Eds.), *Suicide and attempted suicide* (pp. 205–213). Stockholm: Nordiska Bokhandelns Forlag.

Suokas, J., & Lonnqvist, J. (1995). Suicide attempts in which alcohol is involved: A special group in general hospital emergency rooms. *Acta Psychiatrica Scandinavica, 91,* 36–40.

Tanney, B. L. (1992). Mental disorders, psychiatric patients, and suicide. In R. W. Maris, A. L. Berman, J. T. Maltsberger, & R. I. Yufit (Eds.), *Assessment and prediction of suicide* (pp. 277–320). New York: Guilford Press.

Topp, D. O. (1979). Suicide in prison. *British Journal of Psychiatry, 134,* 24–27.

Tsuang, M. T. (1983). Risk of suicide in the relatives of schizophrenics, manics, depressives and controls. *Journal of Clinical Psychiatry, 44,* 396–400.

Veiel, H. O. F., Brill, G., Hafner, H., & Welz, R. (1988). The social support of suicidal attempters: The different roles of family and friends. *American Journal of Community Psychology, 16,* 839–861.

Virkkunen, M. (1974). Suicides in schizophrenia and paranoid psychoses. *Acta Psychiatrica Scandinavica, 250*(Suppl.), 211–219.

Wasserman, D., Varnik, A., & Eklund, G. (1994). Male suicides and alcohol consumption in the former USSR. *Acta Psychiatrica Scandinavica, 89,* 306–313.

Weiden, P., & Roy, A. (1992). General versus specific risk factors in suicide in schizophrenia. In D. Jacobs (Ed.), *Suicide and clinical practice* (pp. 75–100). Washington, DC: American Psychiatric Press.

Weishaar, M. E., & Beck, A. T. (1992). Clinical and cognitive predictors of suicide. In R. W. Maris, A. L. Berman, J. T. Maltsberger, & R. I. Yufit (Eds.), *Assessment and prediction of suicide* (pp. 467–483). New York: Guilford Press.

Weiss, R. D., & Stephens, P. S. (1992). Substance abuse and suicide. In D. Jacobs (Ed.), *Suicide and clinical practice* (pp. 101–114). Washington, DC: American Psychiatric Press.

Westermeyer, J. G., & Harrow, M. (1989). Early phases of schizophrenia and depression: Prediction of suicide. In R. Williams & J. T. Dalby (Eds.), *Depression in schizophrenics* (pp. 153–169). New York: Plenum Press.

Westermeyer, J. G., Harrow, M., & Marengo, J. T. (1991). Risk for suicide in schizophrenia and other psychotic and non-psychotic disorders. *Journal of Nervous and Mental Disease, 179,* 259–266.

Williams, C. L., Davidson, J. A., & Montgomery, I. (1980). Impulsive suicidal behavior. *Journal of Clinical Psychology, 36,* 90–94.

Yufit, R. I., & Bongar, B. (1992). Suicide, stress, and coping with life cycle events. In R. W. Maris, A. L. Berman, J. T. Maltsberger, & R. I. Yufit (Eds.), *Assessment and prediction of suicide* (pp. 553–573). New York: Guilford Press.

Estimate of Suicide Risk (ESR)

Name _____   Examiner _____ Date _____
Age ___   Sex _____   Institution _____

PART 1. ASSESSMENT

Score each item as 0, 1, or 2. Items with asterisks are especially important to risk.

Historical and Actuarial Factors	0	1	2
1. Psychiatric history			
2. History of alcohol or drug abuse			
3. Prior suicide attempt(s)			
4. History of impulsive behavior			
5. Family history of suicide			
6. Age			
7. Marital status			
8. Sentence length			
9. Time served in sentence			
Clinical Factors			
10. Suicidal ideation			
11. Suicidal intent*			
12. Suicidal plan*			
13. Hopelessness*			
14. Sudden change in psychological functioning*			
15. Stress, vulnerability and coping			
16. Depressive symptomatology			
17. Current use of alcohol or drugs			
18. Psychotic symptoms (e.g., delusions)			
19. Physical isolation (e.g., segregation/dissociation)			
20. Psychosocial isolation			
Column Totals			

Total (Columns 0, 1, and 2)

PART 2. ACTION

Security supervisor notified?   Yes ___ No ___
Monitoring recommended?   Yes ___ No ___
  If yes, indicate frequency: Continuous ___   15 minutes ___   30 minutes ___
                       Other _____
Referral made to another mental health professional?   Yes ___ No ___
  If yes: Psychiatrist _____ Other _____
Other recommendations _____
_____

Date of exam _____   Time _____   Examiner's signature _____

16

Assessing Risk of Violence in Wife Assaulters: The Spousal Assault Risk Assessment Guide

P. RANDALL KROPP

STEPHEN D. HART

As Webster, Douglas, Eaves, and Hart illustrate effectively in Chapter 14 of this volume, risk assessment research has a colorful and controversial history. There have been "generations" of thinking about violence prediction (Monahan, 1984), and there appears to be renewed, albeit cautious, optimism about the relatively new field of risk assessment. This optimism and this wealth of inherited knowledge have fueled the development of the Spousal Assault Risk Assessment Guide (SARA; Kropp, Hart, Webster, & Eaves, 1995). In constructing the SARA, we attended to theoretical and methodological issues highlighted in the past. These included, among others, (1) base rates of spousal violence; (2) heterogeneity of the target group (i.e., spouse assaulters); (3) specificity of the prediction criterion; and (4) links to risk management. After we reviewed these factors (each of which is discussed below), it became apparent that there is considerable potential for predicting repeated violence in spousal assaulters.

Accurate and reliable base rates for violence are often difficult to obtain; they are nonetheless critical to determining whether prediction efforts are feasible. To put it in grossly simplified terms, given the imperfect accuracy of any prediction instrument published to date, it is not worth our time trying to predict high- or low-rate behaviors (this typically results in unacceptable false-negative or false-positive determinations). Our efforts are best focused on behaviors with a moderate base rate. It appears that spousal assault meets this criterion: Estimates of recidivism in men arrested for spousal assault range from 10% to 50% (Dutton, 1988; Hamberger & Hastings, 1990). A "best-guess" base rate estimate is approximately one-third, which is sufficiently high (and low) to justify risk prediction.

It was next necessary to address the degree of heterogeneity in the target population. There now exists a substantial body of literature delineating typologies of spousal assaulters. Various studies have distinguished among spousal assaulters on the basis of (1) scope of violence—that is, family-only versus general or "mixed" violence (Cadsky & Crawford, 1988; Saunders, 1992b); (2) the presence of personality disorders as defined in the revised third or the fourth edition of the *Diagnostic and Statistical Manual of Mental Disorders* (Hamberger & Hastings, 1988; Dutton, 1995); and (3) specific violent behaviors and/or psychosocial profiles (Follingstad, Laughlin, Polek, Rutledge, & Hause, 1991; Gondolf, 1988). An unavoidable conclusion from this literature is that important distinctions can be made within the spouse assaulter cohort; it is not a homogeneous group. This is necessary knowledge to have before developing an instrument intended to assist clinicians in determining levels of risk.

Recently, Monahan and Steadman (1994) have made recommendations "toward a rejuvenation of risk assessment research" (p. 1). Their discussion highlights the traditional limitation of weak criterion variables that are either too broadly defined (e.g., "all violent behavior") or unreliably measured. They note that there may be unique sets of predictors for various subtypes of violence. Importantly, these authors cite the National Institute of Mental Health's (1991) national plan of research to improve services, which states: "In examining dangerous behavior, it would be desirable to examine violence in the family and in public separately, because each implies different strategies for clinical intervention and regulatory policy" (p. 44). We add that these two types of violence also imply different predictors and information sources. An advantage of having a circumscribed criterion such as spousal assault is that risk assessment can focus on specific victims and measures of violence. Moreover, in spousal assault cases, the assessor often has access to the past and possible future victim(s)—a rich source of information that is seldom available for predictions of general violence.

A final consideration was the need to link risk assessment to risk management; again, we are echoing concerns raised elsewhere (Monahan & Steadman, 1994; Webster, Eaves, Douglas, & Wintrup, 1995). Risk assessment should inform others about effective management strategies in a given case. We believe that the next generation of risk assessment tools will allow clinicians, case managers, probation officers, and so forth to understand not only which risk factors might change, but also how they might change them. We intended the SARA to belong to this generation of instruments. Once again, the specificity of the criterion enhances our ability to make specific management recommendations. This issue is revisited later in this chapter.

In sum, our choice to develop the SARA followed careful consideration of the state of knowledge in the risk assessment field. We concluded that spousal assault is well suited as a prediction criterion. The bulk of this chapter thus describes the development, content, and administration of the SARA.

THE PROBLEM OF SPOUSAL ASSAULT

The physical and psychological damage resulting from violence in intimate relationships has been well documented in recent years. We use the term "spousal assault" to refer to such violence. More specifically, our definition of "spousal assault" is any actual, attempted, or threatened physical harm perpetrated by a man or woman against someone with whom he or she has, or has had, an intimate sexual relationship.[1] This definition is inclusive: It is not limited to acts that result in physical injury; it is not limited (despite the usual meaning of "spousal") to relationships where the partners are or have been legally married; and it is not limited by the gender of the victim or perpetrator. Also, it is consistent with the observation that violence between intimate partners is pandemic in North American society, regardless of the nature of their relationship (Gelles & Straus, 1988; Island & Letellier, 1991; Kurz, 1993; Renzetti, 1992; Straus, 1993). Having said this, we recognize that husband-to-wife assault, hereinafter referred to as "wife assault," can be considered the most serious form of spousal assault because of its prevalence, its repetitive nature, and its high risk of morbidity and mortality (Canadian Centre for Justice Statistics [CCJS], 1994a; Canadian Panel on Violence Against Women, 1993; Kurz, 1993; O'Leary et al., 1989; Walker, 1989). For this reason, the majority of our comments focus on wife assault, although they also apply to other forms of spousal assault.

Over the past decade, increased awareness of spousal assault has led to changes in criminal justice policy. Many jurisdictions in the United States now have domestic violence laws that provide special penalties for spousal assault and other forms of family violence (Ford & Regoli, 1993). Similarly, many Canadian and U.S. jurisdictions have developed policing and prosecutorial policies that encourage or even mandate the arrest of spousal assaulters (CCJS, 1994b; Sherman, 1992). In Canada, one apparent consequence of these changes has been a marked increase in the number of men charged with assaulting female partners (CCJS, 1993). Correctional policy is also being revised in light of the large number of spousal assaulters who are incarcerated or who are residing in the community on bail, probation, or parole. The Correctional Service of Canada started a

Family Violence Initiative in 1993, based in part on research indicating that at least 25% of incarcerated male offenders have a documented history of physical or sexual assault against family members (e.g., Dutton & Hart, 1992a, 1992b).

APPLICATIONS OF THE SARA

The increasing number of spousal assaulters being formally processed by the criminal justice system has resulted in a growing demand for assessments of risk for future violence. This demand is felt in most provinces and states in North America. Such risk assessments are typically conducted in one of four major contexts: pretrial, presentencing, correctional intake, and correctional discharge.

Pretrial

When someone is arrested for offenses related to spousal assault, the nature of the alleged acts or the defendant's history may raise the question of whether he should be denied pretrial release on the grounds that he poses an imminent risk of harm to identifiable persons (i.e., his spouse, his children), or of whether he should have pretrial release conditions that include no-contact orders.

Presentencing

A risk assessment is sometimes requested when a defendant's case has proceeded to trial. If he has not yet been convicted, the results may assist the judge who is considering the diversion or the conditional or unconditional discharge of the defendant. If he has already been convicted, the findings may help the judge to decide between alternative sentences (e.g., probation vs. incarceration), and to set or recommend conditions for community supervision (e.g., "no-contact" orders).

Correctional Intake

After conviction, risk assessments can be helpful to correctional staff members who conduct "front-end" assessments in institutional or community settings. They can be used to develop treatment plans, as well as to determine suitability or set conditions for conjugal visits, family visits, and temporary absences.

Correctional Discharge

In the case of an offender who has been incarcerated, risk assessment prior to discharge can help corrections officials or parole boards to determine suitability or set conditions for conditional release, as well assisting in the development of a postrelease treatment or management plan. For an offender residing in the community who is nearing the end of his supervisory period, a final risk assessment may indicate that correctional staff members should communicate formal warnings to at-risk individuals in an effort to discharge any ethical and legal obligations before the case file is officially closed.

A major problem in conducting risk assessments in these four contexts has been the lack of a systematic, standardized, clinically useful, and empirically based framework for collecting, weighting, and reporting background data and professional judgments. Considering the importance of the matter, it is rather odd that until very recently, there have been no guidelines concerning how to conduct spousal assault risk assessments: what factors need to be considered, what type of information is helpful in making decisions, and where and how to get information. As part of a coordinated effort by the British Columbia Institute on Family Violence, Forensic Psychiatric Services Commission the British Columbia, the of British Columbia Ministry of Women's Equality, and other government and community agencies, we decided to develop such a framework in the form of the SARA.

We did not want the SARA to be a psychological test in the usual sense of these terms (e.g., American Education Research Association, American Psychological Association, & National council on Measurement in Education, 1985). That is, its intended purpose was not to provide an absolute or relative measure of risk by means of cutoff scores or norms. A psychological test of this sort would no doubt be very useful, but the appropriate construction and validation studies would require considerable resources and time. Another reason for not making the SARA a psychological test is that the use of such tests is typically restricted under provincial or state law to registered or licensed professionals with graduate-level training in assessment and psychometric theory. We wanted the SARA to be accessible—and therefore useful—to the full range of individuals engaged in, or affected by, spousal assault risk assessments. Accordingly, the SARA was developed as an assessment guide or checklist (i.e., a framework, guideline, or *aide-mémoire*); it is a means of ensuring that pertinent information will be considered and weighed by evaluators.[2]

We should emphasize that our decision to make the SARA a checklist, rather than a psychological test, was not an attempt to circumvent the need for research. Indeed, we and others are using the SARA to examine the degree of correspondence between different evaluators' opinions (i.e., interrater reliability) and the accuracy of risk assessment in regard to the actual subsequent behavior of those evaluated (i.e., predictive validity). It is our hope that over time, the SARA will be revised in light of such research. Nevertheless, we believe that the existing literature concerning spousal assault is sufficiently mature to be used as the basis for informing and guiding the day-to-day practice of risk assessment.

Although our immediate motivation for the development of the SARA was to facilitate spousal assault risk assessment in the criminal justice system, we would like to note—and encourage—three other potential uses:

Civil Justice Matters

There has been an increased recognition of family violence within the civil justice system. Spousal assault risk assessments now occur frequently in the context of separation/divorce and custody/access hearings. Proper assessments have the potential to protect and enhance the well-being of women and children, given that many separations are precipitated by spousal violence, and given that estrangement increases the risk for repeated and even escalated violence (e.g., Solicitor General of Canada, 1985). In contrast, poorly conducted assessments may expose women and children to undue risk or may infringe on parental or other civil rights. We hope that the SARA may help to prevent these latter problems.

Warnings to Third Parties

Virtually every jurisdiction has numerous statutory and/or common-law duties to warn or advise. These apply to mental health professionals, counselors, and social service providers (Dickens, 1985). Generally, the duty to warn or advise comes into effect when the service provider has "reasonable and probable" or some such grounds to believe that an individual has the intent and the means to engage in behavior harmful to self or others. The SARA can be used in situations where, during the course of voluntary or court-ordered assessment or treatment, a service provider is concerned that an individual poses an imminent risk of physical harm to his spouse and/or children. The presence of several SARA factors—or of one or more "critical items" (as discussed later)— would tend to support the existence of reasonable and probable grounds. Results obtained with the SARA may act as an "independent check" of the professional judgment of providers and may help them to explain to others the basis for their judgments.

Routine Quality Control or Critical-Incident Review

As we discuss later, the SARA represents a distillation of professional and scientific knowledge and experience in the area of spousal assault risk assessment. We have taken great pains to ensure that the items included in the SARA are easy to comprehend (i.e., they provide clear definitions and conceptual clarity), respectful of constitutional and other civil rights (i.e., they do not discriminate on the basis of age, sex, ethnicity, or other grounds), clinically useful (i.e., they can be completed on the basis of a reasonably thorough assessment), and empirically valid (have demonstrated a robust ability to predict violence). We believe that the SARA can be used by mental health professionals, correctional staff members, lawyers, and victims' advocates to check the thoroughness and quality of spousal assault risk assessments conducted by others, in two ways. First, did the evaluator fail to recognize or to give adequate consideration to a risk factor that appears on the SARA? The SARA is not exhaustive, in the sense that there are numerous specific factors not included in the instrument that may be associated with risk for violence. However, in our opinion, it does contain a basic or minimal set of factors that should be considered. Second, did the evaluator consider factors not included in the SARA? Although the SARA is not exhaustive, it seems fair and reasonable that evaluators be asked to provide a clear rationale for basing their judgments on such factors.

DEVELOPMENT OF THE SARA

Content

Our first step was to undertake a careful review of the clinical and empirical literatures on risk for violence, with particular emphasis on spousal assault (Cooper, 1993). The review identified many studies that reported risk factors discriminating those who were violent toward their spouses from those who were not (e.g., Hotaling & Sugarman, 1986; Tolman & Bennet, 1990). Other studies reported factors associated with risk for recidivistic violence among known spousal assaulters—those arrested, convicted, or in treatment (e.g., Gondolf, 1988; Saunders, 1992a, 1992b, 1993).[3] Many of the risk factors in both types of studies were the same as those reported in more general discussions of risk for violence (e.g., Hall, 1987; Monahan, 1981; Monahan & Steadman, 1994; Webster, Harris, Rice, Cormier, & Quinsey, 1994). This supported the belief that constructing a checklist of key risk factors was feasible.

The literature review also identified several key references that discussed the assessment of risk for future violence in spousal assaulters, sometimes described as assessment of "lethality" or "need to warn" (e.g., Goldsmith, 1990; Saunders, 1992a; Sonkin, 1987; Sonkin, Martin, & Walker, 1985).[4] After considerable discussion, we concluded that the guidelines proposed in these references were inadequate for our purposes, for a number of reasons. First, some were simply too long or too complex. For example, Sonkin et al. (1985) identified 15 general dimensions and more than 80 specific factors. Second, some contained factors that seemed to be counterintuitive or only indirect relevant. Examples include "Victim was in a previous battering relationship" (Sonkin et al., 1985) and "Victim has attempted suicide" (Goldsmith, 1990). Both these factors focus on the victim and her past behavior, rather than on the offender and his past behavior, and potentially would be difficult to justify in many circumstances.[5] Third, some contained factors that were vague and insufficiently precise. Examples include "Abuser is moody" (Goldsmith, 1990) and "Jealousy" (Saunders, 1992a). Finally, some included factors that seemed redundant. Examples here include "Contemplation of suicide," "Attempted suicide," and "Threats of suicide" (Sonkin et al., 1985). We attempted to keep our list of factors relatively short and to aim at a moderate level of specificity (i.e., at the level of traits, characteristics, or incidents, rather than the level of isolated or specific behavioral acts). The results was a list of 20 factors, referred to on the SARA as "items," grouped into five content areas, referred to as "sections." The sections and items are presented in the Appendix to this chapter.

Next, we provide a brief rationale for the inclusion of each item; a complete rationale is provided in the SARA manual (Kropp et al., 19950.

Criminal History

Numerous studies indicated that a prior criminal record for offenses unrelated to spousal assault was associated with an increased risk for violence in general and for recidivistic spousal assault more specifically. The factors in the first section of the SARA cover past history of violence, as well as failure to abide by conditions imposed by the courts or criminal justice agencies. We included three specific items related to past criminal record. "Past assault of family members" refers to violence directed against members of the individual's family of origin or against his own children. It does not cover past spousal assaults, which are coded in a different section. "Past assault of strangers or acquaintances" refers to violence directed against people who are not biological or legal family members. "Past violation of conditional release or community supervision" refers to past failures to abide by the conditions of bail, recognizances, court orders, probation, and parole or mandatory supervision. It is irrelevant whether the conditions were imposed following an incident or allegation of spousal assault; any failure is considered a poor prognostic indicator.

Psychosocial Adjustment

Two SARA items reflect the observation that recent or continuing social maladjustment is linked with violence. "Recent relationship problems" refers to separation from an intimate partner or severe conflict in the relationship within the past year. "Recent employment problems" refers to unemployment and/or extremely unstable employment in the past year. It is unclear, and perhaps unimportant for the purpose of risk assessment, whether social maladjustment is the result of more chronic psychopathology or the cause of acute situational financial and interpersonal stress; regardless of their origins, these factors appear to be important predictors.

One item in this section, "Victim of and/or witness to family violence as a child or adolescent," is historical in nature and refers to maladjustment in the individual's family of origin. This is one of the most robust risk factors for spousal assault identified in the literature. Why this factor is associated with violence so strongly is unclear, although some research suggests that social learning mechanisms may be involved (Widom, 1989).

There is now a considerable body of evidence supporting the link between certain forms or symptoms of mental disorder and violent behavior (e.g., Monahan, 1992). This evidence was the basis for four SARA items related to psychological adjustment: "Recent substance abuse/dependence," "Recent suicidal or homicidal ideation/intent," "Recent psychotic and/or manic symptoms," and "Personality disorder with anger, impulsivity, or behavioral instability." Please note that we do not make any assumptions here that a mental disorder is responsible for or "causes" violent behavior. Rather, mental disorder is assumed to be associated with poor coping skills and increased social/interpersonal stress; thus, individuals with mental disorders may be prone to making and acting on bad decisions.

Spousal Assault History

The third section of the SARA includes seven items related to spousal assaults in the past. Risk factors based on the alleged or current offense are included in a different section, so that evaluators can more easily separate the quantum of perceived risk attributed to formally documented events (which are likely to be accepted as factual) from that attributed to alleged events (which are likely to be contended).

The first four items concern the nature and extent of past assaults. "Past physical assault" is an obvious risk factor, based on the axiom—one supported by research—that past behavior predicts future behavior (e.g., Monahan, 1981). "Past sexual assault/sexual jealousy" refers to physical assaults that are of a sexual nature or occur in the context of extreme sexual jealousy. "Past use of weapons and/or credible threats of death" refers to behavior that explicitly or implicitly threatens serious physical harm or death. "Recent escalation in frequency or severity of assault" refers to situations where the "trajectory" of violence (Greenland, 1985) seems to be escalating over time.

The next three items concern behavior or attitudes that accompany assaultive behavior. "Past violation of 'no-contact' orders" covers situations where the individual has failed to comply with the orders of a court or criminal justice agency prohibiting contact with the victim(s) of past spousal assault(s). Although it overlaps to some extent with the third item in the "Criminal History" section, we felt that such a violation is so directly relevant to spousal assault risk assessment that it deserves special attention. "Extreme minimization or denial of spousal assault history" may occur as part of a more general pattern of deflection of personal responsibility for criminal behavior, or it may be specific to past spousal assaults. "Attitudes that support or condone spousal assault" covers a wide range of beliefs or values—personal, social, religious, political, and cultural—that encourage patriarchy (i.e., the male prerogative), misogyny, and the use of physical violence or intimidation to resolve conflicts and enforce control.

Alleged (Current) Offense

The fourth section of the SARA consists of three items, similar in content to those appearing in the preceding section, that are scored solely on the basis of the alleged or current offense: "Severe and/or sexual assault," "Use of weapons and/or credible threats of death," and "Violation of 'no-contact' order."

Other Considerations

The final section does not contain any specific items. It allows the evaluator to note risk factors not included in the SARA that are present in a particular case and that lead the evaluator to describe an individual as at high risk for violence. Examples of rare but important risk factors include a history of stalking behavior (e.g., Cooper, 1994); a history of disfiguring, torturing, or maiming intimate partners; a history of sexual sadism; and so forth.

ASSESSMENT PROCEDURE

Consistent with other proposals, we decided to recommend an assessment procedure based on multiple sources of information and multiple methods of data collection (e.g., Goldsmith, 1990; Saunders, 1992a; Sonkin et al., 1985; Sonkin, 1987). This decision was based on the recognition that victims, offenders, and other collateral sources (e.g., children, neighbors) may tend to underreport violence (albeit for different reasons), but that their reports often provide crucial information that is otherwise difficult or impossible to obtain. Also, we recognized that in many cases, structured assessment procedures (self-report inventories, semistructured interviews) are useful adjuncts to unstructured procedures ("clinical" interviews, reviews of police reports or other case history information). In general, the assessment should include (1) interviews with the accused and victim(s); (2) standardized measures of physical and emotional abuse; (3) standardized measures of substance abuse or dependence; (4) review of collateral records, including police reports, victim statements, criminal records, and so forth; and (5) other assessments as required. If the information is incomplete, the evaluator should postpone undertaking or completing the risk assessment until the missing information becomes available. If it is impossible to track down the missing information, the evaluator should proceed with the risk assessment and emphasize in the final report the ways in which conclusory opinions need to be limited. We now discuss certain aspects of the assessment procedure in more detail.

Interviews with the Accused and Victim(s)

As indicated by a perusal of the SARA items, interviews with the offender or defendant should cover the following areas: childhood abuse and neglect experiences (item 6); occupational and social history (item 5); relationship history (item 4); physical and mental health history (items 7–10); current mental status (items 7–10); history of assaultive/abusive behavior (items 1, 2, and 11–20); criminal history (items 1–3 and 11–20); current life stressors ("Other Considerations"); and current social support network (item 4 and "Other Considerations"). We recommend the use of structured or semistructured interviews to ensure that information is collected in a systematic and time-efficient manner.

It is important to recognize that the legal context of spousal assault risk assessments may interfere with the interview process. For example, the assessment results are usually not confidential (or at least there are serious limits to their confidentiality); the individual knows that almost anything he says may become a matter of public record. Also, it is possible that any statements made by him concerning past, current, or alleged offenses may be used against him in court at some time in the future. For reasons such as these, the offender may be somewhat reluctant to report current and/or past violence, and may fail to comply with the assessment altogether. For this reason, collateral reports of the offender's behavior, including interviews with the victim(s), are critical. Such reports can also be obtained from children or other witnesses to the violence; from criminal justice personnel (police, probation, or parole officers) who are familiar with the accused; or from past therapists.[6]

Physical and Emotional Abuse

We recommend the use of structured interviews, self-report questionnaires, or both to supplement clinical interviews whenever possible. Structured interviews and self-reports help to ensure that the assessment is systematic, standardized, and free of bias (i.e., that everyone is asked the same questions in the same way); also, standardized measures often provide norms that allow the assessor to compare the responses of the individual to those of a reference group (Kazdin, 1992).

There are several good reviews of standardized procedures for the assessment of emotional and physical abuse in intimate relationships (e.g.,

Goldsmith, 1990; Hotaling & Sugarman, 1986; Saunders, 1992a). We favor the scales developed by Marshall (1992) to measure actual, attempted, and threatened violence, as these scales appear to provide a more comprehensive assessment than do most other self-reports (particularly in the area of sexual violence). A scale developed by Tolman (1989) is helpful to measure more general emotional and psychological abuse. We recommend asking an accused person to rate his own past abusive behavior toward a victim, and the victim to rate the accused's past abusive behavior toward her. In addition to indicating the extent and severity of past abuse (SARA items 11–14, 18–20), these responses suggest the extent to which the accused may be minimizing or denying his abusive behavior (item 16).

Substance Abuse or Dependence

We recommend the use of standardized self-report scales to screen for alcohol abuse or dependence (Selzer, 1971) and drug abuse or dependence (Skinner, 1982). Both Selzer's and Skinner's scales are brief, yet research suggests that they are extremely useful indicators of substance use problems. The offender/accused should be asked to describe his own substance use; whenever possible, his substance use should also be rated by the victim(s).

Collateral Records

Every effort should be made to obtain copies of police reports, criminal records, and victim impact statements. If these documents are not routinely provided to the evaluator as part of the referral process, they can usually be obtained through the criminal justice agencies involved with the case. Police reports often contain important comments regarding physical evidence of assault (e.g., cuts and bruises); statements by eyewitnesses or by those who have seen or heard an incident; the arresting officers' observations of an accused individual's behavior; and comments made about a victim's safety at the time of arrest. Criminal records are helpful in determining past arrests or convictions for assault,[7] as well as breaches of conditions of bail, probation, parole, and so forth. Finally, victim impact statements provide a measure of the physical and emotional effects on the victim(s).

Other Assessments

Interviews with relatives or children of the offender/accused and victim(s) can provide valuable information concerning the individual's pattern of assaultiveness. Such interviews may help to establish whether or not the accused is generally assaultive—that is, whether he has abused other family members or acquaintances. As discussed in the rationale for SARA items 1 and 2, this may have implications for risk.

Similarly, interviews with probation officers or other criminal justice personnel can provide information concerning the day-to-day activities of the offender/accused. Often such personnel have spoken with key witnesses, relatives, and community contacts (e.g., employers) in order to prepare presentencing reports or simply as a routine part of case management. Moreover, the probation officer can often address the history of the offender/accused with respect to his compliance with release conditions. This information is essential for scoring SARA items 3 and 20.

Psychological, psychiatric, or medical assessments can provide information that is useful to the spousal assault risk assessment. For example, items 7–10 of the SARA make specific reference to symptoms of mental disorders. Standardized measures of personality and psychopathology can provide valuable information regarding the presence of substance abuse or dependence (item 7), other major Axis I mental illness (e.g., thought disorder, suspicious thinking, depression/suicidal thoughts—items 8 and 9), and personality disorder (item 10).[8] Information regarding cognitive and intellectual functioning may also be useful, because deficits in this area may increase risk or preclude an offender from participating in, or benefiting from, treatment programs.

CODING JUDGMENTS

As discussed earlier, the SARA is not "scored" in the manner of most psychological tests. Rather, the evaluator is called upon to make three kinds of judgments, which are coded on a summary form (see the Appendix).

Presence of Individual Items

The presence of individual items is coded according to a 3-point response format (0 = "absent," 1 = "subthreshold," and 2 = "present"). The SARA manual (Kropp et al., 1995) presents detailed criteria for defining and coding each item.

The presence of individual items is a relatively objective indicator of risk: In general, and especially in the absence of critical items (see below), risk can be expected to increase with the number of items coded present. Of course, completing the SARA does require some degree of professional, subjective judgment on the part of the evaluator; however, it is important to remember that the items were selected on the basis of their demonstrated validity, and that considerable pains have been taken to ensure that the coding of items is simple and clear.

Presence of Critical Items

"Critical items" are those that, given the circumstances in the case at hand, are sufficient on their own to compel the evaluator to conclude that the individual poses an imminent risk of harm. They are included in recognition of the fact that risk, as perceived by the evaluator, is not a simple linear function of the number of risk factors present in a case. This is why we do not simply sum the numerical scores on individual SARA items to yield a total "score;" it is conceivable that an evaluator could judge an individual to be at high risk for violence on the basis of a single critical item. Critical items are coded according to a 2-point format (0 = "absent," 1 = "present").

Summary Risk Judgments

Evaluators are frequently required to address two separate issues: imminent risk of harm to spouse (which is generally the issue that prompted the risk assessment), and imminent risk of harm to some other identifiable person (e.g., the individual's children, other family members, or the new partner of an ex-spouse). With the SARA, such risk is coded according to a 3-point response format (1 = "low," 2 = "moderate," and 3 = "high"). If the individual is deemed to be at risk for harming "others," the evaluator must identify the potential victims. These summary risk judgments capture the evaluator's overall professional opinion in a straightforward manner that permits comparison with the opinions of other evaluators.

WHO SHOULD CONDUCT EVALUATIONS?

Who conducts spousal assault risk assessments is determined in most cases by relevant law and custom, and by the policies and procedures of the civil and criminal justice agencies involved. Evaluators should note that several SARA items tap aspects of mental health and may require the completion of a psychodiagnostic assessment. For this reason, the SARA manual (Kropp et al., 1995) recommends that assessments should be conducted by qualified mental health professionals (e.g., forensic psychiatrists and psychologists). However, evaluators who are not mental health professionals can also complete the SARA, as long as they have access to the requisite psychological or psychiatric reports.

LIMITATIONS OF THE SARA

In its present form, the SARA represents a distillation of relevant clinical and empirical knowledge and is a potentially useful tool in a variety of criminal and civil justice contexts. However, it is also clear from our description that the SARA is a work in progress, and we must emphasize two major limitations of the guide.

The SARA Is Not a Test

As discussed earlier, the SARA is not a psychological test. A positive consequence of this fact is that use of the SARA is not restricted to a particular professional group. A negative consequence is that the SARA has less structure than a psychological test with respect to administration and scoring. This means that it may be more susceptible to the various factors that render assessments unreliable. This issue requires further investigation (see below).

Use of the SARA Does Not Abrogate Professional Responsibility

Use of an instrument such as the SARA to aid decision making does not abrogate professional judgment or responsibility. There is sometimes a desire on the part of evaluators to "sanitize" the risk assessment process by arguing that decisions based on tests and checklists are completely objective—unbiased by their own personal opinions, values, and morals, and also made without regard to the possible human consequences of the assessment results. Obviously, this is not necessarily the case, nor should it be. Our view is that evaluators should accept responsibility for risk assessments and judgments, and should recognize the direct effect that assessments may have on the individual being assessed and on his potential victim(s).

THE SARA AND RISK MANAGEMENT

For risk assessments to be maximally useful, they should include strategies for managing any risks posed by the individual (Webster et al., 1994). In general, risk management strategies flow logically from the risk assessment: Individuals with recent substance abuse or dependence may benefit from substance use counseling, those who have used weapons in past assaults may be asked to surrender firearms, and so forth. Evaluators should also comment on the likely success or failure of any management strategies recommended in the report. For example, if court-mandated counseling is recommended for an individual who has attitudes supporting or condoning spousal assault, then the evaluator could address the dropout rate for such treatment (typically about 30%; see Hamberger & Hastings, 1993) and acknowledge that although such treatment probably helps, its efficacy is unknown (Hamberger & Hastings, 1993; Rosenfeld, 1992). Table 16.1 illustrates further examples of risk management strategies that might be dictated by SARA items. The table includes a column denoting whether an item is static and/or dynamic, for this influences the degree to which change is possible.

EVALUATION OF THE SARA

Interevaluator Agreement

We tested the interevaluator agreement of SARA judgments on 14 spousal assaulters referred to a community forensic clinic. Each subject was interviewed in the presence of two clinicians trained in the use of the SARA. Following the interview, each clinician completed the SARA independently. Pearson correlation coefficients for individual items ranged from .64 (item 10, "Personality disorder . . . ") to .95 (item 11, "past physical assault"). Perfect correlations were observed for two items (item

TABLE 16.1. Examples of Risk Management Strategies Suggested by SARA Items

SARA items	Static and/or dynamic?	Management strategies
Past violation of conditional release or community supervision	Static	Intensive supervision or monitoring
Past violation of "no-contact" orders	Static	Intensive supervision or monitoring
Personality disorder with anger, impulsivity, or behavioral instability	Primarily static	Intensive supervision (static) Long-term individual therapy? (dynamic)
Extreme minimization or denial of spousal assault history	Primarily static	Intensive supervision (static) Group treatment (dynamic)
Attitudes that support or condone spousal assault	Primarily static	Intensive supervision (static) Psychoeducation (dynamic)
Recent relationship problems	Static and/or dynamic	Interpersonal treatment—group or individual (static) Legal counsel or dispute resolution (dynamic)
Recent employment problems	Static and/or dynamic	Vocational counseling
Recent substance abuse/dependence	Dynamic	Court-ordered abstinence or urinalysis Alcohol/drug treatment
Recent suicidal or homicidal ideation/intent	Dynamic	Crisis counseling Hospitalization Court-ordered weapons restrictions

8, "Recent suicidal or homicidal ideation/intent," and item 9, "Recent psychotic and/or manic symptoms") because of the infrequency of their presence. It was expected that there would be less agreement for the coding of items requiring raters to use clinical intuition. This prediction was supported, with the lowest observed correlations for item 10 (see above) and item 17, "Attitudes that support or condone spousal assault" ($r = .66$). In general, we conclude that raters can agree on ratings for individual items. This suggests that the directions for scoring items are relatively unambiguous and understandable.

We also computed interevaluator agreement statistics for four methods of determining risk: sum of item scores ($r = .92$), number of items present (i.e., scored as "2"; $r = .86$), number of critical items ($r = .66$), and summary risk level ($r = .80$). We expected lower agreement for coding critical items and summary risk judgments, as reliability seems to decrease whenever professionals make complex judgments in the absence of formal, structured decision-making rules (e.g., Goldberg, 1991). The relatively low correlation for number of critical items may also be explained by the absence of any discussion of critical item scoring in the original SARA manual. This is an oversight that we have since attempted to correct in our revised version of the manual (Kropp et al., 1995). In sum, these preliminary findings are encouraging and suggest that the SARA can produce reliable risk judgments.

Criterion-Related Validity

Two research studies are currently underway to evaluate the validity of the SARA. The first type is retrospective in nature. As part of continuing research examining the long-term efficacy of court-mandated treatment for spousal assaulters, we have identified groups of recidivists and nonrecidivists. We are coding the SARA on the basis of the original assessment and treatment files to determine whether the SARA can differentiate between the two groups. The second type of research is prospective in nature. We have access to SARA data that were collected in the course of court-ordered risk assessments since 1995, and we will conduct a followup using criminal history data to determine whether the SARA predicts recidivism. This research may also help to determine (1) whether some SARA items are more strongly related to recidivism than others, and (2) which coding methods yield the most accurate predictions.

SARA Profiles of Reference Groups

We have noted earlier that the SARA does not yield norm-referenced or criterion-referenced scores. That is, each SARA item is important in and of itself; item codes do not have to be combined or transformed according to mathematical algorithms for the purpose of making decisions. In contrast, with psychological tests, scores on individual items and untransformed summary scores are typically of very limited interest; rather, transformed summary scores are analyzed and interpreted. The transformations are based on norms (e.g., standard scores, T scores, percentile ranks) or on some criterion (e.g., pass–fail scores).

Notwithstanding these comments, knowledge of the typical SARA profiles of various groups of spousal assaulters might aid considerably in risk assessment and management. For example, the presence or absence of a certain number or combination of SARA items, or of critical items, might characterize highly recidivistic offenders, offenders who are responsive to court-mandated treatment, offenders who abide by the conditions of "no-contact" orders, and so forth. We hope to generate reference profiles in the course of our other research using the SARA.[9]

CONCLUSION

Risk assessment of spousal assaulters is an extremely important activity—one with the potential for doing considerable good (by protecting the safety of women and children) or considerable evil (by exposing these same people to the threat of serious harm, or by infringing on the rights of [alleged] offenders). The SARA seems to be a useful guide or checklist for conducting such risk assessments in a variety of contexts. Like most schemes of its sort, it has some advantages over existing methods, but comes with its own acknowledged limitations and weaknesses. Our hope is that the SARA will prove useful to service providers and researchers working in this important and expanding area.

ACKNOWLEDGMENTS

The activities described in this chapter were funded in part by the British Columbia Ministry of Women's Equality as part of the Project for the Protection of Victims of Spousal Assault. However, the opinions expressed are our own and do not necessarily reflect those of the Ministry.

Copies of the second edition of the SARA manual (Kropp et al., 1995) are available at a nominal cost from the British Columbia Institute on Family Violence, Suite 551, 409 Granville Street, Vancouver, British Columbia V6C 1T2, Canada.

NOTES

1. Our definition is very similar to that used by researchers (e.g., Canadian Centre for Justice Statistics, 1994a; Gelles & Straus, 1988; Straus, Gelles, & Steinmetz, 1980) and by policy makers (e.g., Canadian Panel on Violence Against Women, 1993; Ministry of the Attorney General of British Columbia, 1993).

2. In this respect, the SARA is similar to other commonly used forensic assessment instruments (Grisso, 1986).

3. A more recent study (Cooper, 1994) suggests that factors associated with spousal assault are also associated with spousal homicide.

4. Several of the articles incorporated factors identified in studies of battered women who kill—that is, factors associated with the "justifiable homicide" of wife assaulters by victims acting in self-defense.

5. Imagine, for example, that a psychologist conducting a pretrial spousal assault risk assessment concluded that the defendant is at high risk for imminent, physically harmful behavior directed toward his spouse, at least in part on the grounds that his wife is terrified of him. The psychologist is now on the witness stand, being cross-examined by the defendant's lawyer, who asks: "So, Doctor, my client is at risk for violence simply because his wife says she is afraid? Isn't it possible, Doctor, that she could be exaggerating her fear, or even lying? If so, wouldn't your conclusions be invalid? Isn't it also possible that my client's wife has an emotional problem, and that her fears are completely unfounded? And what if my client's wife was afraid of you, or afraid of the judge? Would this mean that you, or the judge, were at high risk for violence?"

6. When an interviewer is talking with a victim, it is important to remember that the *accused's* behavior, rather than the victim's behavior, should be the primary focus of the interviews. However, if the victim has not sought counseling or advocacy services, then the interviewer may need to provide her with basic emotional support or referral information; similarly, interviews with child witnesses require special sensitivity. Prior to conducting any interviews, evaluators should familiarize themselves with relevant legal and professional standards (e.g., Committee on Ethical Guidelines for Forensic Psychologists, 1991).

7. There may be charges/convictions indicative of past abusive behavior that are not labeled "assault." For example, incidents of mischief, destruction of property, and so forth may be related to the mistreatment of others. The exact nature of these possible abuse-related crimes can be explored in the interviews with the accused and victim(s).

8. There are a number of self-report personality inventories available, including the Millon Clinical Multiaxial Inventory—II (Millon, 1987) and the Personality Assessment Inventory (Morey, 1991). The latter is particularly useful in this context, as it contains three indices of aggression and a measure of receptiveness to treatment. If psychopathy is suspected, we recommend the Hare Psychopathy Checklist—Revised (Hare, 1991). Other inventories are available that measure jealousy, dependence, intrusiveness, anger, and so forth.

9. Note that the use of reference profiles is intended to help inform evaluators about the base rates of risk factors, recidivism, and so forth, in spousal assaulters; their use is based on the assumption that such information improves clinical judgments of risk (Monahan, 1981; Webster et al., 1994). We do not recommend that reference profiles be used in an actuarial manner to override or supplant the expert judgment of the evaluator; if this is the case, then the SARA becomes a *de facto* psychological test.

REFERENCES

American Education Research Association, American Psychological Association, & National Council on Measurement in Education. (1985). *Standards for educational and psychological testing*. Washington, DC: American Psychological Association.

Cadsky, O., & Crawford, M. (1988). Establishing batterer typologies in a clinical sample of men who assault their female partners. *Canadian Journal of Community Mental Health, 7*(2), 119–127.

Canadian Centre for Justice Statistics (CCJS). (1993). Common assault in Canada. *Juristat Service Bulletin, 13*(6), 1–21.

Canadian Centre for Justice Statistics (CCJS). (1994a). Wife assault: The findings of a national survey. *Juristat Service Bulletin, 14*(9), 1–22.

Canadian Centre for Justice Statistics (CCJS). (1994b). The Winnipeg Family Violence Court. *Juristat Service Bulletin, 14*(12), 1–15.

Canadian Panel on Violence Against Women. (1993). *Changing the landscape: Ending violence—achieving equality*. Ottawa: Minister of Supply and Services Canada.

Committee on Ethical Guidelines for Forensic Psychologists. (1991). Specialty guidelines for forensic psychologists. *Law and Human Behavior, 15,* 655–666.

Cooper, M. (1993). *Assessing the risk of repeated violence among men arrested for wife assault: A review of the literature.* Vancouver: British Columbia Institute on Family Violence.

Cooper, M. (1994). *Criminal harassment and potential for treatment: Literature review and annotated bibliography.* Vancouver: British Columbia Institute on Family Violence.

Dickens, B. (1985). Prediction, professionalism, and public policy. In C. D. Webster, M. H. Ben-Aron, & S. J. Hucker (Eds.), *Dangerousness: Probability and prediction, psychiatry and public policy* (pp. 177–207). New York: Cambridge University Press.

Dutton, D. G. (1988). *The domestic assault of women: Psychological and criminal justice perspectives.* Boston: Allyn & Bacon.

Dutton, D. G. (1995). *The domestic assault of women: Psychological and criminal justice perspectives* (rev. ed.). Vancouver: University of British Columbia Press.

Dutton, D. G., & Hart, S. D. (1992a). Evidence for long-term, specific effects of childhood abuse on criminal behavior in men. *International Journal of Offender Therapy and Comparative Criminology, 36,* 129–137.

Dutton, D. G., & Hart, S. D. (1992b). Risk markers for family violence in a federally incarcerated population. *International Journal of Law and Psychiatry, 15,* 101–112.

Follingstad, D. R., Laughlin, J. E., Polek, D. S., Rutledge, L. L., & Hause, E. S. (1991). Identification of patterns of wife abuse. *Journal of Intgerpersonal Violence, 6*(2), 187–204.

Ford, D. A., & Regoli, M. J. (1993). The criminal prosecution of wife assaulters: Process, problems, and effects. In N. Z. Hilton (Ed.), *Legal responses to wife assault: Current trends and evaluation* (pp. 127–164). Newbury Park, CA: Sage.

Gelles, R. J., & Straus, M. A. (1988). *Intimate violence: The causes and consequences of abuse in the American family.* New York: Simon & Schuster.

Goldberg, L. R. (1991). Human mind versus regression equation: Five contrasts. In D. Cicchetti & W. Grove (Eds.), *Thinking clearly about psychology: Vol. 1. Matters of public interest* (pp. 173–184). Minneapolis: University of Minnesota Press.

Goldsmith, H. R. (1990). Men who abuse their spouses: An approach to assessing future risk. *Journal of Offender Counseling, Services and Rehabilitation, 15,* 45–56.

Gondolf, E. W. (1988). Who are those guys?: Toward a behavioral typology of batterers. *Violence and Victims, 3,* 187–203.

Greenland, C. (1985). Dangerousness, mental disorder, and politics. In C. D. Webster, M. H. Ben-Aron, & S. J. Hucker (Eds.), *Dangerousness: Probability and prediction, psychiatry and public policy* (pp. 25–40). New York: Cambridge University Press.

Grisso, T. (1986). *Assessing competencies: Forensic assessments and instruments.* New York: Plenum Press.

Hall, H. V. (1987). *Violence prediction: Guidelines for the forensic practitioner.* Springfield, IL: Charles C Thomas.

Hamberger, L. K., & Hastings, J. E. (1988). Characteristics of male spouse abusers consistent with personality disorders. *Hospital and Community Psychiatry, 39,* 763–770.

Hamberger, L. K., & Hastings, J. E. (1990). Recidivism following spouse abuse abatement counseling: Treatment program implications. *Violence and Victims,* 5(3), 157–170.

Hamberger, L. K., & Hastings, J. E. (1993). Court-mandated treatment of men who assault their partner: Issues, controversies, and outcomes. In N. Z. Hilton (Ed.), *Legal responses to wife assault: Current trends and evaluation* (pp. 188–229). Newbury Park, CA: Sage.

Hare, R. D. (1991). *Manual for the Hare Psychopathy Checklist—Revised..* Toronto: Multi-Health Systems.

Hotaling, G. T., & Sugarman, D. B. (1986). An analysis of risk markers in husband-to-wife violence: The current state of knowledge. *Violence and Victims, 1,* 101–124.

Island, D., & Letellier, P. (1991). *Men who beat the men who love them: Battered gay men and domestic violence.* Binghamton, NY: Harrington Park Press.

Kazdin, A. E. (1992). *Research design in clinical psychology* (2nd ed.). Boston: Allyn & Bacon.

Kropp, R. P., Hart, S. D., Webster, C. D., & Eaves, D. (1995). *Manual for the Spousal Assault Risk Assessment Guide* (2nd ed.). Vancouver: British Columbia Institute on Family Violence.

Kurz, D. (1993). Physical assaults by husbands: A major social problem. In R. J. Gelles & D. R. Loseke (Eds.), *Current controversies in family violence* (pp. 88–103). Newbury Park, CA: Sage.

Marshall, L. (1992). The Severity of Violence Against Women Scales. *Journal of Family Violence, 7,* 189–203.

Millon, T. (1987). *Manual for the Millon Clinical Multiaxial Inventory—II.* Minneapolis: National Computer Systems.

Ministry of the Attorney General of British Columbia. (1993). *Policy on the criminal justice system response to violence against women and children: Part I. Violence against women in relationships policy.* Victoria: Queen's Printer.

Monahan, J. (1981). *Predicting violent behavior: An assessment of clinical techniques.* Beverly Hills, CA: Sage.

Monahan, J. (1984). The prediction of violent behavior: Toward a second generation of theory and policy. *American Journal of Psychiatry, 141,* 10–15.

Monahan, J. (1992). Mental disorder and violent behavior. *American Psychologist, 47,* 511–521.

Monahan, J., & Steadman, H. J. (1994). Toward a rejuvenation of risk assessment research. In J. Monahan & H. J. Steadman (Eds.), *Violence and mental disorder: Developments in risk assessment* (pp. 1–17). Chicago: University of Chicago Press.

Morey, L. C. (1991). *Personality Assessment Inventory professional manual.* Odessa, FL: Psychological Assessment Resources.

National Institute of Mental Health. (1991). *Caring for people with severe mental disorders: A national plan of research to improve services.* Washington, DC: U.S. Government Printing Office.

O'Leary, K. D., Barling, J., Arias, I., Rosenbaum, A., Malone, J., & Tyree, A. (1989). Prevalence and stability of physical aggression between spouses. *Journal of Consulting and Clinical Psychology, 57,* 263–268.

Renzetti, C. M. (1992). *Violent betrayal: Partner abuse in lesbian relationships.* Newbury Park, CA: Sage.

Rosenfeld, B. D. (1992). Court-ordered treatment of spouse abuse. *Clinical Psychology Review, 12,* 205–226.

Saunders, D. G. (1992a). Woman battering. In R. T. Ammerman & M. Hersen (Eds.), *Assessment of family violence: A clinical and legal sourcebook* (pp. 208–235). New York: Wiley.

Saunders, D. G. (1992b). A typology of men who batter women: Three types derived from cluster analysis. *American Journal of Orthopsychiatry, 62,* 264–275.

Saunders, D. G. (1993). Husbands who assault: Multiple profiles requiring multiple responses. In N. Z. Hilton (Ed.), *Legal responses to wife assault: Current trends and evaluation* (pp. 9–34). Newbury Park, CA: Sage.

Selzer, M. (1971). The Michigan Alcoholism Screening Test: The quest for a new diagnostic instrument. *American Journal of Psychiatry, 127,* 1653–1658.

Sherman, L. W. (1992). *Policing domestic violence: Experiments and dilemmas.* New York: Free Press.

Skinner, H. A. (1982). The Drug Abuse Screening Test. *Addictive Behavior, 7,* 363–371.

Solicitor General of Canada. (1985). *Canadian urban victimization survey: Female victims of crime* (Bulletin No. 4). Ottawa: Solicitor General.

Sonkin, D. J. (1987). The assessment of court-mandated male batterers. In D. J. Sonkin (Ed.), *Domestic violence on trial: Psychological and legal dimensions of family violence* (pp. 174–196). New York: Springer.

Sonkin, D. J., Martin, D., & Walker, L. (1985). *The male batterer: A treatment approach.* New York: Springer.

Straus, M. A. (1993). Physical assaults by wives: A major social problem. In R. J. Gelles & D. R. Loseke (Eds.), *Current controversies in family violence* (pp. 67–87). Newbury Park, CA: Sage.

Straus, M. A., Gelles, J. R., & Steinmetz, S. (1980). *Behind closed doors: Violence in the American family.* Garden City, NY: Doubleday/Anchor.

Tolman, R. M. (1989). The development of a measure of psychological maltreatment of women by their male partners. *Violence and Victims, 4,* 159–178.

Tolman, R. M., & Bennett, L. W. (1990). A review of research on men who batter. *Journal of Interpersonal Violence, 5,* 87–118.

Walker, L. E. (1989). Psychology and violence against women. *American Psychologist, 44,* 695–702.

Webster, C. D., Eaves, D., Douglas, K., & Wintrup, A. (1995). *The HCR-20 scheme: The assessment of dangerousness and risk.* Vancouver: Simon Fraser University and Forensic Psychiatric Services of British Columbia.

Webster, C. D., Harris, G. T., Rice, M. E., Cormier, C., & Quinsey, V. L. (1994). *The Violence Prediction Scheme: Assessing dangerousness in high risk men.* Toronto: University of Toronto, Centre of Criminology

Widom, C. S. (1989). The cycle of violence. *Science, 244,* 160–166.

The Spousal Assault Risk Assessment Guide (SARA) Coding Form

Name of Accused _____ DoB _____
Name of Assessor _____ Title _____
Signature _____ Date _____

	Rating			Critical
Criminal History	0	1	2	Item
1. Past assault of family members				
2. Past assault of strangers or acquaintances				
3. Past violation of conditional release or community supervision				
Psychosocial Adjustment				
4. Recent relationship problems				
5. Recent employment problems				
6. Victim of and/or witness to family violence as a child or adolescent				
7. Recent substance abuse/dependence				
8. Recent suicidal or homicidal ideation/intent				
9. Recent psychotic and/or manic symptoms				
10. Personality disorder with anger, impulsivity, or behavioral instability				
Spousal Assault History				
11. Past physical assault				
12. Past sexual assault/sexual jealousy				
13. Past use of weapons and/or credible threats of death				
14. Recent escalation in frequency or severity of assault				
15. Past violation of "no-contact" orders				
16. Extreme minimization or denial of spousal assault history				
17. Attitudes that support or condone spousal assault				
Alleged (Current) Offense				
18. Severe and/or sexual assault				
19. Use of weapons and/or credible threats of death				
20. Violation of "no contact" order				
Other Considerations				
_____				
_____				

The Spousal Assault Risk Assessment Guide (SARA) Coding Form *(cont.)*

SUMMARY RISK RATINGS

	Low	Moderate	High
1. Imminent risk toward partner			
2. Imminent risk toward others			

Specify:_____

Note. From Kropp, Hart, Webster, and Eaves (1995, pp. 65–66). Copyright by the British Columbia Institute on Family Violence. Reprinted by permission.

17

Assessing Risk of Sexual Violence: Guidelines for Clinical Practice

DOUGLAS P. BOER
ROBIN J. WILSON
CLAUDINE M. GAUTHIER
STEPHEN D. HART

Although it would be a mistake to characterize all sexually violent offenders as impulsive, anyone who works with them is aware of the importance of impulsivity in understanding their criminal behavior (McGrath, 1991; Pithers, 1990). Many sex offenders have "automatic," poorly controlled thoughts and urges, which appear to be a proximal cause of sexual misbehavior (Pithers, Marques, Gibat, & Marlatt, 1983; Segal & Stermac, 1990). Others exhibit a general tendency toward behavioral disorganization and instability that extends beyond the sexual realm into many different areas of psychosocial functioning—a disposition that has been referred to as "lifestyle impulsivity" (Prentky, Knight, Lee, & Cerce, 1995). Typologies based on motivational factors recognize explicitly that some sex crimes are "situational" or "opportunistic" in nature (e.g., Douglas, Burgess, Burgess, & Ressler, 1992; Knight & Prentky, 1990).

Those who work with impulsive clients need systematic methods to assess their risk for all types of violence, including sexual violence. It seems clear that unaided clinical judgment represents as best only a marginal improvement over chance in the prediction of sexual violence (Webster, Harris, Rice, Cormier, & Quinsey, 1994). Also, despite some success in the development of actuarial methods for assessing risk for general violence (e.g., Harris, Rice, & Quinsey, 1993), and despite excellent reviews of risk factors associated with status as a sex offender or with recidivistic sexual violence (Cooper, 1994; Furby, Weinrott, & Blackshaw, 1989; Hall, 1990; Hanson & Bussière, 1996; Hanson, Scott, & Steffy, 1995; Pithers, Beal, Armstrong, & Petty, 1989; Proulx, Pellerin, McKibben, Aubut, & Ouimet, in press; Quinsey, 1984, 1986; Quinsey, Lalumière, Rice, & Harris, 1995), there are at present no well-validated actuarial scales of risk for sexual violence. Perhaps the best attempt to date was made by Quinsey et al. (1995). From several long-term follow-up studies of rapists and child molesters assessed at a maximum-security forensic hospital in Penetanguishene, Ontario, these authors identified a set of 13 variables— including the Hare Psychopathy Checklist—Revised (PCL-R; Hare, 1991; see also Hart & Dempster, Chapter 12, this volume) and a phallometric index of sexual deviation—that was about 77% accurate in identifying recidivistic sex offenders. However, some of the scale's items did not perform well in cross-validation samples, and two of the authors recently recommended abandoning it in favor of an actuarial scale of risk for general violence (Rice & Harris, 1997).

If unaided clinical judgment is to be avoided, and if there are no well-validated actuarial scales, how should one assess the risk for sexual violence? One possibility is structured clinical judgment—that is, risk assessments conducted according to explicit guidelines that are grounded in the scientific literature. Clinical guidelines can improve unaided clinical judgment in several ways. First, they can make risk assessments more systematic, and hence can increase agreement among evaluators. Second, to the extent that such guidelines are informed by empirical research, they can improve the accuracy of violence predictions. Third, guidelines can be developed in a way that assists the planning and delivery of interventions, such as treatment and supervision. And finally, guidelines can be used in the course of routine quality assurance or critical-incident reviews as a relatively objective means of evaluating the adequacy of risk assessments.

In this chapter, we present a set of clinical guidelines for the assessment of risk for sexual violence. Similar guidelines have been recommended by others in recent years (see especially Atkinson, Kropp, Laws, & Hart, 1995; Colorado Sex Offender Treatment Board, 1996; Greer, 1991; McGovern & Peters, 1988; McGrath, 1991; Murphy, Haynes, & Page, 1992; Revitch & Schlesinger, 1989; Ross & Loss, 1991), although all of these attempts appeared to us to have important limitations. The philosophy underlying the selection of our guidelines is similar to that which guided the development of the Spousal Assault Risk Assessment Guide (SARA; Kropp, Hart, Webster, & Eaves, 1995; see also Kropp & Hart, Chapter 16, this volume). We have attempted to identify risk factors that are (1) empirically related to future sexual violence, according to the scientific and professional literatures; (2) clinically useful (i.e., they can be used to make decisions about the institutional and community management of sex offenders, and changes in the status of dynamic risk factors can be taken into account); (3) not discriminatory (i.e., they do not include factors that might violate constitutional or human rights); and (4) parsimonious (i.e., the factor set is long enough to be reasonably comprehensive, yet short enough to minimize redundancy). In addition to specifying *which* risk factors should be assessed, we also attempt to specify *how* a risk assessment should be conducted.

We caution readers from the outset that our recommended guidelines should be considered a first step toward the establishment of minimum standards of practice; the guidelines are neither exhaustive nor fixed. In any given evaluation, there may be case-specific factors that are crucial to professional judgments concerning risk. Also, as the scientific literature matures, new risk factors for sexual violence may be identified, or those previously considered important may be proven to be of little value. With this proviso in mind, we turn now to a discussion of (1) the definition of sexual violence; (2) procedural guidelines for conducting sexual violence risk assessments; (3) the basic risk factors that should be considered; and (4) key questions to address when making judgments about risk.

DEFINITION OF SEXUAL VIOLENCE

Our working definition of "sexual violence" is actual, attempted, or threatened sexual contact with a person who is nonconsenting or unable to give consent. This definition has two major elements. The first element concerns the nature of the act. We have construed "sexual contact" broadly to include such acts as sexual battery (e.g., rape, sexual touching), communications of a sexual nature (e.g., exhibitionism, obscene letters or phone calls, distribution of pornography), and violations of property rights for sexual purposes (e.g., voyeurism, theft of fetish objects). The second element concerns the victim of the act. In most cases of sexual violence, victims are aware of the acts perpetrated against them, but do not consent to the acts. That is, the sexual contact is coerced. In other cases, victims may assent to the acts, but are unable to give consent (i.e., true, full, legal consent) by reason of youth or mental disability. Finally, some victims are unable to give consent because they are not aware of the acts perpetrated against them (e.g., victims of voyeurism).

Although our definition is broad, we believe it is a useful one. It is similar to those used by many researchers and clinicians, and it is also consistent with legal and social policy definitions. Also, we should point out that although it is possible to break down sexual violence into many specific categories (e.g., frotteurism, toucherism, piquerism), this ignores the fact that to the best of our knowledge, most individuals who have committed acts of sexual violence have engaged in many different kinds of violence (Abel, Mittelman, & Becker, 1985; Abel & Rouleau, 1990; Freund, 1990). Finally, we note that research on sexual violence conducted by Quinsey et al. (1995) finds that in general, factors associated with recidivism in one major category of offenders (e.g., rapists) also predict recidivism in another (e.g., child molesters).

PROCEDURAL GUIDELINES

Risk assessment differs from other forms of assessment, such as assessment of mental disorder or assessments for treatment, in several ways. First, it does not fall within the domain of any particular profession or discipline. For example, risk assessments are routinely conducted by correctional, psychological, and medical professionals, as well as by multidisciplinary teams. Second, sexual violence risk assessment requires evaluators to become familiar with factors associated with general crime and violence, as well as with those associated specifically or uniquely with sexual violence. Third, risk assessment is by its very nature a forensic concern. In most cases, evaluators work for the court itself, or for correctional or mental health agencies that provide consultation to the court. In other situations, evaluators recognize that some individuals being assessed may pose a degree of risk to public safety, and that the task requires them to balance the legal rights of the individuals and the public. On the basis of these and other considerations, we suggest six general principles that should guide the conduct of sexual violence risk assessments. These are summarized in Table 17.1, and analyzed in some detail below.

1. *Sexual violence risk assessments should gather information concerning multiple domains of the individual's functioning.* Such domains include

TABLE 17.1. Guiding Principles for Conducting Sexual Violence Risk Assessments

1. Sexual violence risk assessments should gather information concerning multiple domains of the individual's functioning.
2. Sexual violence risk assessments should use multiple methods to gather information.
3. Sexual violence risk assessments should gather information from multiple sources.
4. Sexual violence risk assessments should gather information concerning both static and dynamic factors.
5. Sexual violence risk assessments should explicitly evaluate the accuracy of information gathered.
6. Sexual violence risk assessments should be repeated at regular intervals.

sexual (e.g., sexual preference and sexual deviation), intrapersonal (e.g., antisocial attitudes, mental disorder, substance use), interpersonal (e.g., intimate and familial relationships), social (e.g., social skills, educational and vocational achievement), and biological (e.g., neurological and endocrine disease) functioning. This principle recognizes that sexually violent offenders are a very heterogeneous group, and that sexual violence itself is a complex and multifaceted phenomenon. For a discussion of general issues in the assessment of sex offenders, see Coleman and Dwyer (1990), Colorado Sex Offender Treatment Board (1996), Cooper (1994), Earls (1992), Langevin and Watson (in press), and Quinsey and Lalumière (1996).

2. *Sexual violence risk assessments should use multiple methods to gather information.* Such methods include interviews; behavioral observations; reviews of case records (e.g., medical, psychological, and correctional reports); psychological tests (e.g., self-reports of personality factors, performance tests of intellectual ability); physiological assessments (e.g., phallometry, polygraphy); and medical examinations (e.g., neurological and biochemical tests). This principle recognizes that each method of information is prone to certain weaknesses, and that overreliance on a particular method can result in an evaluation that is incomplete and systematically biased (Colorado Sex Offender Treatment Board, 1996). The literature on sex offenders contains many useful discussions of specific assessment methods (e.g., Abrams, 1991; Association for the Treatment of Sexual Abusers, 1993; Coleman & Dwyer, 1990; Cooper, 1994; Day, Miner, Sturgeon, & Murphy, 1989; Farrall, 1992; Freund & Watson, 1991; Langevin, 1992; Murphy, 1990).

3. *Sexual violence risk assessments should gather information from multiple sources.* These sources should include, but are not limited to, the following: the offender; the victim(s); the offender's family, friends, and coworkers; and law enforcement, corrections, and mental health professionals familiar with the offender. This principle recognizes that sex offenders typically minimize or deny their sexual deviations and misbehaviors (Barbaree, 1991), and that overreliance on a particular source of information can also result in an evaluation that is incomplete and systematically biased (Coleman & Dwyer, 1990; Colorado Sex Offender Treatment Board, 1996; Cooper, 1994; McGovern & Peters, 1988). The same point has been made concerning forensic assessments more generally (e.g., Committee on Ethical Guidelines for Forensic Psychologists, 1991).

4. *Sexual violence risk assessments should gather information concerning both static and dynamic aspects of risk.* This principle recognizes that static factors may be the best long-term predictors of sexual violence, but that dynamic factors are associated reliably with short-term fluctuations in risk and are important in developing rational intervention programs. This issue has been discussed in relation to risk for sexual violence, as well as

risk for other kinds of criminal and violent behavior (Andrews & Bonta, 1994; Kropp & Hart, Chapter 16, this volume; Quinsey & Walker, 1992; Webster et al., 1994).

5. *Sexual violence risk assessments should evaluate explicitly the accuracy of information gathered.* This principle recognizes that forensic examiners must routinely make judgments about the credibility of various sources of information, attempt to reconcile contradictory information, and determine whether the information is sufficiently comprehensive to permit valid decision making. Important judgments concerning the accuracy of information gathered should be admitted and discussed in oral or written reports (Committee on Ethical Guidelines for Forensic Psychologists, 1991; Kropp & Hart, Chapter 16; Webster et al., 1994).

6. *Sexual violence risk assessments should be repeated at regular intervals.* This principle recognizes that the status of risk factors, both static and dynamic, changes over time (e.g., Colorado Sex Offender Treatment Board, 1996). For offenders living in the community, these changes can occur quite rapidly, and so we suggest that risk for sexual violence should be reassessed at least every 6–12 months or whenever there is an important change in the status of a case.

CONTENT GUIDELINES

We have identified a set of 20 factors that, in our opinion, should be considered in any minimally comprehensive sexual violence risk assessment (see Table 17.2). For the sake of convenience, we refer to these risk factors here as the Sexual Violence Risk—20 (SVR-20).

The SVR-20 factors were identified via a comprehensive review of the literature on sex offenders. As noted earlier, we reviewed empirical studies on factors discriminating between sexual and nonsexual offenders, and on those associated with recidivistic violence or sexual violence in sex offenders. Space limitations prohibit a complete listing of the studies in this chapter; instead, we refer readers to the excellent reviews by Furby et al. (1989), Hanson and Bussière (1996), Quinsey (1984, 1986), and Quinsey et al. (1995). We also reviewed the sexual violence risk assessment guidelines proposed by others (e.g., Colorado Sex Offender Treatment Board, 1996; see also Cooper, 1994, for a helpful review of several such schemes).

Our literature review resulted in a rather long list of risk factors. The next step was to shorten the list by eliminating redundant factors; by combining related but highly specific factors into a single, more general factor; and by eliminating items that discriminated on the basis of age, sex, race, and so forth. During this process, it became clear to us that the factors could be divided into three major sections. The first section comprises factors relating to the individual's psychosocial adjustment.

TABLE 17.2. The Sexual Violence Risk—20 (SVR-20): 20 Factors to Consider When Assessing Risk for Sexual Violence

Psychosocial Adjustment

1. Sexual deviation	7. Relationship problems
2. Victim of child abuse	8. Employment problems
3. Psychopathy	9. Past nonsexual violent offenses
4. Cognitive impairment	10. Past nonviolent offenses
5. Substance use problems	11. Past supervision failure
6. Suicidal/homicidal ideation	

Sexual Offending

12. High density offenses	16. Escalation in frequency/severity
13. Multiple offense types	17. Extreme minimization/denial of
14. Physical harm to victim(s)	offenses
15. Uses weapons or threats of death	18. Attitudes that support or condone
	offenses

Future Plans

19. Lacks realistic plans	20. Negative attitude toward intervention

Most of these factors are historical in nature, reflecting fixed or relatively stable characteristics, whereas others reflect both past and current functioning. The factors in the second section all relate to the individual's history of sexual offending. Once again, these factors are primarily historical in nature, although some also have dynamic aspects. The third section contains two risk factors that reflect the individual's future plans. These factors are unusual, in that they reflect current functioning as much as past functioning.

It is interesting to note that many factors included in the first and third sections of the SVR-20 appear in many schemes for the assessment of risk for general violence; that is, they predict general violence, as well as sexual violence. In contrast, those in the second section tend to be associated specifically with risk for sexual violence. This point is made clear in Table 17.3, which summarizes the correspondence between the SVR-20 and three measures associated with risk for general violence: the Violence Prediction Scheme (VPS; Webster et al., 1994); the 20-item Historical/Clinical/Risk Management (HCR-20) scheme (Webster, Eaves, Douglas, & Wintrup, 1995; see also Webster, Douglas, Eaves, & Hart, Chapter 14, this volume); and the PCL-R (Hare, 1991; see also Hart & Dempster, Chapter 12, this volume, and Hart & Hare, 1996). The table also summarizes the correspondence between the SVR-20 and the risk factors for sexual violence identified by McGovern and Peters (1988), Murphy et al. (1992), Ross and Loss (1991), and Greer (1991). For each SVR-20 factor, we have indicated whether the correspondence is direct or indirect (i.e., partial).

TABLE 17.3. Content Overlap between the SVR-20 and Other Schemes for Assessing Risk for General or Sexual Violence

SVR-20 risk factor	General violence			Sexual violence			
	VPS[a]	HCR-20[b]	PCL-R[c]	M&P[d]	MH&P[e]	R&L[f]	G[g]
Psychosocial Adjustment							
1. Sexual deviation	✓	[✓]	—	✓	✓	✓	✓
2. Victim of child abuse	✓	—	—	✓	—	✓	✓
3. Psychopathy	✓	✓	✓	—	—	—	—
4. Cognitive impairment	✓	✓	—	✓	✓	—	[✓]
5. Substance use problems	[✓]	✓	[✓]	✓	✓	[✓]	[✓]
6. Suicidal/homicidal ideation	✓	[✓]	—	—	—	—	—
7. Relationship problems	✓	✓	✓	✓	[✓]	[✓]	[✓]
8. Employment problems	✓	✓	✓	✓	—	✓	—
9. Past nonsexual violent offenses	[✓]	✓	[✓]	✓	✓	✓	—
10. Past nonviolent offenses	✓	—	✓	[✓]	✓	✓	—
11. Past supervision failure	✓	✓	✓	[✓]	—	—	—
Sexual Offending							
12. High density of offenses	—	—	—	✓	[✓]	✓	✓
13. Multiple offense types	—	—	—	✓	—	✓	—
14. Physical harm to victim(s)	—	[✓]	[✓]	✓	✓	✓	✓
15. Uses weapons or threats of death	—	[✓]	[✓]	[✓]	✓	✓	✓
16. Escalation in frequency/severity	—	—	—	—	—	✓	—
17. Extreme minimization/denial of offenses	[✓]	[✓]	[✓]	✓	✓	✓	✓
18. Attitudes that support/condone offenses	[✓]	—	[✓]	✓	—	—	[✓]
Future Plans							
19. Lacks realistic plans	✓	✓	✓	—	[✓]	✓	[✓]
20. Negative attitude toward intervention	✓	✓	—	✓	[✓]	[✓]	✓

Note. ✓, SVR-20 factor corresponds directly to a factor in that scheme; [✓], factor corresponds partially or indirectly; —, no corresponding factor.
[a]Violence Prediction Scheme (Webster et al., 1994).
[b]Historical/Clinical/Risk Management 20-item scheme (Webster et al., 1995).
[c]Hare Psychopathy Checklist—Revised (Hare, 1991).
[d]McGovern and Peters (1988).
[e]Murphy et al. (1992).
[f]Ross and Loss (1991).
[g]Greer (1991).

We are currently working on a document that contains a detailed definition of each factor and a review of the empirical support for its inclusion in the SVR-20. In addition, we are developing a system for coding the presence versus absence of each factor, as well as any recent changes (attenuation or exacerbation) in risk related to each factor. We turn now to a brief discussion of the 20 risk factors.

Psychosocial Adjustment

Two factors reflect an individual's psychosexual adjustment: "Sexual deviation" and "Victim of child abuse." The first of these refers to the presence of a paraphilia (i.e., a pattern of abnormal and dysfunctional sexual arousal). It is important to note here that not all sex offenders have paraphilias, and not all paraphiles are sex offenders; however, paraphiles are at risk for acting out their sexual impulses and fantasies. Indeed, it is common for sex offenders to have multiple paraphilias, including arousal to violent or nonconsensual sex (Abel et al., 1985; Abel & Rouleau, 1990). The presence of a paraphilia can be inferred from the individual's self-reports, from psychophysiological assessments, or from a clear pattern of sexual misbehavior. "Victim of child abuse" is included because it appears that victimization is a general risk factor for criminality and violence and, more importantly, because sexual victimization in childhood often predicts sexual violence, in adolescence or adulthood.

There is now a considerable body of evidence supporting the link between certain forms or symptoms of mental disorder and violent behavior (Monahan & Steadman, 1994). The SVR-20 includes four factors related to psychological adjustment: "Psychopathy," as assessed by the PCL-R; "Cognitive impairment," as indicated by the presence of psychosis, mania, mental retardation, or serious neuropsychological impairment; "Substance use problems," including misuse of alcohol, prescription drugs, and illicit drugs; and "Suicidal/homicidal ideation," which includes urges, images, and stated intentions to harm oneself or others. Of the four, the last factor has the weakest empirical support as a predictor of sexual violence; however, it may be related to the severity (lethality) of any future violence, and it would be entirely unreasonable to disregard homicidal ideation when conducting any violence risk assessment.

Two SVR-20 factors reflect a failure to function appropriately in important social roles. "Relationship problems" refers to an individual's failure to maintain stable, long-term intimate (i.e., romantic sexual) relations as an adult. This includes failing ever to establish such relations. "Employment problems" refers to the individual's failure to achieve and maintain stable employment. In the case of juveniles, one should consider the quality of their relationships with their families of origin rather than their intimate relationships, and the stability of their educational history rather than their employment.

Three factors that reflect an individual's predisposition toward general antisocial behavior are also predictive of sexual violence: "Past nonsexual violent offenses," such as robbery or common assault; "Past nonviolent offenses," such as theft or fraud; and "Past supervision failure," including any failure to abide by conditions imposed by the courts or criminal justice agencies, such as bail, recognizance, probation, or parole. These risk factors should be assessed on the basis of the individual's self-reported behavior and case history information, in addition to any formal criminal record.

Sexual Offending

The second section comprises seven items related to past sexual violence. "High density of offenses" concerns the frequency of past misbehaviors, taking into account time at risk. "Multiple offense types" reflects the degree to which an individual targets different categories of victims (e.g., male vs. female, prepubescent minors vs. postpubescent minors vs. adults, family members vs. strangers) and commits varied misbehaviors (e.g., physical coercion vs. psychological manipulation, physical contact vs. exhibitionism vs. voyeurism). This factor is presumably related to the severity of the individual's sexual deviation. The severity of physical and psychological harm to victims in past sex offenses is reflected by "Physical harm to victim(s)," "Uses weapons or threats of death," and "Escalation in frequency/severity of sexual violence." Although empirical support for these factors is sometimes weak or mixed, they may be more predictive of the lethality of future sexual violence than of the probability of violence. The last two factors in this section concern psychological aspects of sexual violence. "Extreme minimization/denial of offenses" may occur as part of a more general pattern of deflection of personal responsibility for criminal behavior, or it may be specific to past sexual violence. "Attitudes that support or condone offenses" covers a wide range of beliefs or values—personal, social, religious, political, and cultural—that encourage patriarchy (i.e., the male prerogative), misogyny, or sexual contact between adults and minors.

Future Plans

The third section of the SVR-20 consists of two items that are scored solely on the basis of plans for the future. "Lacks realistic plans" refers to the individual's tendency to make grossly unrealistic plans, or to avoid making plans altogether. "Negative attitude toward intervention" concerns the extent to which the individual is pessimistic, resistant, or uncooperative with assessment, treatment, and supervision programs.

DECISION-MAKING GUIDELINES

The SVR-20 risk factors are not intended to be used as an actuarial scale. In our view, it makes little sense for evaluators to sum the number of risk factors present in a given case, and then to use arbitrary cutoffs to classify an individual as at low, moderate, or high risk. As Kropp et al. (1995; see also Kropp & Hart, Chapter 16) point out on the basis of their experience with the SARA, it is both possible and reasonable for an evaluator to conclude from the presence of a single risk factor that an individual is at high risk for sexual violence—if, for example, that risk factor is SVR-20 item 6 ("Suicidal/homicidal ideation") and reflects the individual's stated intent to commit a sexual homicide. (Interestingly, as Table 17.3 indicates, this factor is not considered explicitly in many risk assessment schemes.) It seems likely that on average, judgments of risk will vary positively and monotonically as a function of the number of factors present in a given case. However, it seems equally likely that the relation between the two is distinctly nonlinear, and that risk depends on the specific combination, not just the number, of risk factors present.

At the present time, then, we cannot recommend a decision-making algorithm to use with the SVR-20 factors. Instead, evaluators should consider the SVR-20 and any other case-specific factors deemed important, and should integrate them in an unstructured or "clinical" manner. It may be helpful, however, to address the following questions during the decision-making process:

1. *What is the likelihood that the individual will engage in sexual violence?* In our experience, it is best to communicate this likelihood as a crude estimate of relative risk—that is, as a low, moderate, or high probability relative to some specific comparison group of patients or offenders. It may also be helpful to provide information concerning the base rate of recidivism over specific time periods in that comparison group.

2. *What is the probable severity of any future sexual violence?* The assumption in most cases is that any future misbehavior will mirror the index offense. However, this assumption may be untenable if the individual has committed multiple types of offenses in the past, or if the risk assessment gives the evaluator good reason to believe that the individual's "trajectory" of sexual violence may be changing (Greenland, 1985). Perhaps most important to consider is the likelihood that the individual will commit acts of extreme violence, such as sadistic assault or sexual homicide.

3. *Who are the likely victims of any future sexual violence?* There are some cases in which it is possible to identify potential victims by name, because of their relationship to the offender or because of the role they play in the offender's sexual fantasies. Even if this is not possible, any information concerning victim preference may be helpful to those who must manage the offender while he lives in the community.

4. *What steps could be taken to manage the individual's risk for sexual violence?* In light of the risk factors present in the case at hand, the evaluator should make concrete and practical suggestions for risk management. These could include recommendations concerning custodial sentences, place of residence, mental health treatment, vocational training, parole supervision, and so forth.

5. *What factors might exacerbate the individual's risk for sexual violence?* Once again, the risk factors present in a given case may allow the evaluator to identify some "warning signs" that, if they occur, should prompt the offender or case management professionals to consider a formal reassessment of risk.

Here is an example of a "risk message" that adheres quite closely to the guidelines presented above. It is taken from the parole assessment of a pseudonymous Mr. Steele, a 45-year-old man serving a 60-month sentence for sexual assault and nearing his release eligibility date. The body of the report summarizes the case history information and outlines the risk factors present; the concluding opinion reads as follows:

> Based on a comprehensive risk assessment, it is my opinion that, should he be released into the community, Mr. Steele poses a high risk for sexual violence relative to other sex offenders incarcerated in the Correctional Service. Follow-up studies indicate that about 10% of sex offenders in the Correctional Service are arrested for new sex offenses within 1 year of their release from prison; by 10 years after release, the figure is about 35%. If my risk assessment is accurate, Mr. Steele's likelihood of sexually violent recidivism is substantially higher than these estimates.
>
> According to the available information, all Mr. Steele's sexual offenses have been pedophilic in nature, involving noncoercive sexual touching of young boys with whom he was acquainted through casual contact. There is no information that leads me to believe that his offenses will change in nature or escalate in severity in the future. If he reoffends, his victims are most likely to be boys between the ages of 6 and 12 who live within a few miles of his residence.
>
> Given the long-standing nature of Mr. Steele's paraphilia, its resistance to treatment, and his extensive history of offending, the most effective way to manage his risk for sexual violence is through incapacitation—that is, by denying his request for parole. Should Mr. Steele be released into the community, risk management strategies should focus on intensive supervision. Frequent meetings with a parole officer, polygraph interviews, and psychological treatment for sexual deviation might be effective means of monitoring his behavior. Release conditions should also include a stipulation not to be alone with children and to stay away from schoolyards, parks, or other public places frequented by children. If Mr. Steele should begin to abuse alcohol again, or if he fails to obtain full-time employment, his risk for sexual violence may be exacerbated and should be reassessed as soon as possible.

DISCUSSION

Although they are in need of further refinement, the guidelines proposed in this chapter may help to improve assessments of risk for sexual violence. They attempt to systematize the way in which evaluators collect information, the risk factors that should be considered, and the way in which evaluators make and report decisions about risk. Although many of the procedures recommended here are admittedly imprecise or subjective, leaving considerable room for individual judgment, we believe that they represent an improvement over the status quo. We do not expect that the use of clinical guidelines will necessarily result in perfect, near-perfect, or even good agreement between evaluators concerning an individual's risk for sexual violence. However, if evaluators use similar procedures and consider the same risk factors, agreement should be enhanced. Also, as noted above, to the extent that the factors considered by evaluators are related empirically to future violence, the validity or accuracy of judgments should be improved.

Following the lead of the SARA's creators (see Kropp & Hart, Chapter 16), we can suggest interesting lines of research that can be pursued once the SVR-20 is finalized. The first concerns interevaluator agreement. It will be important to determine the reliability of judgments concerning the presence of individual risk factors, as well as judgments of overall risk. Another interesting question is whether reliability is influenced by such things as an evaluator's training and level of experience, or the nature and extent of assessment information available.

The second major topic for future research concerns the accuracy of the SVR-20. One crucial issue concerns whether structured clinical judgments of risk based on the SVR-20 have any predictive validity. One way to address this issue would be to conduct a long-term follow-up of a large sample of sex offenders who were released into the community after being evaluated with the SVR-20. The problem is that the base rates of (officially detected) sexually violent recidivism are quite low, at least relative to those for any recidivism or for violent recidivism in general; they may be as low as 30–50% over 25 years (Hanson, Steffy, & Gauthier, 1993; Rice & Harris, 1995). Another method of evaluating accuracy would be to conduct a follow-back (or retrospective) study using a case–control design. A group of recidivistic sex offenders could be identified and compared to another group of nonrecidivistic offenders released from the same institution. The groups could be matched on important variables, such as age, race, date of release, and so forth. The SVR-20 would then be coded, by evaluators unaware of offenders' status, on the basis of institutional file information as it existed at the time the offenders were released. Although this design would be much more statistically powerful than a true prospective study (because the sampling method would ensure a mathematically optimal base rate of violence), as well as being less complex and expensive to conduct, the results might be limited by the nature of the information contained in the files.

A third research topic concerns "reference group" profiles on the SVR-20. Information concerning the typical profiles of various groups of sex offenders could aid considerably in risk assessment and management. For example, it might be helpful to have separate reference profiles for incest offenders, extrafamilial child molesters, and rapists. Similarly, the presence or absence of a certain number or combination of SVR-20 factors might characterize highly recidivistic offenders, offenders who are responsive to court-mandated treatment, and so forth. Finally, the SVR-20 may prove useful for describing a sample of sex offenders as part of program evaluation or other research.

CONCLUSION

Risk assessment professionals cannot wait for the release of validated actuarial risk scales; they need help to do their jobs well, and the help must come sooner rather than later. Fortunately, we can learn much from the existing clinical and empirical literatures on sexual violence. The SVR-20, like the SARA, represents a distillation of current professional and scientific wisdom, and may be a useful guide or checklist for conducting sexual violence risk assessments in a variety of contexts. Like most schemes of its sort, it has some advantages over existing methods, but comes with its own acknowledged limitations and weaknesses. Our hope is that the SVR-20 will prove useful to service providers in the short term, and that in the long term it will help to stimulate research in this important and expanding area.

ACKNOWLEDGMENTS

The opinions expressed in this chapter are our own and do not necessarily reflect the views or policies of the Correctional Service of Canada. Thanks to Drs. Randy Kropp, David Cooke, and Brian Judd for their helpful comments.

REFERENCES

Abel, G. G., Mittelman, M. S., & Becker, J. V. (1985). Sexual offenders: Results of assessment and recommendations for treatment. In M. H. Ben-Aron, S. J. Hucker, & C. D. Webster (Eds.), *Clinical criminology: The assessment and treatment of criminal behavior* (pp. 191–206). Toronto: Clarke Institute of Psychiatry.

Abel, G. G., & Rouleau, J. (1990). The nature and extent of sexual assault. In W. L. Marshall, D. R. Laws, & H. E. Barbaree (Eds.), *Handbook of sexual assault: Issues, theories, and treatment of the offender* (pp. 9–21). New York: Plenum Press.

Abrams, S. (1991). The use of polygraphy with sex offenders. *Annals of Sex Research,* 4, 239–263.

Andrews, D. A., & Bonta, J. (1994). *The psychology of criminal conduct.* Cincinnati, OH: Anderson.

Association for the Treatment of Sexual Abusers. (1993). *The ATSA practitioner's handbook.* Lake Oswego, OR: Author.

Atkinson, R. L., Kropp, P. R., Laws, D. R., & Hart, S. D. (1995). *The sex offender risk assessment guide.* Unpublished manuscript.

Barbaree, H. E. (1991). Denial and minimization among sex offenders: Assessment and treatment outcome. *Forum on Corrections Research, 3*(4), 30–33.

Coleman, E., & Dwyer, M. (1990). Proposed standards of care for the treatment of adult sex offenders. *Journal of Offender Rehabilitation, 16,* 93–106.

Colorado Sex Offender Treatment Board. (1996). *Standards and guidelines for the assessment, evaluation, treatment, and behavioral monitoring of adult sex offenders.* Denver: Colorado Department of Public Safety, Division of Criminal Justice.

Committee on Ethical Guidelines for Forensic Psychologists. (1991). Specialty guidelines for forensic psychologists. *Law and Human Behavior, 15,* 655–665.

Cooper, M. (1994). *Setting standards and guiding principles for the assessment, treatment, and management of sex offenders in British Columbia.* Vancouver: British Columbia Institute on Family Violence.

Day, D. M., Miner, M. H., Sturgeon, V. H., & Murphy, J. (1989). Assessment of sexual arousal by means of physiological and self-report measures. In D. R. Laws (Ed.), *Relapse prevention with sex offenders* (pp. 115–123). New York: Guilford Press.

Douglas, J. E., Burgess, A. W., Burgess, A. E., & Ressler, R. K. (1992). *Crime Classification Manual: A standard system for investigating and classifying violent crimes.* New York: Lexington Books.

Earls, C. D. (1992). Clinical issues in the psychological assessment of child molesters. In W. O'Donohue & J. H. Geer (Eds.), *The sexual abuse of children: Vol. 2. Clinical issues* (pp. 232–255). Hillsdale, NJ: Erlbaum.

Farrall, W. R. (1992). Instrumentation and methodological issues in the assessment of sexual arousal. In W. O'Donohue & J. H. Geer (Eds.), *The sexual abuse of children: Vol. 2. Clinical issues* (pp. 188–231). Hillsdale, NJ: Erlbaum.

Freund, K. (1990). Courtship disorder. In W. L. Marshall, D. R. Laws, & H. E. Barbaree (Eds.), *Handbook of sexual assault: Issues, theories, and treatment of the offender* (pp. 195–207). New York: Plenum Press.

Freund, K. & Watson, R. (1991). Assessment of the sensitivity and specificity of a phallometric test: An update of "Phallometric diagnosis of pedophilia." *Psychological Assessment, 3,* 254–260.

Furby, L., Weinrott, M. R., & Blackshaw, L. (1989). Sex offenders' recidivism: A review. *Psychological Bulletin, 105,* 3–30.

Greenland, C. (1985). Dangerousness, mental disorder, and politics. In C. D. Webster, M. H. Ben-Aron, & S. J. Hucker (Eds.), *Dangerousness: Probability and prediction, psychiatry and public policy* (pp. 25–40). New York: Cambridge University Press.

Greer, W. C. (1991). Aftercare: Community integration following institutional treatment. In G. D. Ryan & S. L. Lane (Eds.), *Juvenile sex offending: Causes, consequences, and corrections* (pp. 377–390). New York: Lexington Books.

Hall, G. C. N. (1990). Prediction of sexual aggression. *Clinical Psychology Review, 10,* 229–245.

Hanson, R. K., & Bussière, M. T. (1996). *Predictors of sexual recidivism: A meta-analysis.* Ottawa: Public Works and Government Services Canada.

Hanson, R. K., Scott, H., & Steffy, R. A. (1995). Comparison of child molesters and non-sexual criminals: Risk predictors and long-term recidivism. *Journal of Research in Crime and Delinquency, 32,* 325–337.

Hanson, R. K., Steffy, R. A., & Gauthier, R. (1993). Long-term recidivism of child molesters. *Journal of Consulting and Clinical Psychology, 61,* 646–652.

Hare, R. D. (1991). *Manual for the Psychopathy Checklist—Revised.* Toronto: Multi-Health Systems.

Harris, G. T., Rice, M. E., & Quinsey, V. L. (1993). Violent recidivism of mentally disordered offenders: The development of a statistical prediction instrument. *Criminal Justice and Behavior, 20,* 315–335.

Hart, S. D., & Hare, R. D. (1996). Psychopathy and risk assessment. *Current Opinion in Psychiatry, 9,* 380–383.

Knight, R. A., & Prentky, R. A. (1990). Classifying sexual offenders: The development and corroboration of taxonomic models. In W. L. Marshall, D. R. Laws, & H. E. Barbaree (Eds.), *Handbook of sexual assault: Issues, theories, and treatment of the offender* (pp. 23–52). New York: Plenum Press.

Kropp, P. R., Hart, S. D., Webster, C. D., & Eaves, D. (1995). *Manual for the Spousal Assault Risk Assessment Guide* (2nd ed.). Vancouver: British Columbia Institute on Family Violence.

Langevin, R. (1992). Biological factors contributing to paraphilic behavior. *Psychiatric Annals, 22,* 307–314.

Langevin, R., & Watson, R. J. (in press). Major factors in the assessment of paraphilics and sex offenders. In E. Coleman (Ed.), *Sex offender treatment: Biological dysfunction, intrapsychic conflict, interpersonal violence.* Binghamton, NY: Haworth Press.

McGovern, K., & Peters, J. (1988). Guidelines for assessing sex offenders. In L. A. Walker (Ed.), *Handbook on sexual abuse of children* (pp. 216–246). New York: Springer.

McGrath, R. J. (1991). Sex offender risk assessment and disposition planning: A review of empirical and clinical findings. *International Journal of Offender Therapy and Comparative Criminology, 35,* 328–350.

Monahan, J. A., & Steadman, H. J. (Eds.). (1994). *Violence and mental disorder: Developments in risk assessment.* Chicago: University of Chicago Press.

Murphy, W. D. (1990). Assessment and modification of cognitive distortions in sex offenders. In W. L. Marshall, D. R. Laws, & H. E. Barbaree (Eds.), *Handbook of sexual assault: Issues, theories, and treatment of the offender* (pp. 331–342). New York: Plenum Press.

Murphy, W. D., Haynes, M. R., & Page, I. J. (1992). Adolescent sex offenders. In W. O'Donohue & J. H. Geer (Eds.), *The sexual abuse of children: Vol. 2. Clinical issues* (pp. 394–429). Hillsdale, NJ: Erlbaum.

Pithers, W. D. (1990). Relapse prevention with sexual aggressors: A method for maintaining therapeutic gain and enhancing external supervision. In W. L. Marshall, D. R. Laws, & H. E. Barbaree (Eds.), *Handbook of sexual assault: Issues, theories, and treatment of the offender* (pp. 343–361). New York: Plenum Press.

Pithers, W. D., Beal, L. S., Armstrong, J., & Petty, J. (1989). Identification of risk factors through clinical interviews and analysis of records. In D. R. Laws (Ed.), *Relapse prevention with sex offenders* (pp. 77–87). New York: Guilford Press.

Pithers, W. D., Marques, J. K., Gibat, C. C., & Marlatt, G. A. (1983). Relapse prevention with sexual aggressives: A self-control model of treatment and maintenance of change. In J. G. Greer & I. R. Stuart (Eds.), *The sexual aggressor: Current perspectives on treatment* (pp. 214–239). New York: Van Nostrand Reinhold.

Prentky, R. A., Knight, R. A., Lee, A. F., & Cerce, D. D. (1995). Predictive validity of lifestyle impulsivity for rapists. *Criminal Justice and Behavior, 22,* 106–128.

Proulx, J., Pellerin, B., McKibben, A., Aubut, J., & Ouimet, M. (in press). Static and dynamic predictors of recidivism in sexual offenders. *Sexual Abuse.*

Quinsey, V. L. (1984). Sexual aggression: Studies of offenders against women. In D. N. Weisstub (Ed.), *Law and mental health: International perspectives* (Vol. 1, pp. 84–121). Elmsford, NY: Pergamon Press.

Quinsey, V. L. (1986). Men who have sex with children. In D. N. Weisstub (Ed.), *Law and mental health: International perspectives* (Vol. 2, pp. 140–172). Elmsford, NY: Pergamon Press.

Quinsey, V. L., & Lalumière, M. L. (1996). *The assessment of sexual aggressors against children.* Thousand Oaks, CA: Sage.

Quinsey, V. L., Lalumière, M. L., Rice, M. E., & Harris, G. T. (1995). Predicting sexual offenses. In J. C. Campbell (Ed.), *Assessing dangerousness: Violence by sexual offenders, batterers, and child abusers* (pp. 114–137). Thousand Oaks, CA: Sage.

Quinsey, V. L., & Walker, W. D. (1992). Dealing with dangerousness: Community risk management strategies with violent offenders. In R. DeV. Peters, R. J. McMahon, & V. L. Quinsey (Eds.), *Aggression and violence throughout the lifespan* (pp. 244–262). Newbury Park, CA: Sage.

Revitch, E., & Schlesinger, L. B. (1989). *Sex murder and sex aggression: Phenomenology, psychopathology, psychodynamics, and prognosis.* Springfield, IL: Charles C Thomas.

Rice, M. E., & Harris, G. T. (1995). Cross-validation and extension of the Violence Risk Appraisal Guide for child molesters and rapists. *Law and Human Behavior, 21,* 231–241.

Ross, J., & Loss, P. (1991). Assessment of the juvenile sex offender. In G. D. Ryan & S. L. Lane (Eds.), *Juvenile sex offending: Causes, consequences, and corrections* (pp. 199–251). Toronto: Lexington.

Segal, Z. V., & Stermac, L. E. (1990). The role of cognition in sexual assault. In W. L. Marshall, D. R. Laws, & H. E. Barbaree (Eds.), *Handbook of sexual assault: Issues, theories, and treatment of the offender* (pp. 161–174). New York: Plenum Press.

Webster, C. D., Eaves, D., Douglas, K. S., & Wingrup, A. (1995). *The HCR-20 scheme: The assessment of dangerousness and risk.* Vancouver: Simon Fraser University and Forensic Psychiatric Services Commission of British Columbia.

Webster, C. D., Harris, G. T., Rice, M. T., Cormier, C., & Quinsey, V. L. (1994). *The Violence Prediction Scheme: Assessing dangerousness in high risk men.* Toronto: University of Toronto, Centre of Criminology.

18

A Guide for Conducting Risk Assessments

CHRISTOPHER D. WEBSTER

The chapters in this section of the volume suggest that there is value in conducting systematic assessments to determine the likelihood of individuals' behaving violently in the future. The authors of all these chapters state or imply that predictive error can possibly be minimized if careful attention is paid to the task and if an appropriate device, scheme, or *aide-mémoire* is used to concentrate attention on factors apt to be particularly salient to the task at hand. Elsewhere, we have argued that a parallel can be drawn to a bicycle chain (Webster & Polvi, 1995). The bicycle becomes inoperable the moment there is a break in just one chain link. No matter how good the condition of the remaining links, the machine is rendered useless as soon as one has failed. Risk assessments follow the same principle: No matter how well the evaluation is conducted, it may take a single error at one stage to render it invalid or indefensible. In what follows, I do not propose that risk assessments can become completely error-free—only that, with effort, some of the most obvious faults can be eliminated. If this is so, it leads to the worthwhile possibility that recent findings may enhance predictive accuracy and improve standards of professional practice. Some of the points covered here are contained in Monahan (1981) and in the American Psychological Association's (1992) *Ethical Principles of Psychologists and Code of Conduct* (especially Section 7). As already noted, we have recently addressed the topic in greater detail elsewhere (Webster & Polvi, 1995).

A secondary purpose of the present chapter is to provide a guide for those who are sometimes called upon to conduct reviews of cases that seemingly went awry. Usually such reexaminations are demanded when a person assessed as "safe" commits a notably violent act. It is a pity that such calls rarely arise when persons have behaved safely according to plan and prediction. Nevertheless, there needs to be some generally agreed-upon method of carrying out such inquiries, reviews, and investigations. It goes without saying that "reassessors" will realize how easy it is to be clear-sighted after the fact.

The present chapter is organized in a slightly unusual way. Rather than attempt the obvious course of explaining how assessors might best succeed in offering accurate predictions of risk, I have opted to do the opposite. My hope in taking this seemingly perverse course is that the material may thus seem a little more interesting than otherwise might have been the case. It is an approach adapted from Jay Haley's (1969) article "The Art of Being a Failure as a Psychotherapist." Thus, I pose the question: How should assessors proceed if the aim is to conduct minimal-effort risk assessments that, though probably offering highly inaccurate opinions, can be vaguely defended in court, before a tribunal, at an inquest, and so on? Twenty points are proposed.

THE ART OF BEING A FAILURE AS AN ASSESSOR: TWENTY SUGGESTIONS

1. Avoid Clarifying the Purpose of the Evaluation

Assessors should always accept the demands for risk evaluations as they are placed on them, and should never query why a particular analysis or examination needs to be completed. An assessment of dangerousness is likely to be what the referring agent wants and expects. It does not make a great deal of difference whether the question has to do with competence to stand trial, involuntary hospitalization, transfer from high to medium prison security, setting of bail, or fitness for execution. It does not matter greatly whether the issue centers on spousal assault, sexual predation, or threats of violence in the workplace. It is of no account whether the issue is civil or criminal. The only qualities that matter are intuition and the willing application of the gift of "gut feeling" to any and all circumstances. If the purpose of an evaluation is left unclear, an assessor can scarcely later be criticized for lack of precision in report writing. Many of those who receive psychiatric and psychological reports on the risk of violence prize the quality of ambiguity very highly. They hope that the clinician will develop for them some kind of fairly plausible theory that might further a case for a light sentence, the allowance of parole, the granting of community privileges, or the like. In some instances, the referring agent's request may be so general that it is not even clear that a statement about risk is expected. This, of course, does not mean that if assessors really want to fail, they should not offer one in any event. The general advice here, then, is never to query the referring agent's intentions. Such laxity and good-natured compliance allowed some practitioners, in earlier years, to complete a full 35-year career without ever seriously being called to task. Although loose, "from-the-hip" assessments still suffice in a remarkable number of cases, professional bodies are misguidedly beginning to insist on at least some minimal standards for assessment practice (e.g., American Psychological Association, 1992).

There is no need to consult the legal or policy definitions of violence at the outset of a new evaluation case. Certainly, it pays to be in ignorance of the potential range of penalties or outcomes that will flow from decisions about dangerousness and risk. It is not the assessor's job to worry about how frequently the case will be reviewed in the future or matters of that sort.

2. Avoid Demanding Adequate Circumstances for Conduct of Assessments

A great many referring agents want assessments to be completed very quickly and with minimal expenditure of funds. Only rarely, and usually only in extremely high-profile cases, are experts given unfettered opportunities to examine clients at leisure and with a full range of resources at hand. Administrators balk when it comes to paying for thorough assessments of dangerousness and risk, in ways they do not when matters of physical health are at stake. This is true despite the fact that slipshod evaluations of risk may result in high costs to society, both economically and in other ways (Dietz, 1985). Day-to-day evaluations are apt to be conducted in prisons, remand centers, emergency wards, and the like (Boyd, 1964). Opportunities for retrieval of past records and for specialized testing and interviewing tend to be scant. Physical settings are often oppressive and lacking in privacy. File information is typically minimal. Such conditions are apt to induce the person being assessed to withhold information that, discreetly given and received, would almost certainly have a constructive bearing on the matter at hand. Since this is the case, the person under assessment should be offered only the most crude of explanations about the purpose of the assessment (if any; see point 1 above) and the uses to which the eventual report will be put. This way, the subject of the assessment may be even more disinclined than usual to divulge any information of possible consequence. The main point for would-be assessors is to hobble themselves at the outset. The prospect of failure is greatly enhanced by accepting conditions almost bound to yield erroneous, spurious, and misleading information.

3. Avoid Establishing and Disclosing Limits of Incompetence

It is a sad mistake for assessors to study the now-vast literature on the topic of the prediction of violence. Particularly to be avoided are texts like Monahan's (1981) survey of the literature. His book quite explicitly demands that assessors consider their general competence to undertake risk assessments, as well as their specific ability with respect to each case at hand. This is touted as an ethical issue. Fortunately, almost no attention is currently paid to educating forensic and correctional clinicians as to how best to conduct assessments. This means that they have little ability even to read the literature as it appears. Such basic terms as "correlation," "false positives," "positive predictive power," "receiver–operator curves," "survival analyses," and the like should be left to researchers (Hart, Menzies, & Webster, 1993). If clinicians elect to remain deliberately unaware of how prediction accuracy is interpreted in research circles, how can their competence be gauged against such standards? Moreover, if they do not understand the basic criteria against which their perform-ance should be judged, how can they improve their predictive power?

The very best way of ensuring failure is to make certain that any remarks that absolutely have to be made in an assessment can never be matched to actual outcome weeks, months, or years later. This does not take much enterprise or effort. Assessors simply go through their careers without having any data collected, and they beat back the attempts of anyone interested in doing this job as a favor. I return to this all-important matter under point 20.

4. Avoid Acknowledging the Possibility of Assessor Bias

One of the easiest and most obvious ways of producing inaccurate and generally misleading assessments is to enter an evaluation with a set bias against the client. The bias may be in the client's favor, but more usually it is against him or her (Lewis & Appleby, 1988; Pfafflin, 1979). The chances of failure are likely to rise as impartiality is abandoned. Assessors who have served as long-time therapists of particular individuals can at times offer singularly error-prone opinions. Their comments, if taken literally in some instances, can help yield the sought-after poor estima-tions of violence risk. Perhaps the most difficult of all bias issues has to do with "illusory correlations" (Monahan, 1981; Webster, Dickens, & Addario, 1985). This simply means the tendency for individual assessors to assume faith in their own predictive powers as a result of a single case or a few cases that proved (in some cases dramatically) the correctness of their opinion. Such cases help solidify an impression of competence—one that, if tested against a fairly large number of cases, would prove to be without grounding. An especially effective way of introducing inaccuracy in predictions can occur within interdisciplinary teams as members vie to construct the concept of "dangerousness" (Pfohl, 1978; Menzies, 1989). This particular technique may contribute substantially to the general problem of overpredicting violence (Webster, Harris, Rice, Cormier, & Quinsey, 1994).

5. Avoid a Systematic Approach to Assessment

In recent years, a number of assessment guides have been published (see, e.g., Bjørkly, 1994; Campbell, 1995; Hall, 1987; Monahan, 1981; Webster, Eaves, Douglas, & Wintrup, 1995; and all of the previous chapters in this section). These should be strictly avoided. There is not, and there never will be, an evaluation scheme that will fit the particular issue or case at hand. The present schemes are underconceptualized, underdeveloped, and undernormed. That their authors even have the temerity to put them into print is unconscionable. Assessments conducted in such a fixed, mechanical fashion are almost certain to miss the unique factors in the particular case under consideration. Allowing points for this or that characteristic not only demeans the individual under evaluation, but discredits professional persons and professional bodies. If an assessor has ever consulted a manual or guide in the distant past, there is no need to refresh the memory about item details. When an edict from on high indicates that evaluators must follow a device, it is important to ensure that the one selected has little (if any) pertinence to the task at hand. If pressed, an evaluator should indicate a reliance on the well-established "triad" of fire setting, enuresis, and cruelty to animals (Hellman & Blackman, 1966). The main aim here is to ensure that there is no point-by-point consideration of the factors likely to be involved in violent recidivism. Such an approach is especially to be eschewed because it renders it possible to think in practical terms of how the institution of particular conditions might attenuate risk of violence. It is important never to consider developing and testing a device specific to the purpose at hand. Such a move might demonstrate existing levels of incompetence all too clearly.

6. Avoid Becoming Familiar with the Files

The assessment task is often greatly complicated by the presence of volu-minous files. Those evaluators who occasionally agree to review a case in retrospect (i.e., to help apportion blame after the occurrence of some tragic, desperate, or brutal event) will know that the courier rarely brings a single box. When decisions have to be made about the release of serious offenders, there is again usually a great weight of file material. Anyone who wishes to fail as an assessor should set these boxes aside and get on right away with the "real job"—namely, interviewing the individual. It will take hours, if not days, to go through the full files and make a systematic historical

outline. In addition, there will be the problem of much conflicting information. The evaluator will find it easy to be able to point out differing opinions
written within the same week. These views will often come from the same
person. So in the face of this ambiguity and inconsistency, and when failure
of prediction is the aim, the files should not be studied obsessively. There
is little point in reading about an individual's quarter-century-distant crime
spree. This is especially so when there is at hand a prison report indicating
that the individual, after decades of incarceration, is beginning to think
about rehabilitating himself or herself.

7. Avoid Checking the Correctness of Data

As already noted under point 6, some assessment cases come with large
files. Some of that information is likely to be factually correct, some of it
will be of doubtful accuracy, and some of it will be dead wrong. If failure
is the aim, no attempt should be made to sort fact from fiction; all reports
and opinions should be accorded equal weight. It is very tiring to
cross-check information, especially if it means calling for reports that
ought to have been on file but are missing. Obtaining the required
consents to speak to relatives, friends, and others is also taxing. Only
rarely will there be actuarially based reports on file that may result in a
probability estimate for future violence. When these are present, they
should never be checked. If they are checked, they may well prove to have
been incorrectly calculated; the error will have perpetuated itself across
files and across years. By now, the purported risk level will have so
solidified in the minds of others that it would be pointless to expose the
error anyway. So the advice here is never to search out new data that
might confirm or disconfirm existing information, and to allow evident
error to retain its formative effects (Konečni, Mulcahy, & Ebbeson, 1980).

8. Avoid an Actuarial Emphasis

Although some current research suggests that clinical judgment in risk
assessments is not without some minimal value (e.g., Lidz, Mulvey, &
Gardner, 1993; Menzies, Webster, McMain, Staley, & Scaglione, 1994),
attention of late has focused mainly on the relative predictive power of
certain fairly basic historical/statistical factors, such as age, previous
violence, Psychopathy Checklist—Revised score, and the like. The very
fact that article after article in the recent literature has pointed to the
unexpected power of the psychopathy construct in prediction (e.g., Harris, Rice, & Quinsey, 1993) gives reason to avoid the idea and the whole
general approach. It seems that the "numbers people" have already
extracted whatever is to be gained from this limited angle. What is called

for, then, is a renewed emphasis on certain clinical notions so conceptually rich that they can never yield to the metric.

9. Avoid Considering Experiential Information

Those who wish to fail in the prediction exercise should show little interest in how the individual experienced the previous main violent incident or incidents. No effort should be made to locate pertinent reports written by police, correctional officials, or mental health workers at these earlier times. It is not important to know how the person felt at the time of conducting antisocial, disruptive, or sadistic acts. An assessor truly bent on failure will pay no heed to what aspects of violence were or are reinforcing to the individual. And only scant attention needs to be directed to how the person responded after the incident was over (i.e., with guilt, with remorse, etc.). These topics are best avoided during interviews with the client. Certainly, it is misguided to think that persons under assessment might have anything of consequence to contribute to an understanding of their own violence potential (Greenland, 1985).

10. Avoid Considering Current Symptomatology

For the best shot at failure in prediction, it is convenient to center thinking around a previous psychiatric diagnosis, preferably one obtained without recourse to the *Diagnostic and Statistical Manual of Mental Disorders* or a similar scheme. Emphasis should be on the single primary diagnosis; it is too complicated to think about comorbid disorders. Fixing firmly on the previous diagnosis should make it possible to avoid almost completely any consideration of current symptomatology (e.g., patterns of hallucinatory thought that could have a bearing on subsequent violence, effects of alcohol or drug abuse on behavior, etc.). It is best to consider such new notions as "threat/control-override" as being at an exploratory stage only (Link & Steuve, 1994).

11. Avoid a Situational Emphasis

An evaluator determined to yield inaccurate projections of violence does well to place disproportionate weight on trait, personality, and dynamic variables at the expense of environmental considerations. One big advantage of this approach is that the assessor rarely has to leave the office or clinic. Clients themselves are well placed to answer these questions. Otherwise, there would be a need to examine the living, work, social, and financial circumstances likely to prevail in the future. Absence of knowledge of the situational realities almost guarantees failure. Without this information, it is often impossible to gauge the similarity of the projected living arrangements against those that applied before the previous incident of main interest. It pays to be ignorant of how much stress the new circumstances will be apt to create, how clients will likely deal with confrontations, and how amenable they will be to incorporation by antisocial persons and groups. Failure is additionally ensured by refusal to consider such ideas as conditional prediction (Mulvey & Lidz, 1995).

12. Avoid Disputing the Relevance of Some Information

In many files the assessor will note a plethora of previous medical, neurological, sexological, neuropsychological, and psychometric reports. Many of these will give detailed data, often to the second or third decimal place. Prediction failure is assured by according such information greater weight than it probably deserves. Negative results from brain scans, psychological tests, and the like should be taken to mean that the individual will almost certainly be violence-free. The essential point is that scores based on exhaustive testing automatically deserve strong weight. It is important, in the interests of inaccuracy, never to question the supposition that the published supporting scientific evidence is weak or nonexistent, or that it has only marginal conceptual links to violence. The seeming accuracy of the information must be allowed to outweigh its actual relevance (e.g., Haynes, 1985).

13. Avoid Considering Risk Management Issues

It is usually easier to offer a projection of risk than to give advice as to how violence might be reduced or eliminated. Once the matter of management comes into play, it brings with it a host of issues having to do with planning. If untoward acts of violence are indeed to be minimized, some kinds of detailed arrangements will probably have to be made with the client. Risk, it will soon become clear, is not immutable. It will vary critically according to how much social support is or is not available, how easily that help can be mobilized in times of crisis, and so on. Decisions will have to be made about the stage at which the plan will be revoked and by whose authority. Information will have to be given to staff members as to how they should react during or after threatened and actual assaultive conduct. Long-range predictions tend to become short-range predictions under these kinds of circumstances. Sustained involvement of assessors in this level of work is apt to be very time-consuming, and it becomes difficult for them to think of the necessary kinds of moment-to-moment strategies (Bolen, 1994). Evaluators of risk will do well to avoid tangling with these kinds of complexities. It will take too long to understand the issues, and, generally speaking, the chances of failure in prediction probably rise in proportion to the absence of knowledge about environmental particulars.

14. Avoid Considering Base Rate Statistics

Treating each and every assessment case as if it were truly unique, without any possible standards for comparison, greatly enhances the chance of erroneous prediction. All that this entails is making the assumption that the individual is unlikely to behave in much the same way as other offenders of the same type, age, and background. The failure-seeking evaluator simply treats the case without reference to similar others. This saves work because it means that colleagues and periodicals do not have to be consulted, and that no time needs to be spent examining data bases. Those assessors determined on more or less perpetual failure will be quick to discourage colleagues who might have an interest in establishing an information retrieval system for the unit or institution. They will also be slow to undertake the amassing of information about their own cases. Certainly, they will rule out the possibility of collecting systematic follow-up information about persons assessed previously. Absence of such knowledge almost guarantees failure (Ziskin & Faust, 1988, pp. 413–419).

15. Avoid Prediction Specificity

Naive and inexperienced assessors—those willing to put themselves on the line—state specifically in their reports estimates of the likelihood of which types of violent behaviors will occur over a set period of weeks, months, or years. This means that both their failures and their successes will be plain for all to examine in due course. Assessors bent on failure and unassailability should take no such step. It is much safer to stick to the tried-and-true approach of offering "predictions" so vague that, regardless of the eventual outcome, the original prognostications can be interpreted to mean almost anything. This technique, which is part of the fortuneteller's bag of tricks, means that forecasts cannot be understood when examined closely, let alone tested. It is a procedure that, in its own way, passes beyond the notion of prediction accuracy or inaccuracy into the realm of existential analysis or even life after the grave.

16. Avoid Justification of Opinion

In some instances, like it or not, assessors will be confronted with actuarially based predictions. Such a projection will state, perhaps, that the individual under consideration stands an 80% chance of recidivating violently in some particular way during the next 3 years. Evaluators who have internalized point 8 above will naturally be disinclined to allow much if any weight to this "number-crunched" estimate. They will have little patience with the view that opinions based on actuarial data are likely to have greater predictive power than those based on clinical or dynamic factors (Dawes, Faust, & Meehl, 1989). The easier course in this respect is to ignore the actuarial data completely, on the assumption that these omissions in the report will go unnoticed by the parties who eventually receive the report. When they do go unnoticed, the chances of failure in prediction will probably rise, if current research is any indication (e.g., Menzies & Webster, 1995). If the failure to deal with actuarial estimates is observed, it can always be argued that, helpful though the numerical estimate may be, it pales into insignificance against some clinical or other factors assumed to be extraordinarily important in the case at hand. The idea is to raise the chance of a failed prediction through placing inordinate weight on some particular variable. This can, of course, be defended on the basis of incomparable clinical experience and acumen. Very few realize how idiosyncratic clinical opinion is (Quinsey, 1981; Quinsey & Ambtman, 1979).

17. Avoid Obtaining Second Opinions

Really failure-prone assessors—those who were never trained for risk assessment in the first place and who, as a result, have probably become increasingly incompetent over the years (Ziskin & Faust, 1988)—will not rush to have their opinions checked by others. Such checking could reveal that some or all of the points so far considered are suspect. If an assessment were to be reworked in the light of remarks arising from these quarters, it is more than possible that the chances of error in prediction would decrease rather than increase. So, if failure is the aim, it is best not to expose draft reports to the opinions of colleagues. There is as well, of course, the attendant problem that the very seeking of such opinions indicates lack of confidence. Since most people will not realize that there is no established connection between the assessors' confidence in their opinions and clients' actual violent outcomes (Lidz et al., 1993), and if failure in prediction is the aim, there is no point in having too much truck with other colleagues.

18. Avoid Probabilistic Reporting

What courts and tribunals want to know is whether certain individuals are, or are not, dangerous. They have enough trouble dealing with their own terms, such as "on the balance of probabilities" and "beyond a reasonable doubt." Judges spend endless hours explaining the meaning of such phrases to jurors, often with very uncertain results. How then can it be expected that judges themselves will adopt with alacrity the meaning of "probability" as understood by statisticians in the social and biological sciences? This arcane knowledge has no place in courts, parole boards, and the like. It is simply too esoteric and complicated. For an assessor bent on yielding failure, it is vital that the referring agent be given what is traditionally expected—namely, a pronouncement to the effect that an individual under assessment is, or is not, dangerous (Webster, 1984). This way, those receiving the opinion do not have to translate it into the kind of yes–no terms they understand and can deal with. Moreover, if failure is the aim, there is no need to stipulate what the probability of violence might be under one set of circumstances rather than another. This only adds a level of unnecessary complexity, something more to keep researchers occupied.

19. Avoid Relevant Reporting

Those who receive reports are busy people. What they are interested in is the "bottom line." They want to know, as noted in the discussion of point 18 above, whether or not certain persons are dangerous. Therefore, very little is to be gained by spending hours laying out the background of a case in an orderly and systematic fashion. The important thing is that a report should *look* authoritative. This may mean including mounds of material already on file or in the word processor, even if its pertinence to the case is marginal. Those assessors who strive for impressive levels of predictive inaccuracy (to be revealed, presumably, in the afterlife) will know intuitively that a good part of their prowess comes from an ability to write reports that contain much misleading and biased information and that omit possibly key data.

20. Avoid Obtaining Outcome Data

In any event, the whole question of success versus failure is largely academic for this simple reason: It is highly unlikely that anyone will ever determine the outcome of assessment opinion in a systematic way. Only occasionally, and often only in highly unusual circumstances (e.g., Steadman & Cocozza, 1974; Thornberry & Jacoby, 1979), are follow-ups obtained in an orderly fashion. This means that, as noted briefly at the outset under point 3, extraordinary levels of incompetence can be maintained over decades at a stretch. Without follow-up data upon which to establish base rates of violence for particular subgroups, it is entirely impossible to determine the predictive accuracy or inaccuracy of assessors. This means that those who are failing never have to confront the possibility that, in the interests of fairness, they should withdraw from this particular professional activity. Some evangelists would argue that assessors should, in their reports, be able to inform the referring agents as to their own predictive acumen (e.g., Webster, 1984). This is patent nonsense. Assessors bent on failure evaluate clients, write reports, and close files. They never arrange follow-up meetings with the clients even when this would be easy to do. It is simple to avoid ever having a knowledge of outcome. The absence of such knowledge pretty much guarantees continual failure.

CONCLUDING COMMENT

The aim of this chapter has, of course, been to draw attention to the fact that in all likelihood, the quality of routine assessments of risk could be improved in terms of both accuracy and procedural fairness. People who suffer from serious problems with impulsivity sometimes tend to receive less-than-optimal consideration from mental health, justice, and correctional officials. There is a tendency to incorporate into a new report the findings from previous assessments without much penetrating analysis. Actuarial information that is easy to obtain and verify is set aside in favor of clinical issues. Clinicians are regrettably impatient with what they see as the reductionistic tendencies of researchers, and researchers are no less accommodating when it comes to recognizing the day-to-day stresses and actualities of life in a clinic. Rarely is there available the support of trained professional staffers whose task it is to play a leading role in assembling and verifying background information, in coding data accurately, and in ensuring that scales and other devices appropriate to the task at hand are administered. Too often the process is left to a harried senior clinician, with little or no division of labor. My point is that assessment of risk must be acknowledged to be a difficult and challenging task. It could well be that the painstaking, systematic approach advocated here and throughout this section of the volume will eventually be shown to be less than ideal. Other approaches, grounded in conceptual frameworks very different from the one advocated here, may eventually prove superior (e.g., Marks-Tarlow, 1993). But for the moment, I would argue that if indeed the aim is (as it should be) to enhance the predictive power of assessors, we should stick to what we know. What we do know is that we currently overpredict violence in persons with disorders involving impulsivity, and that with due attention to the 20 points discussed here, assessments could probably be improved at least a little. Only slight improvements could mean much—both in protecting some individuals' rights to live unfettered lives, and in protecting those in society who are needlessly threatened and assaulted. It seems as if we live unnecessarily in a "Wright brothers" era, when in fact we could be flying with many aspects of current aeronautical technology (including, importantly, simulation training).

My thinking along these lines—influenced, in part, by doing "postmortems" on false-negative cases—has yielded the 20-item list given above. A version of this list that is worded positively, and has been made into a checklist for ease of use, is presented as the Appendix to this chapter. Like most of the several other checklists included in this book, it is at an exploratory level of development. It is intended to be used either as a guide to the conduct of particular evaluations or as a checklist to be employed during the course of "risk assessment autopsies."

REFERENCES

American Psychological Association. (1992). *Ethical principles of psychologists and code of conduct.* Washington, DC: Author.

Bjørkly, S. (1994). The scale for the prediction of aggression and dangerousness in psychotic patients: A prospective pilot study. *Criminal Justice and Behavior, 21,* 341–356.

Bolen, D. E. (1994). *Stupid crimes: A novel.* Toronto: Vintage Books.

Boyd, B. A. (1964). Our jails and the psychiatric examination and treatment of disturbed offenders. *Canadian Journal of Corrections, 6,* 477–479.

Campbell, J. C. (Ed.). (1995). *Assessing dangerousness: Violence by sexual offenders, batterers, and child abusers.* Thousand Oaks, CA: Sage.

Dawes, R. M., Faust, D., & Meehl, P. E. (1989). Clinical versus actuarial judgement. *Science, 243,* 1668–1674.

Dietz, P. E. (1985). Hypothetical criteria for the prediction of individual criminality. In C. D. Webster, M. H. Ben-Aron, & S. J. Hucker (Eds.), *Dangerousness: Probability and prediction, psychiatry and public policy* (pp. 87–102), New York: Cambridge University Press.

Greenland, C. (1985). Dangerousness, mental disorder, and politics. In C.D. Webster, M.H. Ben-Aron, & S.J. Hucker (Eds.), *Dangerousness: Probability and prediction, psychiatry and public policy* (pp. 25–40). New York: Cambridge University Press.

Haley, J. (1969). The art of being a failure as a psychotherapist. *American Journal of Orthopsychiatry, 39,* 691–695.

Hall, H. V. (1987). *Violence prediction: Guidelines for the forensic practitioner.* Springfield, IL: Charles C. Thomas.

Harris, G. T., Rice, M. E., & Quinsey, V. L. (1993). Violent recidivism of mentally disordered offenders: The development of a statistical predictioninstrument. *Criminal Justice and Behavior, 20,* 315–335.

Hart, S. J., Menzies, R. J., & Webster, C. D. (1993). A note on portraying the accuracy of violence predictions. *Law and Human Behavior, 17,* 695–700.

Haynes, R. B. (1985). The reliability of psychiatric diagnosis. In C. D. Webster, M. H. Ben-Aron, & S. J. Hucker (Eds.), *Dangerousness: Probability and prediction, psychiatry and public policy* (pp. 53–64). New York: Cambridge University Press.

Hellman, D., & Blackman, J. (1966). Enuresis, firesetting, and cruelty to animals: A triad predictive of adult crime. *American Journal of Psychiatry, 122,* 1431–1436.

Konečni, V., Mulcahy, E., & Ebbesen, E. (1980). Prison or mental hospital: Factors affecting the processing of persons suspected of being "mentally disordered sex offenders." In P. Lipsitt & B. Sales (Eds.), *New directions in psychological research* (pp. 87–124). New York: Van Nostrand Reinhold.

Lewis, G., & Appleby, L. (1988). Personality disorder: The patients psychiatrists dislike. *British Journal of Psychiatry, 153,* 44–49.

Lidz, C. W., Mulvey, E. P., & Gardner, W. (1993). The accuracy of predictions of violence to others. *Journal of the American Medical Association, 269,* 1007–1111.

Link, B. G., & Steuve, A. (1994). Psychotic symptoms and the violent/illegal behavior of mental patients compared to community controls. In J. Monahan & H. J. Steadman (Eds.), *Violence and mental disorder: Developments in risk assessment* (pp. 137–159). Chicago: University of Chicago Press.

Marks-Tarlow, T. (1993). A new look at impulsivity: Hidden order beneath apparent chaos? In W. G. McCown, J. L. Johnson, & M. B. Shure (Ed.), *The impulsive client: Theory, research, and treatment* (pp. 119–138). Washington, DC: American Psychological Association.

Menzies, R. J. (1989). *Survival of the sanest: Order and disorder in a pretrial psychiatric cllinic.* Toronto: University of Toronto Press.

Menzies, R. J., & Webster, C. D. (1995). The construction and validation of risk assessments in a six-year follow-up of forensic patients: A tri-dimensional analysis. *Journal of Consulting and Clinical Psychology, 63,* 766–778.

Menzies, R. J., Webster, C. D., McMain, S., Staley, S., & Scaglione, R. (1994). The dimensions of dangerousness revisited: Assessing forensic predictions about violence. *Law and Human Behavior, 18,* 1–28.

Monahan, J. (1981). *Predicting violent behavior: An assessment of clinical techniques.* Beverly Hills, CA: Sage.

Mulvey, E. P., & Lidz, C. W. (1995). Conditional prediction: A model for research on dangerousness to others in a new era. *International Journal of Law and Mental Health, 18,* 129–143.

Pfafflin, F. (1979). The contempt of psychiatric experts for sexual convicts: Evaluation of 983 files from sexual offence cases in the State of Hamburg, Germany. *International Journal of Law and Psychiatry, 2,* 485–497.

Pfohl, S. J. (1978). *Predicting dangerousness: The social construction of psychiatric reality.* Lexington, MA: Lexington Books.

Quinsey, V. L. (1981). The long-term management of the mentally abnormal offender. In S. J. Hucker, C. D. Webster, & M. H. Ben-Aron (Eds.), *Mental disorder and criminal responsibility* (pp. 137–155). Toronto: Butterworths.

Quinsey, V. L., & Ambtman, R. (1979). Variables affecting psychiatrists' and teachers' assessments of mentally ill offenders. *Journal of Consulting and Clinical Psychology, 47,* 353–362.

Steadman, H. J., & Cocozza, J. J. (1974). *Careers of the criminally insane: Excessive social control of deviance.* Lexington, MA: Lexington Books.

Thornberry, T. P., & Jacoby, J. E. (1979). *The criminally insane: A community follow-up of mentally ill offenders.* Chicago: University of Chicago Press.

Webster, C. D. (1984). How much of the clinical predictability of dangerousness issue is due to language and communication difficulties?: Some sample courtroom questions and some inspired but heady answers. *International Journal of Offender Therapy and Comparative Criminology, 28,* 159–167.

Webster, C. D., Dickens, B. M., & Addario, S. M. (1985). *Constructing dangerousness: Scientific, legal and policy implications.* Toronto: University of Toronto Centre of Criminology.

Webster, C. D., Eaves, D., Douglas, K., & Wintrup, A. (1995). *The HCR-20 scheme: The assessment of dangerousness and risk.* Vancouver: Simon Fraser University and Forensic Psychiatric Services Commission of British Columbia.

Webster, C. D., Harris, G. T., Rice, M. E., Cormier, C., & Quinsey, V. L. (1994). *The Violence Prediction Scheme: Assessing dangerousness in high risk men.* Toronto: University of Toronto, Centre of Criminology.

Webster, C. D., & Polvi, N. (1995). Challenging assessments of dangerousness and risk. In J. Ziskin (Ed.), *Coping with psychiatric and psychological testimony* (5th ed.): *Vol. 2. Special topics* (pp. 1371–1399). Los Angeles: Law & Psychology Press.

Ziskin, J., & Faust, D. (1988). *Coping with psychiatric and psychological testimony* (4th ed.). Los Angeles: Law & Psychology Press.

Checklist for Conducting Risk Assessments and Retrospective Reviews

Items	Deficiency		
	None	Some	Serious
Preparing	0	1	2
1. Clarification of purpose			
2. Adequate assessment circumstances			
3. Assessor competence			
4. Acknowledgment of assessor bias			
5. Systematic analysis			
Assessing			
6. Familiarity with files			
7. Correctness of data			
8. Actuarial emphasis			
9. Consideration of experiential information			
10. Consideration of current symptomatology			
11. Situational emphasis			
12. Relevance of information			
13. Consideration of risk management			
Reporting			
14. Use of base rate statistics			
15. Prediction specificity			
16. Justification of opinion			
17. Use of second opinions			
18. Probabilistic reporting			
19. Relevant reporting			
20. Use of outcome data			
Totals			
Overall Score			/40

Note. Copyright 1996 by Christopher D. Webster. Reprinted by permission.

IV

PRACTICE: TREATMENT

The books Jack's father had read—all of them paperbacks—were stacked on the bottom shelf of his smoker's stand. *Take Charge of Your Life, Achieving Inner Peace and Better Health, Twenty-Two Days to Increased Effectiveness, Life Crises and How to Make Them Work for You, Living with Passion* . . . From time to time he'd tried to press other books into his father's hands . . .

> —CAROL SHIELDS, *Happenstance, the Husband's Story* (1994, pp. 91–92)

If I would like to be cured of anything, it is the individualism inscribed in me by mass culture, and present always as moralizing, medicalizing scrawls on the wall of my brain. Even after years of therapy, drugs and recurring depressions, and considerable thinking about all of the above or perhaps because of the treatment and thinking—I find ineradicable the idea of what's wrong with me is decaying will.

> —JOHN BENTLEY MAYS, *In the Jaws of the Black Dogs: A Memoir of Depression* (1995, p. 226)

When we can identify our triggers, we set a powerful and freeing process in motion. We can begin the identification with silent questions: What is going on here? Why do I feel out of control? Why am I behaving this way? What am I anxious about? We may be able to trace our feelings back to a chance remark or a stray thought or event that set our anxiety off and running.

> —G. HALVERSON-BOYD and L. K. HUNTER, *Dancing in Limbo: Making Sense of Life after Cancer* (1995, p. 73)

Pharmacotherapy, when looked at closely, will appear to be as arbitrary as much an art, not least in the derogatory sense of being impressionistic where ideally it should be objective as psychotherapy. Like any other serious assessment of human emotional life, pharmacotherapy properly rests on fallible attempts at intimate understanding of another person.

> —PETER D. KRAMER, *Listening to Prozac* (1994, p 6)

19

Mentally Disordered Offenders: What Research Says about Effective Service

GRANT T. HARRIS
MARNIE E. RICE

Several difficulties face those attempting to discern what interventions are effective for mentally disordered offenders. First, the population is not consistently or well defined. One's status as an "offender" depends upon the particular practices of police, prosecutors, and courts in one's home jurisdiction; and one's status as "mentally disordered" depends on the fluctuating formal and informal decisions of clinicians. Although the reliability of psychiatric diagnostic schemes is improving, diagnostic reliability in practice remains modest, or at best unknown (American Psychiatric Association, 1994; Regier, Kaelber, Roper, Rae, & Sartorius, 1994). Just who is a mentally disordered offender varies considerably through time and place, and such offenders are a notoriously heterogeneous population (Rice, Harris, Quinsey, & Cyr, 1990; Silver, Cirincione, & Steadman, 1994). Thus, the literature on mentally disordered offenders lies outside the mainstream of standard clinical work on the effectiveness of interventions for well-defined psychological problems or psychiatric disorders, and outside the domain of effective services for criminal populations. Interventions for psychiatric patients often specifically exclude "forensic" patients, and interventions for offenders often specifically exclude those who suffer from psychotic disorders (e.g., Hildebran & Pithers, 1992).

Second, an examination of modern diagnostic systems (e.g., the *Diagnostic and Statistical Manual of Mental Disorders*, fourth edition [DSM-IV]; American Psychiatric Association, 1994) shows an amazing array of mental disorders. These include those diagnosed in infancy, childhood, or adolescence (e.g., mental retardation, stuttering, selective mutism); deliriums and dementias; substance-related disorders (e.g., alcohol dependence, substance-induced sexual dysfunction); schizophrenia and other psychotic disorders; mood disorders (e.g., major depression, bipolar disorders); anxiety disorders (e.g., panic disorder, posttraumatic stress disorder); somatoform disorders (e.g., hypochondriasis, body dysmorphic disorder); factitious disorders; dissociative disorders; sexual and gender identity disorders (e.g., hypoactive sexual desire disorder, transvestic fetishism); eating disorders; sleep disorders; impulse-control disorders (e.g., intermittent explosive disorder, kleptomania); adjustment disorders; and personality disorders (e.g., antisocial, narcissistic, and borderline personality disorders). As we discuss later, impulsivity (variously conceived) or the failure to inhibit responding has been noted as a feature of many of these disorders. If clinicians had to be able to determine the correct diagnosis and prescribe the indicated treatment for each of these possibilities, treating mentally disordered offenders would be a daunting task indeed.

A third difficulty lies in the question of the appropriate outcome measure for mentally disordered offenders. No one would question the relevance of a reduction in criminal recidivism as at least one critical outcome measure for criminal populations. For mental patients, however, desirable outcomes include reductions in hospitalization and service use, increases in use of certain other services (mostly community), vocational and community adjustment, quality of life, avowed happiness, and decrease in symptom severity (Hargreaves & Shumway, 1989; Lehman, 1988; Wiederanders & Choate, 1994). Large differences in the ability of interventions to effect various outcomes, or results showing that some interventions improved some outcomes (e.g., quality of life) while worsening others (e.g., criminal recidivism), would make conclusions about appropriate service for mentally disordered offenders well-nigh impossible.

Fourth, there are some psychiatric disorders for which there is no effective treatment. For example, there are no credible claims for the effective treatment for the impulsive, exploitative, and irresponsible conduct associated with antisocial personality disorder or psychopathy, and some interventions probably increase the recidivism of such individuals, compared to no intervention (Harris, Rice, & Cormier, 1994; Rice, Harris, & Cormier, 1992). Similarly, there is little evidence that any chemical or psychological treatments reduce the recidivism of paraphilic offenders (Quinsey, Harris, Rice, & Lalumière, 1993; Rice, Harris, & Quinsey, 1996).

Fifth, mentally disordered offenders are heterogeneous in other ways. Some are adults, some juveniles; some are felons, some misdemeanants; some are institutionalized, some are maintained in the community; most are men, but some are women. Little is known about effective interventions for mentally disordered offenders specifically, and almost nothing is known about how these other demographic and status variables moderate any treatment effects. In sum, mentally disordered offenders are heterogeneous in a number of different ways: They have a variety of disorders, which are sometimes hard to classify; they have committed a wide variety of antisocial acts; they live in a wide variety of circumstances, including prisons, psychiatric hospitals, boarding houses, nursing homes, family homes, and cardboard boxes on city streets; and they vary in age, gender, and ethnic background. In addition, there are various outcomes by which one could judge the effectiveness of service for mentally disordered offenders: repetition of the index offense, any criminal or violent recidivism, rehospitalization, exacerbation of symptoms, the amount and quality of social contact, vocational adjustment, income, academic achievements, and happiness. Finally, most of these outcomes may be determined either by official records, self-reports, or the reports of collaterals.

In the face of this nearly bewildering diversity, it is little wonder that even experienced forensic clinicians show no agreement about what is appropriate for mentally disordered offenders (Quinsey & Maguire, 1983). The thesis of this chapter is that knowledge of the empirical and scientific literature on effective service for offenders and for persons with mental disorders can greatly reduce this uncertainty and guide intervention for mentally disordered offenders. Elsewhere (Rice et al., 1996; Rice, Harris, Quinsey, & Cyr, 1990) we have extensively reviewed the outcome research for the clinical problems experienced by mentally disordered offenders. Such an extensive review is beyond the scope of the present work. Rather, our purpose is to abstract from the existing empirical literature some clear principles that, when applied to services for mentally disordered offenders, will give such services the best chance of being effective.

CLINICAL ASSESSMENT AND RISK APPRAISAL

We have examined the clinical presentation of mentally disordered offenders in several studies (Rice & Harris, 1988; Rice, Harris, Quinsey, & Cyr, 1990; Rice et al., 1996; see also Quinsey, Cyr, & Lavallee, 1988). Beginning with an extensive list of psychiatric symptoms, psychological problems, problem behaviors, and personal difficulties, these studies showed that patients' clinical presentation was well captured by a small number of factors or problem domains. The important problem domains were as follows: institutional misconduct, positive schizophrenic symptoms, social withdrawal, life skills deficits, depression, substance abuse, and aggression. The key implication of these findings is that many important problems were not psychiatric symptoms (at least as these are usually conceived), and were not problems that were typically addressed in the assessment and treatment of mentally disordered offenders. Even such problems as depression and substance abuse showed low correspondence with formal diagnostic criteria. We concluded that an exclusive focus on symptoms and diagnosis would lead clinicians working with mentally disordered offenders to neglect many factors relevant both to future antisocial conduct and to community adjustment.

In these studies of mentally disordered offenders, we also used cluster analyses to identify homogeneous subgroups. Regardless of the particular population studied, essentially the same clusters emerged. Some clusters resembled offenders one would expect in correctional institutions: a well-behaved group of subjects who were nonetheless likely to reoffend violently if released;[1] and another group of subjects who were impulsive, aggressive, disruptive, and noncompliant within the institution, and also likely to reoffend violently if released. Some clusters resembled patients one would find among the inpatients or outpatients of an ordinary psychiatric hospital (Harris & Rice, 1990): disturbed, disruptive patients with many positive psychotic symptoms, but not at high risk for violent recidivism; and another group of disturbed, withdrawn patients who lacked the interpersonal skills associated with everyday life, but were not highly likely to reoffend violently. Finally, there was a group that seemed to resemble both populations simultaneously: disturbed, disruptive, impulsive offenders/patients with positive psychotic symptoms who were assaultive and noncompliant within the institution, had many interpersonal and functional skill deficits, and were likely to reoffend violently if released.[2] These studies indicated that services for mentally disordered offenders needed to be able to address the clinical needs of criminal offenders *and* of the population usually labeled as persons suffering from serious mental illness.

One somewhat surprising finding of these studies was that diagnosis (especially as assigned by institutional clinicians) was largely unrelated to risk, clinical presentation, or identifiable clinical needs. For example, among a cluster of individuals who presented as pervasively sad, withdrawn, and hopeless, only a small minority had been diagnosed as depressed and were receiving antidepressant medications. At the same time, only a few of the individuals receiving antidepressant medications were described as sad and withdrawn. Of course, this could be partly because the medications were effective in relieving the symptoms of persons for whom they were prescribed (Rice et al., 1996). Nevertheless, clinical needs are captured not by diagnosis, but by current symptoms, skill deficits, and other psychosocial needs (see also Uttaro & Mechanic, 1994).

Studies of the recidivism of mentally disordered offenders clearly indicate that the same variables predict recidivism in these offenders as in offenders without mental disorders (Harris & Rice, 1994; Harris, Rice, & Quinsey, 1993; Klassen & O'Connor, 1989; Quinsey, 1984; Quinsey & Maguire, 1986; Quinsey, Pruesse, & Fernley, 1975; Quinsey, Warneford, Pruesse, & Link, 1975; Rice & Harris, 1992; Rice, Harris, Lang, & Bell, 1990). Thus, such variables as criminal history, childhood criminality, marital status, and age are related to subsequent crime and violent crime in both populations. We (Harris et al., 1993) constructed an actuarial instrument for the prediction of violent recidivism. The instrument was developed in a follow-up study that combined 332 mentally disordered offenders (insanity acquittees) with 286 convicted offenders. A long follow-up period (about 7 years) was used to determine which personal characteristics were related to subsequent violent offending. Twelve variables, in combination, showed considerable accuracy in predicting which subjects would fail violently: score on Hare's (1991) Psychopathy Checklist—Revised, elementary school maladjustment, age (younger age indicating higher risk), separation from parents before age 16, failure on a prior conditional release, the number and severity of prior nonviolent offenses, DSM-III diagnosis (schizophrenia indicating lower risk and personality disorder indicating higher risk), never having married, history of alcohol abuse, amount of victim injury in the index offense (greater injury indicating lower risk), and having a female victim in the index offense (female victim indicating lower risk). This list is noteworthy because almost every variable identified has been found to be related to recidivism in studies of criminal offenders without mental disorders. Few of the 12 variables pertain to mental disorder or to psychiatric constructs. We also examined variables pertaining to the severity of mental disorder, insight, Minnesota Multiphasic Personality Inventory results, type of schizophrenia, and history of psychiatric treatment, and none bore a strong relationship with violent outcome. The only exception was diagnosis: Severe mental disorder (schizophrenia) was *negatively* related to subsequent violence. The actuarial instrument performed equally well in mentally disordered offenders and offenders who had been convicted. Clinicians are sometimes surprised at this finding, and often assert that psychotic symptomatology, though obviously irrelevant for offenders in general, is a strong predictor of violence among mentally disordered offenders.

In fact, there is evidence that among the general population, persons who show particular active psychotic symptoms are at higher risk for violent behavior than other persons (e.g., Link, Andrews, & Cullen, 1992). Similarly, among mentally disordered offenders, there may be certain cases in which the symptomatology is related to violent behavior, and treating the symptomatology may reduce the risk of subsequent violent or criminal behavior (Taylor, 1985; Taylor et al., 1994). Yet the data for mentally disordered offenders in general are clear: Schizophrenia and positive psychotic symptomatology are unrelated or negatively related to subsequent violence. These results strongly suggest that treatments to reduce the risk of subsequent criminal behavior among mentally disordered offenders will be more similar to treatments that reduce risk of criminal recidivism among offenders in general than to treatments designed to reduce psychotic symptomatology. Of course, a comprehensive treatment program for mentally disordered offenders will be targeted at increasing community adjustment as well as reducing criminal recidivism, and therefore will include both treatment targets.

Among the risk appraisal tools for criminal offenders, the Level of Supervision Inventory (Andrews, 1982), the Wisconsin Needs Assessment (Baird, 1981), and the Community Risk/Needs Management Scale (Motiuk, 1993) stand out because, in addition to being good instruments for the prediction of future criminal behavior, they include among their predictor variables some that have to do with criminogenic needs. "Criminogenic needs" are empirically related to criminal behavior, and are changeable (or potentially so) over time or with treatment. Thus, unlike most risk prediction instruments, tools that assess such needs offer the potential that risk can be reduced over time and the instruments can be systematically readministered to measure changes resulting from intervention. Among the available instruments, the Level of Supervision Inventory currently has the greatest amount of empirical support for the assessment of criminogenic needs (Bonta, 1996).

In addition to violence toward others, the possibility of suicide is an important risk appraisal concern for mentally disordered offenders. Some investigators have hypothesized a link between suicidal behavior and impulsivity (Virkkunen, DeJong, Bartko, & Linnoila, 1989). Again, the available research suggests that the most accurate identification of high-risk patients would be achieved through an actuarial approach. Factors with an empirical relationship to suicidal behavior are as follows: a history of suicide attempts, being unmarried and living alone, unemployment, insomnia, alcohol abuse, threats of or plans for suicide, family history of suicide, terminal illness, and of course the symptoms of depression (see Roy, 1994). Again, a systematic approach to appraising the risk of suicide, in which several factors are evaluated and added independently, is indicated (Sainsbury, 1986).

In summary, then, risk appraisal for mentally disordered offenders should be accomplished with the same actuarial tools validated for offenders (or patients) in general. Needs assessment should proceed by identifying skills, psychosocial strengths and deficits, and symptomatology, regardless of diagnosis. We now turn to a consideration of two separate literatures relevant to the treatment of mentally disordered offenders: what is currently known about effective interventions for reducing criminal and violent recidivism among offenders, and what is known about improving desirable outcomes for persons with serious mental disorders. First, however, we briefly consider the meanings of "impulsivity" in the present context.

IMPULSIVITY AND MENTALLY DISORDERED OFFENDERS

As several other chapters in this book show, impulsivity is indicated in many kinds of criminal and antisocial behavior. Indeed, as noted several times already, impulsivity (or the failure to control impulses) has been advanced as an encompassing theory of crime in general (Gottfredson & Hirschi, 1990). In this context, we note that there are two somewhat distinct senses to the concept of "impulsivity." The first is the idea of behaving in response to instinctive forces suddenly and without reflection. In that sense, persons suffering from psychotic disorders sometimes engage in dangerous or antisocial actions without due consideration of the consequences. For example, persons with bipolar I disorder who are experiencing a manic episode may engage in foolish, risky conduct because they ignore or minimize the probable consequences of their actions. Persons with schizophrenia may exhibit disorganized interpersonal behaviors that could be characterized as a failure to inhibit inappropriate or irrelevant responses. Indeed, the failure of selective attention has been proposed as a core schizophrenic characteristic (Neale & Oltmanns, 1980). Persons suffering from mental retardation may commit dangerous or antisocial actions because their intellectual handicap interferes with careful consideration of consequences. Some organic disorders (e.g., Huntington's disease and Tourette's syndrome) seem to entail a kind of automatic uncontrolled response that might be thought of as impulsivity. Thus, many Axis I disorders may be characterized by a tendency to act without reflection. Of course, on Axis II, antisocial personality disorder or psychopathy includes this sense of impulsivity (failure to plan ahead) as a defining property. Again, the characteristic actions can seem reckless and negligent. Zamble and Quinsey (1997) have reported, for example, that many criminal offenses occurred with amazingly little planning or foresight—at least as later reported by incarcerated offenders.

There is another sense of "impulsivity," however. In this second sense, impulsivity is simply the failure to resist impulses. These failures to resist can seem anything but sudden or unplanned. Thus, for example, some of the devious, Machiavellian schemes of psychopathic offenders certainly represent the failure to resist the impulse to lie, cheat, and steal, but they also entail considerable planning and reflection. Similarly, some sex offenses may spring forth fully formed with little or no planning. But it is undeniable that many sexual aggressors, while failing to resist their sexual impulses, engage in enormous amounts of stalking, prowling, cruising, "grooming," and outright conscious planning to find and set up their victims and to minimize the chances that they will be apprehended afterwards.

In this book, both senses of "impulsivity" are alluded to. Is "impulsivity" a single clinical entity that can be tackled directly in treatment? As the foregoing implies, we think that the answer to this question is negative. Consequently, the following discussion does not focus on treating impulsivity directly (because we do not think that this is yet possible). Rather, we address the issue of what interventions make empirical sense for criminal offenders and what clinical services are likely to be effective for persons with serious mental disorders.

INTERVENTIONS FOR REDUCING CRIMINAL RECIDIVISM

There have been very few controlled outcome studies of the effects of treatment of any kind on the subsequent criminal recidivism of mentally disordered offenders. What little empirical evidence exists suggests that the treatments evaluated to date do little to alter the likelihood of future criminal and violent behavior, although there may be positive effects (compared to spending time in prison) for psychotic offenders (Rice et al., 1992). Fortunately, as we have discussed, there is considerable evidence that interventions that reduce criminal recidivism in offenders without mental disorders can also be expected to reduce criminal recidivism in mentally disordered offenders.

In examining what kinds of treatment approaches show the most promise in reducing criminal recidivism, we must first ask the question of whether any kind of treatment has been shown to be effective. This question has been debated at length over the years since Martinson (1974) published his highly influential review, which came to be associated with the position that "nothing works." Many of those charged with setting correctional policy in the United States have adopted the view that rehabilitation does not work and that deterrence is a more effective strategy (Gendreau, 1996a). Deterrence policies have entailed higher incarceration rates, increasing criminal sanctions, more determinate sentencing, and novel punishments (e.g., boot camps and shock incarceration).

Nevertheless, studies showing positive effects of treatment have continued to appear in the literature (e.g., Basta & Davidson, 1988; Cullen & Gendreau, 1989; Gendreau, 1996b; Gendreau & Ross, 1979; Kazdin, 1987; Palmer, 1992; Van Voorhis, 1987). In general, these reviews have concluded that there is considerable evidence that treatment for offenders can not only reduce recidivism, but can have other positive effects. However, critics have dismissed much of the evidence because almost every study had serious flaws; because there were also many negative studies; because it was difficult to discern a clear pattern in the results;

and because the magnitude of effects, when found, was modest (Sechrest, White, & Brown, 1979).

Fortunately, a significant methodological advance has made it possible to examine the evidence for the effects of interventions more objectively than had been possible in the past. The advent of meta-analysis has made it possible to address directly many of the criticisms that have been lodged against narrative reviews. Meta-analysis provides a method of combining data from many different studies so that one can examine the magnitudes of effects, and, in addition, can examine what variables influence the effect sizes obtained. In the area of offender treatment, for example, meta-analyses have examined whether treatment has an effect on recidivism or other outcomes, as well as whether such variables as amount or type of treatment influence the magnitude of the effect. The effect size is the statistic used in meta-analysis to estimate the amount by which the treated group differs from a control group (whose members may be untreated or, in some cases, received an alternate treatment). Although there are different ways of calculating effect sizes, the measure we use in this chapter is Cohen's d, which refers to the difference (in standard deviation units) between the means of the treatment and control groups. According to Cohen (1969), a d of .20 is a small effect size, a d of .50 is moderate, and a d of .80 is large.

There have now been several meta-analyses of the effectiveness of treatments for juvenile and adult offenders. These meta-analyses are quite consistent with one another in finding positive effects of treatment. More recent meta-analyses have become more comprehensive and more sophisticated, and have allowed exploration of the factors that might be responsible for variability in the findings across studies. We discuss the meta-analyses further, in chronological order of their appearance, below.

Garrett (1985) conducted a meta-analysis of 111 studies of the effects of treatment published since 1960. Garrett included studies with a comparison group or ones that examined pre–post treatment changes. Outcome measures included criminal recidivism, institutional adjustment, psychological adjustment, and academic performance. All studies included adjudicated delinquents age 21 or under. Treatments were provided either in institutions or in community residential settings. Evaluations of diversion, probation, and parole were not included. Garrett found an overall effect size of .37. The effect size for recidivism (.13) was smaller than for the other outcomes, and the effect size for community adjustment was the largest (.63). Studies with relatively weak designs yielded larger effect sizes, and effect sizes for behavioral programs (.63) were larger than for cognitive-behavioral programs (.58), Outward Bound programs (.38), or psychodynamic programs (.17).

The second series of meta-analyses to appear was conducted by a single team of investigators (Gensheimer, Mayer, Gottschalk, & Davidson, 1986; Gottschalk, Davidson, Gensheimer, & Mayer, 1987; Gottschalk,

Davidson, Mayer, & Gensheimer, 1987; Mayer, Gensheimer, Davidson, & Gottschalk, 1986). There was a high degree of overlap among the studies included in the four reports. All examined studies published between 1967 and 1983 (or between 1967 and 1981 in one paper) listed in *Psychological Abstracts*, as well as unpublished material solicited from prominent authors in the field. All included only studies that had at least some adjudicated juvenile delinquents as subjects, and included only studies that examined outcome (including criminal recidivism) after the end of treatment. The samples in all four meta-analyses were primarily male (percentages ranged from 73% to 81%) and the mean (or, in one case, median) ages of the delinquents ranged from 14.5 to 16 years.

The first meta-analysis (Gensheimer et al., 1986) included only studies that involved diversion (i.e., the channeling of youths away from the juvenile justice system to alternative, nonjudicial programs). The overall effect size obtained was .40, and the effect for recidivism was .44. Effect sizes were bigger for younger subjects (the product–moment correlation between effect size and age was −.35). Programs that involved more contact hours yielded bigger effect sizes ($r = .69$). But the biggest relationship was found with the investigator's involvement in the treatment program: The greater the investigator's involvement, the bigger the effect size ($r = .76$). The authors examined possible explanations for this finding and concluded that it had to do with program integrity—an issue we return to later in this chapter.

The second study (Gottschalk, Davidson, Gensheimer, & Mayer, 1987) examined just community-based interventions (90 studies). The obtained effect size was .56 overall, and .39 for recidivism. Among the variables found to be related to effect size were number of hours of treatment (more hours yielded higher effect sizes), and type of treatment (behavioral, educational/vocational, and group psychotherapy interventions yielded higher effect sizes than individual psychotherapy, casework, or nonspecific intervention).

The third (Gottschalk, Davidson, Mayer, & Gensheimer, 1987) and fourth (Mayer et al., 1986) studies examined 30 and 39 studies, respectively, of behavioral and social learning interventions (how these differed was not completely specified), with almost total overlap in the studies included. Treatment was provided in the institution in just over one-third of the cases, and the remainder were conducted in either residential or nonresidential community settings. The overall mean effect sizes for all outcomes combined were .57 and .92, respectively, and the effect sizes for recidivism were .31 and .52, respectively.

Although all of the effect sizes obtained in these studies were positive, the confidence intervals around the effect sizes for recidivism all included 0, and so in no case could the null hypothesis that treatment had no effect on recidivism be rejected. The authors were most pessimistic in the case of the behavioral studies: "No substantial outcome evidence exists for the efficacy of behavioral techniques in affecting violence and antisocial behavior as represented by juvenile offenders" (Gottschalk, Davidson, Mayer, & Gensheimer, 1987, p. 418). Although their conclusions were less pessimistic in each of the other chapters (where effect sizes and sample sizes were larger), the results and conclusions of these studies would do little to alter the view of those who believe that "nothing works."

Whitehead and Lab (1989) contributed further to the pessimistic view of treatment with their meta-analysis of 50 studies evaluating treatment for juvenile delinquents and published from the beginning of 1975 to the end of 1984. All studies had control groups. Programs included diversion, community corrections, institutional or residential treatment, and specialty programs such as Scared Straight and Outward Bound. Recidivism was defined differently across the studies, but all reflected subsequent contact with the juvenile justice system. The overall effect size was .27. Interestingly, Whitehead and Lab found the highest effect size for diversion programs that operated as an extension of, rather than in place of, the formal justice system. They argued that programs involving a degree of coercion, but avoiding the negative consequences of normal criminal justice system processing, might have positive effects on recidivism. They also noted that effect sizes were negative in a number of cases, suggesting that treatment actually increased recidivism. The authors concluded: "The results are far from encouraging for advocates of correctional intervention" (p. 289), and "the results clearly support [the conclusion] that correctional treatment has little effect on recidivism" (p. 291). In one of the few studies to examine the issue, Whitehead and Lab found no differential effects for gender. Like Garrett, they also reported smaller effect sizes for more rigorous studies.

The findings and conclusions of the Whitehead and Lab (1989) study led to a clever subsequent reanalysis of mostly the same studies (but with a few deleted for various reasons and a few more, including studies with adult offenders, added) by Andrews et al. (1990). What made this study an improvement over earlier studies was that prior to examining effect sizes, the authors classified the studies according to variables they believed on clinical and theoretical grounds to be related to effectiveness. These authors proposed three main principles of effective correctional treatment (Andrews et al., 1990; Andrews & Bonta, 1994). First, they argued that more intensive service should be reserved for higher-risk cases, and they presented data supporting the view that treatment effects are greater for higher-risk than for lower-risk cases. Second, the authors argued that treatment designed to reduce recidivism must be targeted to criminogenic needs—that is, to those factors that are empirically related to recidivism and are changeable. They argued that the most promising treatment targets include changing antisocial attitudes and peer associations; promoting family affection, parental monitoring, and parental supervision; promoting identification with prosocial role models; reducing chemical dependence; reducing impulsivity and increasing self-control; and increasing prosocial skills. Less promising treatment targets, they argued, include increasing self-esteem and working on unspecified personal and emotional problems in therapy. Traditional psychodynamic and nondirective client-centered therapies, relationship-oriented milieu approaches, and unstructured, peer-oriented group counseling are to be especially avoided. Finally, they argued that treatment must be responsive to the learning styles of offenders and capable of meeting the criminogenic needs identified above. For example, Gendreau (1996b) has argued that psychiatrically disturbed offenders will be more responsive to treatments provided in low-pressure sheltered-living environments than in high-pressure institutional environments. Generally speaking (i.e., for most offenders), the treatments indicated are behavioral and social learning approaches, skill enhancement, and cognitive change. They must also be applied by using authority in a firm but fair manner; by modeling anticriminal styles of thinking, feeling, and acting; and by engaging in concrete problem solving and systematic skill training. Service providers must relate to offenders in a warm, flexible, and enthusiastic manner, while being careful not to support criminal attitudes or behaviors. Highly verbal, evocative, and relationship-dependent therapies should, they argued, be reserved for those few offenders who show a high level of interpersonal maturity.

Keeping these principles in mind, then, Andrews et al. (1990) classified the studies according to whether or not they heeded the principles of risk, need, and responsivity. Overall, they obtained a small treatment effect size of .21, very similar to that obtained by Whitehead and Lab (1989). However, when they examined how effect sizes varied in relation to how well the treatments adhered to the principles of effective service, they found that the overall effect size for appropriate services was .63—significantly greater than those for services that were clearly inappropriate, for services that were not sufficiently well described to be classified, and also for criminal sanctions (e.g., variations among restitution, probation and custody; or variations in the duration of probation, etc.). Furthermore, they found that services offered in the community were more effective than services offered in residential settings. Although they had only a few studies of adult offenders, they found no difference in effect size between treatments offered to adults and those offered to juvenile offenders.

Izzo and Ross (1990) conducted a meta-analysis of 46 studies of the effects of cognitive and noncognitive treatments on the recidivism of adjudicated juvenile delinquents. All studies were published between 1970 and 1985, and subjects (the majority of whom were males) ranged from 11 to 18 years of age, with an average age of 13. The authors hypothesized that cognitive programs would be more effective than noncognitive programs. Cognitive programs were those employing one or more of the following: problem solving, negotiation skills training, interpersonal skills training, rational–emotional therapy, role playing and modeling, or cognitive behavior modification. Although no overall effect size was given, the effect size for cognitive treatments was significantly greater than that for noncognitive treatments, and effect sizes were greater for treatments provided in the community than for treatments provided in the institution.

In by far the most ambitious and comprehensive meta-analysis of offender treatment, Lipsey (1992) conducted a meta-analysis of 443 studies of the effects of treatments on the recidivism of juvenile delinquents aged 12 to 21. Lipsey included published and unpublished studies that had been conducted since 1950, that included a control or comparison group, and that had been conducted in English-speaking industrialized countries. Lipsey's study demonstrated quite clearly that it is simply not true that "nothing works." Although the average overall effect size was a small .17, the confidence interval did not include 0, and thus Lipsey could assert with confidence that intervention can have a significant positive impact. Because his study included so many studies and so many subjects, he could convincingly rule out the null hypothesis that nothing works, even though the effect size he obtained for recidivism was one of the lowest of all those obtained in the meta-analyses reviewed above. Another great strength of Lipsey's study was that he was able to examine the effects of a great number of possible moderator variables. He confirmed many of the findings found in smaller meta-analytic studies. First, like Andrews et al. (1990), he found a tendency for treatments targeted to higher risk juveniles to yield larger effect sizes. As Andrews et al. had also done, he found that the type of intervention was extremely important. The most successful treatments were those that were more structured and specific (e.g., behavioral or skills training approaches). Treatments that involved employment (but not vocational counseling) were effective for older adolescents. Interventions that enhanced involvement with prosocial peers were notably effective. Also in line with the findings of Andrews et al., some programs were found to be ineffective or even harmful, including traditional counseling and casework, special tutoring and school classes, and deterrence- or fear-based programs (e.g., shock incarceration). Another important variable had to do with the involvement of the researchers in mounting an intervention: The more highly involved the researchers, the more effective was the intervention. Lipsey attributed this to the high commitment of involved researchers to ensuring that the program was carried out as carefully and vigorously as planned. In a related vein, Lipsey also found that more intensive interventions (i.e., more hours of programming over a longer time period) were more effective than less intensive ones.

Lipsey and Wilson (1993) recently undertook an even more ambitious study, in which they reviewed the evidence from meta-analyses regarding the efficacy of psychological, educational, and behavioral treatments for all populations and all types of outcomes. They found 290 meta-analytic studies they could include in their review, which included published and unpublished studies in the areas of mental health interventions (treatment programs for offenders were considered under this heading), work setting or organizational interventions (e.g., programs intended to increase worker productivity or job satisfaction), and educational interventions (e.g., programmed instruction, tutoring, interventions for test taking). They found a dramatic overall pattern of positive effects that could not be explained as artifact or placebo. They also concluded that the effects were large enough to have both practical and clinical significance. The effect sizes were lower for unpublished than for published studies; one group, pre–post treatment designs, overestimated treatment effects; and some of the effect size could be accounted for as a placebo effect. Nevertheless, the overall mean effect size was .50, which is generally considered to be moderate. The overall mean effect for the delinquency studies was .36.

Lipsey and Wilson compared the average effect sizes obtained for psychological treatments with average effect sizes obtained in meta-analyses of medical treatments. The average obtained effect size for medical treatments (e.g., chemotherapy for breast cancer, coronary bypass surgery, and drug treatments for mental disorders) was .40, very close to the overall effect size for delinquency treatments and somewhat lower than the overall effect size for psychological treatments in general. Although the effect sizes for recidivism outcomes in the delinquency studies have been somewhat lower, the effects are still of meaningful practical magnitude. The more effective treatments (those defined as "clinically relevant" in the meta-analysis of Andrews et al.) represent decreases of 20–40% in recidivism (Lipsey, 1992).

In summary, then, there is now sufficient evidence to support the strong statement that treatment for offenders can both reduce criminal recidivism and have other positive effects. Programs that are highly structured and behavioral or cognitive-behavioral, that are run in the community rather than in an institution, that are run with integrity and enthusiasm, that target higher-risk rather than lower-risk offenders, and that are intensive in terms of number of hours and overall length of program can be expected to be considerably more effective than others. Programs that are based on fear or punishment, as well as traditional psychotherapy or casework, can be expected to be considerably less effective with offenders than other programs; some of these programs may even be harmful for certain offenders (McCord, 1978; Rice et al., 1992). Finally, there is little evidence that factors such as age, sex, or race of offender make a difference to outcome, although at present few studies have examined the effects of these factors. Future work needs to examine these factors further. The biggest question for future studies, however, will be how to maximize treatment effectiveness, rather than to ask whether treatment for offenders works.

TREATMENT FOR PERSONS WITH MENTAL DISORDER

A complete review of all pharmacological and psychological interventions for all difficulties associated with mental disorders is beyond the scope of this chapter. Recent compilations have attempted to synthesize what is known about treatments for such disorders (Hersen & Ammerman, 1994) and even about treatments for antisocial behavior (Ammerman, Hersen, & Sisson, 1994). As mentioned above, the meta-analyses by Lipsey and Wilson (1993) showed that well-developed psychological and behavioral treatments for a wide variety of disorders are effective, and that the magnitude of their effectiveness is roughly equal to that of pharmacological treatments for mental disorders and of medical treatments in general. However, Lipsey and Wilson's (1993) work indicates neither that everything works nor that all treatments are equally effective. They note that poorly developed interventions, and therapies that are well developed but poorly implemented, are probably ineffective.

Given the array of "mental disorders" listed in this chapter's introduction, how could clinicians and agencies hope to meet the needs of each mentally disordered offender the legal system might send their way? In practice, schizophrenia and mood disorders—together often called "serious mental illness" or "functional psychoses"—are the types of disorders most likely to result in an accused person's becoming a mentally disordered offender (Rice & Harris, 1990).[3] Although, as also discussed in the introduction, the personal problems of mentally disordered offenders are not well captured by diagnosis alone, in the following review we confine our attention to the empirical literature on interventions for the problems experienced by persons with "serious mental illness." In the treatment of such persons, there is no doubt of the following:

1. Some drugs are powerfully effective in relieving the symptoms of psychotic and mood disorders. Although effective neither for all symptoms nor for all patients, neuroleptics and antidepressants have profoundly altered the treatment of mental patients. Because there is no effective drug for many problems and symptoms, however, and because some patients resist taking or are unimproved by known drugs, drug treatment cannot represent a complete solution to the difficulties experienced by persons diagnosed with mental disorders.

2. Effective services for persons with serious mental illness need to be comprehensive. Comprehensive services entail an emphasis on teach-

ing and learning; opportunities for patients to share responsibility; efforts to prevent social isolation through active client–clinician interaction; clarity of staff roles and purpose; and stable staffing.

3. Four main outcomes have been studied: symptom number and severity; rehabilitative outcome (social, vocational functioning); humanistic outcome (happiness); and public safety (violence, antisocial conduct). Although these outcomes do not march in lockstep, comprehensive services have been shown to make improvements in each of these outcomes.

4. The principles of effective service apply both to institutional and to community-based programs. However, effective community programs also employ assertive approaches to service delivery, give practical advice and training for families, and help with money and housing. Much has been written about case management for mental patients in the community. It is clear that case management is not a single clinical entity and is manifested in a number of different styles or models, ranging from the "advocate and service broker" model to the "full service and support" model. It is also clear that case management depends for its effectiveness on the interventions arranged for or provided directly by case managers. To the extent that "case-managed" interventions embody the characteristics of effective service in general and eschew ineffective or counterproductive activities, case management can enhance treatment effectiveness.

Let us now consider the evidence for these assertions about effective service in more detail.

Medication

The abundant research demonstrating the effectiveness of antipsychotic and antidepressant drugs does not mean that all clients who receive them derive maximal benefit. This happens for several reasons. First, the specific mechanisms responsible for therapeutic effectiveness are not fully known, so that it is generally unclear when changing dose or drug or adding a second drug will lead to a better or worse clinical condition. Second, many clients who would benefit from neuroleptics, for example, resist taking them. Third, customary practice (and the advice given physicians) is sometimes inconsistent with empirical findings. As an example of this last point, Harris (1989) showed that some psychotic mentally disordered offenders in a secure facility responded quickly to neuroleptic drugs, while others did not. Among those who did not, clinical improvement was sought through many subsequent drug and dose changes. These strategies, however, were completely unrelated to improvements in patients' conditions. The empirical evidence is clear that from the standpoint of clinical efficacy, traditional neuroleptics all have the same effects (Wittlin, 1988). There is some evidence, however, that the newer, atypical antipsychotics (e.g., clozapine and risperidone) may be more effective (Heinrich, Klieser, Lehmann, Kinzler, & Hruschka, 1994; Reid, Mason, & Toprac, 1994). Similarly, the evidence seems clear that megadoses of neuroleptics are not more effective than standard doses even for resistant patients. Why then would physicians switch from drug to drug or attempt very-high-dose treatment, and why would they be advised to do so (e.g., Anderson, Vaulx-Smith, & Keshavan, 1994)?

The answer lies in the profound difference between systematic empirical research and the impressions created by everyday experience. Even if variations in the prescription of megadoses (or switching drugs or adding a particular second drug) and fluctuations in clients' conditions were, in reality, completely independent and unrelated to each other, a clinician who employed such a strategy when clients did poorly would experience many occasions when an improvement in a client's condition followed. Such coincidences often lead to a mistaken belief that the megadose or drug combination has *caused* the clinical improvement when it has not.[4] The purpose of research methods is to prevent such mistaken conclusions. The point, however, is that advice based on clinical experience can (and often does) differ from advice based on systematic research.

The most empirically sound approach is well described by Wittlin (1988; see also Liberman, Van Putten, et al., 1994). It is to prescribe the drug indicated (if any) for the diagnostic group to which the patient seems to belong. One or two other drugs from the same class should be tried if the first fails or produces intolerable side effects. For example, clozapine or risperidone may be indicated if standard neuroleptics fail. The effects of the medication on symptoms should be monitored by means of a standardized instrument such as the Brief Psychiatric Rating Scale (Overall & Gorham, 1988) or its extended version (Lukoff, Liberman, & Nuechterlein, 1986).

Wittlin's (1988) advice is specific and well grounded in the available research. He advises that the physician and client should collaborate to help the client determine the appropriate balance between therapeutic response and side effects, and to anticipate and prevent relapse. The use of antipsychotics should be flexible; the physician should be aware that the appropriate dose in a hospital setting may be relatively low (or may even be unnecessary), compared to the appropriate dose in an overstimulating family environment. It is necessary to be patient, because not all symptoms will respond to drugs, and several weeks of drug administration are required to tell when the optimal response has been achieved. The approach must include step-by-step skills training to teach clients how to self-administer drugs, recognize and cope with side effects, anticipate relapse, and negotiate drug matters with professionals. Wittlin points out that the importance of medication is reduced when program requirements are clear and reasonable, with lavish positive feedback and encouragement for small improvements. When chronic patients who have been on medication for many years move from custodial, understimulating settings to more stimulating, demanding program environments, antipsychotic drugs may hinder learning because of excessive sedation or akinetic, apathetic effects. He also reminds us: "Medication cannot teach a patient how to make and keep friends, get a job, or live in the community. Other forms of rehabilitation, such as behavior therapy, psychotherapy, and family and social therapy . . . are necessary in combination with medication to produce the best results" (p. 122).

Opportunities for Teaching and Learning

The second most important development in the treatment of mental disorders has been the use of psychoeducational or behavioral methods to develop and strengthen patients' repertoire of skills. The most convincing demonstration of the value of these methods was the work of Paul and Lentz (1977), who demonstrated that specific contingency management techniques could equip very chronic psychotic mental patients with the behaviors necessary to leave hospital and live in the community, where the vast majority were maintained free of psychotropic drugs. The behavioral program was no more costly to operate (though it required very different training for its staff) than the traditional custodial institution, and was shown to be much more cost-effective. Paul and Lentz (1977; see also Rhoades, 1981) also demonstrated that the positive effects they achieved were directly attributable to changes they made in the ways staff members interacted with patients. The key features of the behavioral program were its focus on systematically providing positive consequences for independent, prosocial behaviors, while decreasing or eliminating attention for dependent, symptomatic behavior. Paul and Lentz developed a comprehensive technology for measuring clinician–client interactions and showed how making changes in the ways staff members behaved resulted in improved outcomes for the chronic patients.

More recently, the work of Liberman (1988, 1992) and his colleagues (Lukoff et al., 1986; Wallace, 1993; Wallace & Liberman, 1985; see also Benton & Schroeder, 1990; Payne & Halford, 1990) has demonstrated that a faithfully delivered combination of social skills training, vocational training, and training for patients' families (together with appropriately delivered neuroleptic medication) was responsible for profound improvements in all outcome areas (symptoms, social adjustment, public safety, and happiness). Liberman and his colleagues (Wallace, Liberman, MacKain, Blackwell, & Eckman, 1992) have also developed a package of skills training materials that they have shown to be readily transferable to new clinicians and to new settings, where they can be used to teach patients skills that they can generalize to new situations.

Others have also demonstrated that skills training for clients' families can positively affect a variety of outcomes. Training gives information about serious mental disorders, shows how to recognize and ameliorate stresses that may induce relapse, encourages acceptance of the clients, teaches effective communication, teaches problem-solving skills, trains family members in the use of reward and encouragement as means to effect behavior change, and shows how family members can help maximize the therapeutic effects of drugs (Glick et al., 1990; Hogarty et al., 1991; Liberman, Falloon, & Aitchison, 1984; Tarrier et al., 1989). Family skills training seems especially effective when implemented with families high in "expressed emotion" (overinvolvement and criticism), and when provided on an ongoing basis with refresher and consultation sessions (Liberman, 1988).

Community Case Management

As mentioned above, case management is not a single clinical entity; it may best be conceived of not as an intervention, but as a means to deliver interventions. As such, case managers can help ensure that clients receive medication, participate in skills training, make social contact, receive financial assistance, find employment and housing, and/or live with family members who have necessary skills in managing the clients' problems. Alternatively, case management can be provided by a team of individuals with sufficient expertise among them to provide all the necessary services themselves, rather than arranging for them to be provided by others (see, Test, 1992). To the extent that case managers ensure the delivery of this training and these other services (or deliver them themselves), case management can be more cost-effective than traditional community support services and hospitalization. Several individual studies and reviews have attempted to evaluate the effectiveness of case management (Bond, Miller, Krumwied, & Ward, 1988; Hammaker, 1983; Rubin, 1992; Solomon, 1992; Solomon, Draine, & Meyerson, 1994). This literature shows that some case management services or styles have little or no effect on quality of life, symptoms, social adjustment, or antisocial behavior, compared to leaving clients alone. Most studies show that case management can reduce the frequency and duration of hospitalization, but some indicate that case management may result in worse outcomes than doing nothing may. It is also clear that steps must be taken to ensure that case management services do not "devolve" into essentially custodial community care or traditional casework. At their best, however, case management services can be effective.

To be effective, however, it seems that case management must first be assertive. That is, case managers cannot wait in their offices for clients to make and keep appointments; rather, effective case managers seek out their clients in the clients' environments. Second, effective case management seems to depend on the quality of the relationship between case manager and client. That is, effective case managers tailor the intensity of each client's social interaction to his or her fluctuating ability to handle social stimulation; give clients responsibility and permission to make some mistakes; and employ positive (praise, reward, reinforcement, encouragement) rather than negative (scolding, withdrawal, punishment, sanctions) means to effect changes in clients' behavior. Finally, effective case managers minimize rather than emphasize their professional status, and maintain long-term contact (either as individual clinicians or as small cohesive teams) with clients.

Just as the prescription of drugs can fall short of what research shows is possible, the delivery of psychological therapies, psychosocial programs, and case management services often falls short of the ideal program that the research has already identified as effective (Harris & Rice, 1992; McGrew, Bond, Dietzen, & Salyers, 1994; Rice, Harris, Quinsey, & Cyr, 1990; Solomon et al., 1994). The loss of program integrity shares some causes with the nonoptimal use of drugs—inconsistency between clinical lore and the empirical evidence. On the other hand, there are problems typically encountered in the implementation of psychosocial programs that are unique to nondrug treatment.

IMPLEMENTING BEHAVIORAL OR PSYCHOSOCIAL PROGRAMS

Despite the clear evidence in their favor, many investigators have reported on how difficult it is to implement psychosocial or behavioral programs for mental patients, offenders, and mentally disordered offenders. Leitenberg (1987) remarked: "What is most likely to be done in the name of delinquency prevention is least likely to be effective, and what is most likely to be effective is least likely to be done" (p. 312). He added:

> What is not likely to work for preventing delinquency is individual and group counselling, recreation, social casework, street work with gangs, vocational programs that contain no chance of advancement, scared straight programs, diversion programs (unless carefully implemented), remedial education, Outward Bound wilderness programs, tougher law enforcement, community involvement programs and incapacitation of career offenders. (p. 312)

With very few exceptions, Leitenberg could have applied the same generalization to interventions for mental patients, offenders, and mentally disordered offenders. The real-world practice of service delivery, and consequently the outcomes achieved, fall far short of what the scientific and empirical literature says is possible. Why?

Several barriers to effective intervention have been identified. The most fundamental is that most programs, in any human service field, do not measure outcome. The reasons for this are partly technical (most service providers do not know how to measure outcomes) and partly philosophical and organizational (the rationale for most service agencies is the delivery of some service rather than the achievement of some ultimate goal). For example, the real goal of public education is to provide classroom instruction for children; measurable long-range outcomes are often not specified. Most clinicians (including those whose clients are mentally disordered offenders) work in environments where explicit and specific outcome goals have never been articulated. In such environments, there can be no incentive for staff members to adopt the most effective clinical technology, because "effective" presupposes the articulation of an ultimate outcome goal.

The lack of articulated outcomes leads to several other barriers to the adoption of effective interventions. Politics, both public and organizational, can get in the way. In an environment without articulated outcomes, no politician can afford to be "soft on crime." In the absence of articulated outcome goals, the kinds of services delivered by an organization depend greatly upon what services the most powerful or most numerous clinician groups are trained to deliver. In correctional systems, correctional officers hold political sway, and they are trained to provide custody, supervision, and security. In health care systems, physicians and nurses hold political sway, and most are trained to provide primarily medication and supportive counseling.

A related problem is that of training and education for service providers in the first place. Gendreau (1988) refers to the "MBA syndrome," in which managers and administrators are construed as a generic entity—as leaders who need to know how to manage, but need to know nothing about the theory or practice of treatment for the clients over whom they have ultimate authority. Burdened by this sort of ignorance, no leaders could determine what their staffers should do or how they should do it. Such managers are unlikely to gather the right kind of information on how staff members are performing their jobs. Similarly, most staffers in institutions and many in community agencies receive training that formally or informally emphasizes a custodial approach to service delivery. As mentioned above, Paul and Lentz (1977) powerfully demonstrated what can be accomplished when staff members are appropriately trained and supervised. Laws (1974), however, showed how difficult it is to retrain custodially oriented personnel to deliver psychosocial programs. Finally, clinicians (and the public) are ill informed about the causes of crime and antisocial behavior in the first place. For example, one frequently hears that the evils of poverty and racial prejudice are the causes of crime, despite the fact that there are few convincing data to support these views (Andrews & Bonta, 1994). It will be difficult to get correctional and mental health systems to deliver effective services when almost everyone is so misinformed.

The adoption of new pharmacological treatments appears much easier to achieve. Trying a new drug is a behavior with greatly lower response cost than adopting a new psychosocial intervention; drugs can usually be delivered to clients in institutions or the community with minimal disruption to the organization's normal routine. With the exception of some of the newest atypical antipsychotics (e.g., clozapine), drugs are quite cheap. Moreover, because they are commercial products, drugs are effectively marketed by large multinational corporations that can afford to sponsor conferences and buy advertising in journals. Drugs, in addition to their powerful effects in alleviating the suffering of patients, also solve problems for clinicians. Most psychotic patients are quieter, more cooperative, and more socially appropriate when they take neuroleptics than when they do not. Thus, there seems to be less difficulty in persuading clinicians and policy makers to attend to the data supporting the use of psychiatric drugs and to prescribe them for mentally disordered individuals. What can be done, however, to increase the adoption of psychosocial interventions of demonstrated efficacy from both the literature on the treatment of persons with mental disorders and the literature on the treatment of offenders?

Fortunately, there is evidence that some factors can greatly increase the likelihood that psychosocial interventions will be adopted (Gendreau, 1996a; Harris & Rice, 1992). The first consists of authoritative outside consultation and personal assistance for the organization's leaders throughout the implementation, especially in managing psychological and political difficulties. Second, detailed step-by-step materials and staff training packages that allow for active practice also increase the likelihood of adoption. An especially good example is the comprehensive package of staff training materials, patient materials, and personal consultation provided by Liberman and his colleagues (Backer, Liberman, & Kuchnel, 1986; Liberman, Kopelowicz, & Young, 1994). Similarly, an intervention that can be adopted in a series of incremental steps can be much easier to adopt (Glaser, Abelson, & Garrison, 1983). A system to measure and ensure high therapeutic integrity is important. The system should include direct measures of staff behaviors; detailed written descriptions of desired staff behaviors; frequent supervisor approval for enactments of the behaviors, plus a description of what was approved; continual posted feedback describing progress in staff target behaviors; rewards for staff members for superior performance; and monitoring of, and feedback to, supervisors regarding their performance in giving feedback and rewards to their staffers (Andrasik & McNamara, 1977; Burgio, Whitman, & Reid, 1983; Brown, Willis, & Reid, 1981; Ellsworth, 1968; Kuehnel, DeRisi, Liberman, & Mosk, 1984; Paul & Lentz, 1977).

A committed leader inside the organization who will fight to maintain interest, motivation, enthusiasm, and accountability is important as well. Experience from several impressive psychosocial programs indicates that programs often die when their innovators move on. Indeed, as mentioned above, Lipsey (1992) indicated that programs implemented by their researchers/evaluators yielded larger effect sizes, and this was attributed to the leaders' enthusiasm and careful administrative control. Funding for the program should come from the host organization, so that its leaders bear the financial consequences for program success or failure. Finally, the psychosocial program should solve some current problem for the organization and thereby provide immediate rewards to managers contingent upon successful implementation.

PUTTING IT TOGETHER: WE MAY NEVER HAVE SEEN AN IDEAL PROGRAM, BUT WE'D RECOGNIZE IT

In conclusion, a complete empirical literature about what interventions are effective specifically for mentally disordered offenders does not exist. No program or service specifically provided for mentally disordered offenders has been shown to be effective for all relevant outcomes (symptom reduction, criminal and violent recidivism, community and social adjustment, and happiness). Very little is known about how such variables as age, sex, severity of original offense, and ethnic background might moderate the effectiveness of services for mentally disordered offenders. In the absence of specific empirical knowledge, principles of effective service can be abstracted from what *is* known about effective services for persons with serious mental disorders and services aimed at reducing the criminal recidivism of offenders in general. It can be expected that these principles apply regardless of the age, sex, and ethnic background of mentally disordered offenders. That is, we have never seen the ideal treatment program for mentally disordered offenders, but if we ever encountered one, the available empirical literature would allow us to recognize it immediately. It would have the following characteristics:

1. Risk of recidivism would be appraised with actuarial devices, and the intensity of service would be proportional to actuarially appraised risk.[5] Clinical assessment would be individualized, focusing on psychosocial problems and symptoms (rather than diagnosis per se), and would especially concentrate on criminogenic needs (i.e., changeable or potentially changeable personal characteristics empirically related to outcomes, especially recidivism). Identified criminogenic needs would become treatment targets, and for each, an explicit plan would specify how change is to be accomplished and measured.

2. Psychotropic medications would be used conservatively, prescribed for identified treatment targets, and monitored by objective means in order to determine whether they were having the desired effects.

Psychoeducational programs would be used to increase medication compliance.

3. Behavioral and cognitive-behavioral therapies would be used to teach interpersonal skills, vocational skills, skills associated with reducing or eliminating substance abuse, symptom management skills, and the activities of daily living (life skills). Contingency management systems (a token economy) would be used, at least in institutional settings, to extinguish symptomatic dependent and dangerous behavior; to promote prosocial, independent, "noncrazy" behavior; and to encourage attendance at behavioral or cognitive-behavioral training sessions. The available data suggest that such psychoeducational training represents the best option to ameliorate antisocial conduct resulting from the type of impulsivity we have defined as thoughtless response to instinctive urges and situational pressures.

4. Other treatment targets would include altering antisocial, procriminal values and attitudes, and fostering the development of prosocial peer groups. Staff members would be specifically trained for their jobs in the methods of behavioral or cognitive-behavioral therapy, psychoeducational training techniques, and the use of verbal strategies to manage aggression. They would interact frequently with the clients; would model prosocial values and nonaggressive conflict resolution; and would employ warmth, empathy, and a firm but fair use of authority. Though there are few data on the question, we suggest that such attempts to alter procriminal sentiments and peer associations make sense in ameliorating the type of impulsity we have defined as the deliberate, planful failure to resist antisocial, exploitative impulses.

5. Whenever possible, services would be delivered to the clients while they lived in their communities. An assertive approach to case management and supervision would help ensure that the program did not experience the attrition of its neediest clients.

6. The program would be led by a clinician knowledgeable in behavioral and psychoeducational therapies who also had the qualities of an effective leader: intelligence, enthusiasm, clarity of purpose, communication skills, sincerity, and emotional stability. The program would have a system to ensure its own integrity; this would entail measurement of outcomes, objective measurement of clinical gain for each therapeutic activity (including the administration of drugs), and measurement and explicit feedback on the quality of the staff members' performance of their clinical duties. There would also be contingent application of rewards to staffers and managers for appropriate performance in all three areas.

As a final point on the ideal program, readers might conclude that implementation of such services would be forever impossible because of their prohibitive costs. Does it really cost more to do the job right? Paul and Lentz (1977) demonstrated that a faithfully implemented psychosocial program (including its detailed measurement of client and staff behaviors) was less expensive, and much more cost-effective, than tradi-tional custodial hospitalization. Fully measuring the cost-effectiveness of services for mentally disordered offenders would be difficult indeed. Costs are of different types, accrue in many different places, and are borne by different parties. For example, reducing clinical supervision and asser-tive case management for mentally disordered offenders would clearly reduce costs for the state or provincial mental health commission. This, however, might merely shift costs to federally funded health care services, to municipally funded police, to social service or welfare agencies, or to families. If, in addition, the reduction in supervision resulted in an increase in criminal offenses, costs would also be borne by the correctional system, courts, police, jail, and of course victims. By exhaustively moni-toring the real costs, Wolff (1993) demonstrated that implementation of a comprehensive community program for mentally disordered offenders is actually very cost-effective (see also Bigelow, Bloom, & Williams, 1990; Bond, Dincin, Setze, & Witheridge, 1984; Hammaker, 1983; Weisbrod, Test, & Stein, 1980).

Some might view our ideal program as a kind of unattainable dream, never realizable in this era of "just deserts," civil service regulations and collective bargaining, professional credentialism and turf warfare, and patients' and inmates' rights. Each key element, however, of this ideal program already exists (or has existed). We have already discussed the pioneering work of Paul and Lentz (1977; see also Rhoades, 1981) in the application of behavioral techniques, measurement of outcomes, and effective monitoring of staff performance and client behaviors. Also discussed above is the work of Liberman and colleagues (Liberman, 1988; Liberman, Kopelowicz, & Young, 1994) combining the conservative use of neuroleptic drugs and psychosocial training for persons with serious mental disorders and their families. Liberman and his colleagues have produced highly developed and portable training modules that necessi-tate a minimum of specialized clinician training for their use. MacKain and Streveler (1990) have demonstrated that those modules can be pro-vided for mentally disordered offenders in an institution. Stein and Test (1980; Test, 1992) have demonstrated that their comprehensive "Training in Community Living" program can increase community tenure (i.e., can reduce time spent in jails, prisons, or hospitals) for chronic mental pa-tients, a large segment of whom had criminal histories, and who might therefore fit the description "mentally disordered offenders."

Goldstein (Goldstein & Glick, 1987; Goldstein, Sprafkin, Gershaw, & Klein, 1992) has developed a comprehensive skills training package to teach prosocial/anticriminal values, nonviolent anger control, and meth-ods to resist peer pressure for adolescent offenders. A comprehensive program of functional family therapy (including parenting and family living skills) has been developed for disadvantaged juvenile delinquents (Gordon, Graves, & Arbuthnot, 1995). Ross and Fabiano (1985; Ross, Fabiano, & Ewles, 1988) have developed a skills training package to teach interpersonal problem solving to adult offenders. The states of New York, Virginia, Oregon, and Wisconsin (Bloom, Williams, & Bigelow, 1991, 1992; Griffin, Steadman, & Heilbrun, 1991; McGreevy, Steadman, Dvoskin, & Dollard, 1991) have effective conditional release policies for mentally disordered offenders that embody many of the characteristics of effective community case management identified above. And an even more comprehensive case management system has been described for the state of New York (Dvoskin & Steadman, 1994). Some effective means to overcome organizational obstacles to the delivery of effective programs have also been described and developed (Harris & Rice, 1992).

Thus, many of the puzzle's pieces have been found. Of course, many others are as yet undiscovered or unpublished. We await better theories of the interelationships among impulsivity, mental disorder in general, and antisocial conduct. We await more accurate diagnostic schemes and methods to appraise risk. We await even more effective drugs, therapies, methods of supervision, and implementation strategies. We do not, however, need all the pieces to begin assembling the puzzle; we need only the will to do it.

NOTES

1. The likelihood of violent reoffense was assessed with our actuarial instrument for the prediction of violent recidivism, discussed below.

2. In each of our studies of the clinical presentation of mentally disordered offenders, we identified a large cluster of patients who were at very low risk of reoffending violently, and who had few if any identifiable clinical needs. It must be acknowledged that the appropriate service for some mentally disordered offenders is nothing; any intervention will probably worsen symptoms, decrease quality of life, or increase the likelihood of recidivism.

3. One cannot assume, however, that the phrase "serious mental illness" is or can be *defined* as schizophrenia and mood disorders. In our own jurisdiction, for example, government policy has declared those persons diagnosed with posttraumatic stress disorder (an anxiety disorder, according to DSM-IV) and other problems experienced by "survivors" of childhood sexual abuse to be appropriate recipients of services for the seriously mentally ill. As another example, the Canadian Ministry of Justice has recently asserted that dangerous sex offenders who reach the ends of their sentences in federal prisons should then be transferred to provincially operated psychiatric hospitals to receive treatment for what is thought to be a mental health problem. Such a suggestion, if implemented, would bring sex offenders into the population of mentally disordered offenders— a situation that has occurred in other eras and in other jurisdictions (e.g., the states of Massachusetts and Washington).

4. The two main operative sources of error are biased remembering (i.e., noticeable, salient events are more likely to be remembered, and the frequency of events that fit with preconceptions is overestimated) and regression toward the mean (i.e., for most random events, extreme values are less likely than moderate

ones; thus, even in a random process, a moderate observation is always likely to follow an extreme one) (see Paulos, 1988).

5. For a small number of offenders, the actuarially determined level of risk is so high that no realistically achievable intervention could lower it to an acceptable level. Thus, an institutional treatment program that lowered the risk of violent recidivism by 25%, and a community supervision strategy that reduced risk by another third (both powerful effects indeed), would leave offenders whose initial actuarial risk of violent recidivism was 95% still close to 50%. In the case of violent serial rapists or sexual murderers, for example, the public (and courts and policy makers) would probably regard this hypothetical lowered risk as still too high. Incapacitation in the form of indefinite institutionalization is probably warranted in such rare and extreme cases.

REFERENCES

American Psychiatric Association. (1994). *Diagnostic and statistical manual of mental disorders* (4th ed.). Washington, DC: Author.

Ammerman, R., Hersen, M., & Sisson, L. A. (Eds.). (1994). *Handbook of aggressive and destructive behavior in psychiatric patients*. New York: Plenum Press.

Andrasik, F., & McNamara, J. R. (1977). Optimizing staff performance in an institutional behavior change system: A pilot study. *Behavior Modification, 1*, 235–248.

Anderson, S. A., Vaulx-Smith, P., & Keshavan, M. S. (1994). Schizophrenia. In M. Hersen & R. T. Ammerman (Eds.), *Handbook of prescriptive treatments for adults* (pp. 73–94). New York: Plenum Press.

Andrews, D. A. (1982). *The Level of Supervision Inventory (LSI): The first follow-up*. Toronto: Ontario Ministry of Correctional Services.

Andrews, D. A., & Bonta, J. (1994). *The psychology of criminal conduct*. Cincinnati, OH: Anderson.

Andrews, D. A., Zinger, I., Hoge, R. D., Bonta, J., Gendreau, P., & Cullen, F. T. (1990). Does correctional treatment work?: A clinically relevant and psychologically informed meta-analysis. *Criminology, 28*, 369–404.

Backer, T. E., Liberman, R. P., & Kuehnel, T. G. (1986). Dissemination and adoption of innovative psychosocial interventions. *Journal of Consulting and Clinical Psychology, 54*, 111–118.

Baird, C. S. (1981). Probation and parole classification: The Wisconsin model. *Corrections Today, 43*, 36–41.

Basta, J. M., & Davidson, W. S. (1988). Treatment of juvenile offenders: Study outcomes since 1980. *Behavioral Sciences and the Law, 6*, 355–384.

Benton, M. K., & Schroeder, H. E. (1990). Social skills training with schizophrenics: A meta-analytic evaluation. *Journal of Consulting and Clinical Psychology, 58*, 741–747.

Bigelow, D. A., Bloom, J. D., & Williams, M. H. (1990). Costs of managing insanity acquittees under a psychiatric security review board system. *Hospital and Community Psychiatry, 41*, 613–614.

Bloom, J. D., Williams, M. H., & Bigelow, D. A. (1991). Monitored conditional release of persons found not guilty by reason of insanity. *American Journal of Psychiatry, 148*, 444–448.

Bloom, J. D., Williams, M. H., & Bigelow, D. A. (1992). The involvement of schizo-phrenic insanity acquittees in the mental health and criminal justice systems. *Clinical Forensic Psychiatry, 15*, 591–604.

Bond, G. R., Dincin, J., Setze, P. J., & Witheridge, T. F. (1984). The effectiveness of psychiatric rehabilitation: A summary of research at thresholds. *Psychosocial Rehabilitation Journal, 7*, 6–22.

Bond, G. R., Miller, L. D., Krumwied, R. D., & Ward, R. (1988). Assertive case management in three CMHCs: A controlled study. *Hospital and Community Psychiatry, 39*, 411–418.

Bonta, J. (1996). Risk–needs assessment and treatment. In A. Harland (Ed.), *Choosing correctional options that work: Defining the demand and evaluationg the supply* (pp. 18–32). Thousand Oaks, CA: Sage.

Brown, K. M., Willis, B. S., & Reid, D. H. (1981). Differential effects of supervisor verbal feedback and feedback plus approval on institutional staff performance. *Journal of Organizational Behavior Management, 3*, 57–68.

Burgio, L. D., Whitman, T. L., & Reid, D. H. (1983). The reinforcement of behaviour in institutional settings. *Behaviour Research and Therapy, 4*, 157–167.

Cohen, J. (1969). *Statistical power analysis for the behavioral sciences.* New York: Academic Press.

Cullen, F. T., & Gendreau, P. (1989). The effectiveness of correctional rehabilitation. In L. Goodstein & D. MacKenzie (Eds.), *The American prison: Issues in research and policy* (pp. 23–44). New York: Plenum Press.

Dvoskin, J. A., & Steadman, H. J. (1994). Using intensive case management to reduce violence by mentally ill persons in the community. *Hospital and Community Psychiatry, 45*, 679–684.

Ellsworth, R. B. (1968). *Nonprofessionals in psychiatric rehabilitation: The psychiatric aide and the schizophrenic patient.* New York: Appleton-Century-Crofts.

Garrett, C. J. (1985). Effects of residential treatment on adjudicated delinquents: A meta-analysis. *Journal of Research in Crime and Delinquency, 22*, 287–308.

Gendreau, P. (1988, August). *Principles of effective treatments for offenders.* Paper presented at a conference, The Antisocial Personality: Research, Assessment and Treatment Programs, Midland, Ontario.

Gendreau, P. (1996a). Offender rehabilitation: What we know and what needs to be done. *Criminal Justice and Behavior, 23*, 144–161.

Gendreau, P. (1996b). The principles of effective intervention with offenders. In A. Harland (Ed.), *What works in community corrections* (pp. 117–130). Thousand Oaks, CA: Sage.

Gendreau, P., & Ross, R. R. (1979). Effective correctional treatment: Bibliotherapy for cynics. *Crime and Delinquency, 25*, 463–489.

Gensheimer, L. K., Mayer, J. P., Gottschalk, R., & Davidson, W. S. (1986). Diverting youth from the juvenile justice system: A meta-analysis of intervention effi-cacy. In S. J. Apter & A. P. Goldstein (Eds.), *Youth violence: Programs and prospects* (pp. 39–57). Elmsford, NY: Pergamon Press.

Glaser, E. M., Abelson, H. H., & Garrison, K. N. (1983). *Putting knowledge to use.* San Francisco: Jossey-Bass.

Glick, I. D., Spender, J. H., Clarkin, J. F., Haas, G. L., Lewis, A. B., Peyser, J., DeMane, N., Good-Ellis, M., Harris, E., & Lestelle, V. (1990). A randomized clinical trial of inpatient family intervention: IV. Follow-up results for subjects with schizo-phrenia. *Schizophrenia Research, 3*, 187–200.

Goldstein, A. P., & Glick, B. (1987). *Aggression replacement training*. Champaign, IL: Research Press.

Goldstein, A. P., Sprafkin, R. P., Gershaw, N. J., & Klein, P. (1992). *Skillstreaming for the adolescent*. Champaign, IL: Research Press.

Gordon, D. A., Graves, K., & Arbuthnot, J. (1995). The effect of functional family therapy for delinquents on adult criminal behavior. *Criminal Justice and Behavior, 22,* 60–73.

Gottfredson, M. R., & Hirschi, T. (1990). *A general theory of crime*. Stanford, CA: Stanford University Press.

Gottschalk, R., Davidson, W., Gensheimer, L. K., & Mayer, J. P. (1987). Community-based interventions. In H.C. Quay (Ed.), *Handbook of juvenile delinquency* (pp. 266–289). New York: Wiley.

Gottschalk, R., Davidson, W., Mayer, J., & Gensheimer, L. K. (1987). Behavioral approaches with juvenile offenders. In E. K. Morris & C. J. Braukman (Eds.), *Behavioral approaches to crime and delinquency* (pp. 399–422). New York: Plenum Press.

Griffin, P. A., Steadman, H. J., & Heilbrun, K. (1991). Designing conditional release systems for insanity acquittees. *Journal of Mental Health Administration, 18,* 231–241.

Hammaker, R. (1983). A client outcome evaluation of the statewide implementation of community support services. *Psychosocial Rehabilitation Journal, 7,* 1–10.

Hare, R. D. (1991). *Manual for the Hare Psychopathy Checklist—Revised*. Toronto: Multi-Health Systems.

Hargreaves, W. A., & Shumway, M. (1989). Effectiveness of services for the severely mentally ill. In A. Taube, D. Mechanic, & A. Hohmann (Eds.) *The future of mental health services research* (pp. 253–283). Rockville, MD: U.S. Department of Health and Human Services.

Harris, G. T. (1989). The relationship between neuroleptic drug dose and the performance of psychiatric patients in a maximum security token economy program. *Journal of Behavior Therapy and Experimental Psychiatry, 20,* 57–67.

Harris, G. T., & Rice, M. E. (1990). An empirical approach to classification and treatment planning for psychiatric inpatients. *Journal of Clinical Psychology, 46,* 3–14.

Harris, G. T., & Rice, M. E. (1992). Reducing violence in institutions: Maintaining behavior change. In R. DeV. Peters, R. J. McMahon, & V. L. Quinsey (Eds.), *Aggression and violence throughout the life span* (pp. 261–282). Newbury Park, CA: Sage.

Harris, G. T., & Rice, M. E. (1994). The violent patient. In R. T. Ammerman & M. Hersen (Eds.), *Handbook of prescriptive treatments for adults* (pp. 463–486). New York: Plenum Press.

Harris, G. T., Rice, M. E., & Cormier, C. A. (1994). Psychopaths: Is a therapeutic community therapeutic? *Therapeutic Communities, 15,* 283–300.

Harris, G. T., Rice, M. E., & Quinsey, V. L. (1993). Violent recidivism of mentally disordered offenders: The development of a statistical prediction instrument. *Criminal Justice and Behavior, 20,* 315–335.

Heinrich, K., Klieser, E., Lehmann, E., Kinzler, E., & Hruschka, H. (1994). Risperidone versus clozapine in the treatment of schizophrenic patients with acute symptoms: A double blind, randomized trial. *Progress in Neuro-Psychopharmacology and Biological Psychiatry, 18,* 129–137.

Hersen, M., & Ammerman, R. T. (Eds.). (1994). *Handbook of prescriptive treatments for adults*. New York: Plenum Press.

Hildebran, D. D., & Pithers, W. D. (1992). Relapse prevention: Application and outcome. In W. O'Donohue & J. Geer (Eds.), *The sexual abuse of children: Vol. 2. Clinical issues* (pp. 365–393). Hillsdale, NJ: Erlbaum.

Hogarty, G. E., Anderson, C. M., Reiss, D. J., Kornblith, S. J., Greenwald, D. P., Ulrich, R. F., & Carter, M. (1991). Family psychoeducation, social skills training, and maintenance chemotherapy in the aftercare treatment of schizophrenia. *Archives of General Psychiatry, 48*, 340–347.

Izzo, R. L., & Ross, R. R. (1990). Meta-analysis of rehabilitation programs for juvenile delinquents. *Criminal Justice and Behavior, 17*, 134–142.

Kazdin, A. E. (1987). Treatment of antisocial behavior in children: Current status and future directions. *Psychological Bulletin, 102*, 187–203.

Klassen, D., & O'Connor, W. (1989). Assessing the risk of violence in released mental patients: A cross-validation study. *Psychological Assessment, 1*, 75–81.

Kuehnel, T. G., DeRisi, W. J., Liberman, R. P., & Mosk, M. D. (1984). Treatment strategies that promote deinstitutionalization of chronic mental patients. In W.P. Christian, G.T. Hannah, & T.J. Glahn (Eds.), *Programming effective human services* (pp. 245–265). New York: Plenum Press.

Laws, D. R. (1974). The failure of a token economy. *Federal Probation, 1*, 33–38.

Lehman, A. F. (1988). A quality of life interview for the chronically mentally ill. *Evaluation and Program Planning, 11*, 51–62.

Leitenberg, H. (1987). Primary prevention of delinquency. In J. D. Burchard & S. N. Burchard (Eds.), *Prevention of delinquent behavior* (pp. 312–330). Newbury Park, CA: Sage.

Liberman, R. P. (1988). Behavioral family management. In R. P. Liberman (Ed.), *Psychiatric rehabilitation of chronic mental patients* (pp. 200–244). Washington, DC: American Psychiatric Press.

Liberman, R. P. (1992). Future prospects for psychiatric rehabilitation. In R. P. Liberman (Ed.), *Handbook of psychiatric rehabilitation* (pp. 317–325). New York: Macmillan.

Liberman, R. P., Falloon, I. R., & Aitchison, R. A. (1984). Multiple family therapy for schizophrenia: A behavioral, problem-solving approach. *Psychosocial Rehabilitation Journal, 7*, 60–77.

Liberman, R. P., Kopelowicz, A., & Young, A. S. (1994). Biobehavioral treatment and rehabilitation of schizophrenia. *Behavior Therapy, 25*, 89–107.

Liberman, R. P., Van Putten, T., Barringer, D., Mintz, J., Bowen, L., Kuehnel, T. G., Aravagiri, M., & Marder, S. R. (1994). Optimal drug and behavior therapy for treatment-refractory schizophrenic patients. *American Journal of Psychiatry, 151*, 756–759.

Link, B. G., Andrews, H., & Cullen, F. T. (1992). The violent and illegal behavior of mental patients reconsidered. *American Sociological Review, 57*, 275–292.

Lipsey, M. W. (1992). Juvenile delinquency treatment: A meta-analytic inquiry into the variability of effects. In T. D. Cook, H. Cooper, D. S. Cordray, H. Hartman, L. V. Hedges, R. J. Light, T. A. Louis, & F. Mosteller (Eds.), *Meta-analysis for explanation* (pp. 83–127). Newbury Park, CA: Sage.

Lipsey, M. W., & Wilson, D. B. (1993). The efficacy of psychological, educational, and behavioral treatment. *American Psychologist, 48*, 1181–1209.

Lukoff, D., Liberman, R. P., & Nuechterlein, K. (1986). Symptom monitoring in the rehabilitation of schizophrenic patients. *Schizophrenia Bulletin, 12*, 578–602.

MacKain, S. J., & Streveler, A. (1990). Social and independent living skills for psychiatric patients in a prison setting. *Behavior Modification, 14*, 490–518.

Martinson, R. (1974). What works?: Questions and answers about prison reform. *The Public Interest, 35*, 22–54.

Mayer, J. P., Gensheimer, L. K., Davidson, W. S., & Gottschalk, R. (1986). Social learning treatment within juvenile justice: A meta-analysis of impact in the natural environment. In S. J. Apter & A. P. Goldstein (Eds.), *Youth violence: Programs and prospects* (pp. 24–38). Elmsford, NY: Pergamon Press.

McCord, J. (1978). A thirty-year follow-up of treatment effects. *American Psychologist, 33*, 284–289.

McGrew, J. H., Bond, G. R., Dietzen, L., & Salyers, M. (1994). Measuring the fidelity of implementation of a mental health program model. *Journal of Consulting and Clinical Psychology, 62*, 670–678.

McGreevy, M. A., Steadman, H. J., Dvoskin, J. A., & Dollard, N. (1991). New York State's system of managing insanity acquittees in the community. *Hospital and Community Psychiatry, 42*, 512–517.

Motiuk, L. L. (1993). Where are we with our ability to assess risk? *Forum on Corrections Research, 5*, 14–18.

Neale, J. M., & Oltmanns, T. F. (1980). *Schizophrenia.* New York: Wiley.

Overall, J., & Gorham, D. (1988). The Brief Psychiatric Rating Scale (BPRS): Recent developments in ascertainment and scaling. *Psychopharmacology Bulletin, 24*, 97–99.

Palmer, T. (1992). *The re-emergence of correctional intervention.* Newbury Park, CA: Sage.

Paul, G. L., & Lentz, R. J. (1977). *Psychosocial treatment of chronic mental patients: Milieu versus social learning programs.* Cambridge, MA: Harvard University Press.

Paulos, J. A. (1988). *Innumeracy.* New York: Viking.

Payne, P. V., & Halford, W. K. (1990). Clinical section: Social skills training with chronic schizophrenic patients living in community settings. *Behavioural Psychotherapy, 18*, 49–64.

Quinsey, V. L. (1984). Politique institutionelle de liberation: Identification des individus dangereux. Une revue de la littérature [Institutional release policy: The identification of dangerous men. A review of the literature]. *Criminologie, 17*, 53–78.

Quinsey, V. L., Cyr, M., & Lavallee, Y. (1988). Treatment opportunities in a maximum security psychiatric hospital. *International Journal of Law and Psychiatry, 11*, 179–194.

Quinsey, V. L., Harris, G. T., Rice, M. E., & Lalumière, M. L. (1993). Assessing treatment efficacy in outcome studies of sex offenders. *Journal of Interpersonal Violence, 8*, 512–523.

Quinsey, V. L., & Maguire, A. (1983). Offenders remanded for a psychiatric examination: Perceived treatability and disposition. *International Journal of Law and Psychiatry, 6*, 193–205.

Quinsey, V. L., & Maguire, A. (1986). Maximum security psychiatric patients: Actuarial and clinical prediction of dangerousness. *Journal of Interpersonal Violence, 1*, 173–191.

Quinsey, V. L., Pruesse, M., & Fernley, R. (1975). Oak Ridge patients: Prerelease characteristics and postrelease adjustment. *Journal of Psychiatry and Law, 3,* 63–77.

Quinsey, V. L., Warneford, A., Pruesse, M., & Link, N. (1975). Released Oak Ridge patients: A follow-up of review board discharges. *British Journal of Criminology, 15,* 264–270.

Regier, D. A., Kaelber, C. T., Roper, M. T., Rae, D. S., & Sartorius, N. (1994). The ICD-10 clinical field trial for mental and behavioral disorders: Results in Canada and the United States. *American Journal of Psychiatry, 151,* 1340–1350.

Reid, W. H., Mason, M., & Toprac, M. (1994). Savings in hospital bed-days related to treatment with clozapine. *Hospital and Community Psychiatry, 45,* 261–264.

Rhoades, L. J. (1981). *Treating and assessing the chronically mentally ill.* Rockville, MD: U.S. Department of Health and Human Serivces.

Rice, M. E., & Harris, G. T. (1988). An empirical approach to the classification and treatment of maximum security psychiatric patients. *Behavioral Sciences and the Law, 6,* 497–514.

Rice, M. E., & Harris, G. T. (1990). The predictors of insanity acquittal. *International Journal of Law and Psychiatry, 13,* 217–224.

Rice, M. E., & Harris, G. T. (1992). A comparison of criminal recidivism among schizophrenic and nonschizophrenic offenders. *International Journal of Law and Psychiatry, 15,* 397–408.

Rice, M. E., Harris, G. T., & Cormier, C. (1992). Evaluation of a maximum security therapeutic community for psychopaths and other mentally disordered offenders. *Law and Human Behavior, 16,* 399–412.

Rice, M. E., Harris, G. T., Lang, C., & Bell, V. (1990). Recidivism among male insanity acquittees. *Journal of Psychiatry and Law, 18,* 379–403.

Rice, M. E., Harris, G. T., & Quinsey, V. L. (1996). Treatment of forensic patients. In B. Sales & S. Shah (Eds.), *Mental health and the law: Research policy and practice* (pp. 141–189). Durham, NC: Carolina Academic Press.

Rice, M. E., Harris, G. T., Quinsey, V. L., & Cyr, M. (1990). Planning treatment programs in secure psychiatric facilities. In D. Weisstub (Ed.), *Law and mental health: International perspectives* (Vol. 5, pp. 162–230). Elmsford, NY: Pergamon Press.

Ross, R. R., & Fabiano, E. A. (1985). *Time to think: A cognitive model of delinquency prevention and offender rehabilitation.* Johnson City, TN: Institute of Social Science and Arts.

Ross, R. R., Fabiano, E. A., & Ewles, C. D. (1988). Reasoning and rehabilitation. *International Journal of Offender Therapy and Comparative Criminology, 32,* 29–33.

Roy, A. (1994). Affective disorders. In M. Hersen, R. T. Ammerman, & L. A. Sisson (Eds.), *Handbook of aggressive and destructive behavior in psychiatric patients* (pp. 221–235). New York: Plenum Press.

Rubin, A. (1992). Is case management effective for people with serious mental illness?: A research review. *Health and Social Work, 17,* 138–150.

Sainsbury, P. (1986). Depression, suicide, and suicide prevention. In A. Roy (Ed.), *Suicide* (pp. 73–88). Baltimore: Williams & Wilkins.

Sechrest, L., White, S. O., & Brown, E. D. (1979). *The rehabilitation of criminal offenders: Problems and prospects.* Washington, DC: National Academy Press.

Silver, E., Cirincione, C., & Steadman, H. (1994). Demythologizing inaccurate perceptions of the insanity defense. *Law and Human Behavior, 18,* 63–70.

Solomon, P. (1992). The efficacy of case management services for severely mentally disabled clients. *Community Mental Health Journal, 28,* 163–180.

Solomon, P., Draine, J., & Meyerson, A. (1994). Jail recidivism and receipt of community mental health services. *Hospital and Community Psychiatry, 45,* 793–797.

Stein, L. I., & Test, M. A. (1980). Alternative to mental hospital treatment. *Archives of General Psychiatry, 37,* 392–397.

Tarrier, N., Barrowclough, C., Vaughn, C., Bamrah, J., Porceddu, K., Watts, S., & Freeman, H. (1989). Community management of schizophrenia: A two year follow-up of a behavioural intervention with families. *British Journal of Psychiatry, 154,* 625–628.

Taylor, P. J. (1985). Motives for offending among violent and psychotic men. *British Journal of Psychiatry, 147,* 491–498.

Taylor, P. J., Garety, P., Buchanan, A., Reed, A., Wessely, S., Ray, K., Dunn, G., & Grubin, D. (1994). Delusions and violence. In J. Monahan & H. J. Steadman (Eds.), *Violence and mental disorder: Developments in risk assessment* (pp. 161–182). Chicago: University of Chicago Press.

Test, M. A. (1992). Training in community living. In R.P. Liberman (Ed.), *Handbook of psychiatric rehabilitation* (pp. 153–170). New York: Macmillan.

Uttaro, T., & Mechanic, D. (1994). The NAMI consumer survey analysis of unmet needs. *Hospital and Community Psychiatry, 45,* 372–374.

Van Voorhis, P. (1987). Correctional effectiveness: The high cost of ignoring success. *Federal Probation, 51,* 56–62.

Virkkunen, M., DeJong, J., Bartko, J., & Linnoila, M. (1989). Psychobiological concomitants of history of suicide attempts among violent offenders and impulsive fire setters. *Archives of General Psychiatry, 46,* 604–606.

Wallace, C. J. (1993). Psychiatric rehabilitation. *Psychopharmacology Bulletin, 29,* 537–548.

Wallace, C. J., & Liberman, R. P. (1985). Social skills training for patients with schizophrenia: A controlled clinical trial. *Psychiatry Research, 15,* 239–247.

Wallace, C. J., Liberman, R. P., MacKain, S. J., Blackwell, G., & Eckman, T. A. (1992). Effectiveness and replicability of modules for teaching social and instrumental skills to the severely mentally ill. *American Journal of Psychiatry, 149,* 654–658.

Weisbrod, B. A., Test, M., & Stein, L. I. (1980). Alternative to mental hospital treatment. *Archives of General Psychiatry, 37,* 400–405.

Whitehead, J. T., & Lab, S. P. (1989). A meta-analysis of juvenile correctional treatment. *Journal of Research in Crime and Delinquency, 26,* 276–295.

Wiederanders, M. R., & Choate, P. A. (1994). Beyond recidivism: Measuring community adjustments of conditionally released insanity acquittees. *Psychological Assessment, 6,* 61–66.

Wittlin, B. J. (1988). Practical psychopharmacology. In R.P. Liberman (Ed.), *Psychiatric rehabilitation of chronic mental patients* (pp. 118–145). Washington, DC: American Psychiatric Press.

Wolff, N. (1993, June). *Assertive community care for the severely mentally ill: Some economic considerations and concerns.* Paper presented at a conference, Working with the Dangerous Mentally Ill in a Post-Institutional Era, Midland, Ontario.

Zamble, E., & Quinsey, V. L. (1997). *The process of criminal recidivism.* Toronto: Cambridge University Press.

20

Pharmacological Approaches to Impulsive and Aggressive Behavior

G. NEIL CONACHER

Favorable effects upon aggressive behavior have been reported for a number of pharmacological agents over the years (Markowitz, 1995), but few have passed beyond the stage of case reports or small open series to the process of controlled study. Even those agents that have been subjected to properly designed trials have not been tested in large numbers of aggressive persons. Nevertheless, most reviewers agree that three agents or classes of agents have shown promise of a potentially specific antiaggressive effect, and that a fourth class, the selective serotonin reuptake inhibitors (SSRIs), may be the most interesting yet.

Impulsivity has not featured prominently in studies of the treatment of aggression until recently, although in those studies that troubled to define their target behavior, impulsivity or something like it has often been implicit. Over the last decade, impulsivity and the possible therapeutic effect of serotonergic medications have come to dominate research on the treatment of aggression. One major stimulus for this has come from a remarkable series of studies on serotonin metabolite levels in the cerebrospinal fluid (CSF) of completed suicides, fire setters, and impulsively violent criminals (Linnoila et al., 1983; Virkkunen, 1993; Virkkunen, DeJong, Bartko, Goodwin, & Linnoila, 1989). The finding of reduced levels of 5-hydroxyindoleacetic acid (5-HIAA) in the CSF of these groups relative to controls has been very robust (Brown & Linnoila, 1990; Coccaro, 1989).

The three drugs most consistently researched—carbamazepine, propranolol, and lithium—can all have interactions with central serotonin systems (Editorial, 1987), among a whole range of different receptor and cell-membrane-affecting properties, and the emergence of the SSRIs has led to a surge of interest in the therapeutic potential of agents affecting this neurotransmitter. However, problems in the definition of target behaviors still confound the interpretation of results.

CLASSIFYING AGGRESSION

"Aggression," "assault," and "violence" are conceptually related, but what they mean exactly is not always clear (Eichelman, 1992). What then of "anger," "combativeness," "belligerence," "hostility," "irritable mood," "disruptive behavior," "rage outbursts," "episodic dyscontrol," or "intermittent explosive disorder"? All of these terms and others have appeared in the titles of papers relating to the treatment of aggression. Some are near-synonyms and are used interchangeably; some refer to behavior; others refer to an affect or emotion presumed to underlie behavior. The words or phrases form a spectrum—from value judgments in which the element of choice or purpose may be inferred, to terms that carry with them at least an implication of an organic cause in which conscious control is lost or overwhelmed.

Numerous classification systems or nosologies of human aggression have been and are being proposed (Barratt, 1993; Eichelman & Hartwig, 1993). Animal studies suggest that at least two different types of aggression may be regarded as normal species behavior, perhaps served by separate neural substrates: (1) predatory aggression; and (2) defensive, reactive, or affective aggression (Sheard, 1984). Psychoanalysts see human aggression as containing both positive and negative aspects (Storr, 1970), the positive aspects being viewed as the source of creative effort and achievement. The instrumental violence of antisocial personality disorder or psychopathy (Serin, 1991) has conceptual parallels with predatory aggression.

Drug control of violence or aggression has social and political implications (Lion, 1975), and violence as a public health issue (Christoffel, 1994; Golding, 1995) calls for a quite different approach to treatment or prevention (Gil, 1996) than the repetitive or uncontrollable violence that may become the concern of the individual clinician. It is upon this pathological aggression (Bond, 1993; Mak, de Koning, Mos, & Olivier, 1995) or violence that psychopharmacological reports have tended to focus, although this is rarely stated explicitly. Some qualities that have been assumed to distinguish pathological from "normal" aggression are the lack of apparent provocation, its coexistence with mental disorder, its repetitive nature, the lack of apparent control, and the presence of impulsivity or irritability.

AGGRESSION AND MENTAL ILLNESS

Whether an association exists between aggression and mental illness in general is a question that has preoccupied researchers—not simply because it is a meaningful question, but because it continues to be a public concern. In fact, as Gunn (1977) noted, "all in all, it is probably better to concentrate upon specific behavioral problems caused by specific disorders and to avoid too many generalizations" (p. 328). Nonetheless, the most informed modern view is that a small association does exist between mental disorder and violence (Mulvey, 1994). This is a fairly recent shift in expert opinion, and contrasts with the views of Teplin (1985) and others in the 1980s. It is impossible not to wonder whether the change might be attributable to the effect first reported by Penrose (1939). Penrose found an inverse relationship between the number of hospital beds for mental illnesses and the amount of violent crime in European countries. Whatever might be the explanation for this relationship (Conacher, 1996b), there have been marked recent reductions in beds for the mentally ill in most developed countries, and violent crime is often said to be increasing (Golding, 1995).

If antisocial personality disorder is a mental illness, then aggression is associated with it; however, this is recognized to be a circular argument, since aggression is a defining feature of the disorder (Wooton, 1959). Treatment for this disorder is widely understood to be ineffective (Quality Assurance Project, 1991). As a general rule, though, when aggression is found to coexist with mental disorder, the aggression is likely to resolve when the underlying disorder has been treated (Conn & Lion, 1984). This is particularly true of the psychoses. It is now recognized that young paranoid schizophrenic patients are at high risk for violent behavior—a risk that becomes even more marked with the presence of substance abuse (Kar, Wolkenfeld, & Murrill, 1988). This subgroup is also difficult to treat.

Aggressive behavior is common among patients with Alzheimer's disease, affecting some 35% (Aarsland, Cummings, Yenner, & Miller, 1996). The mentally retarded of all ages are at greater risk of violence than the general population (Tardiff & Sweillam, 1982), and for those who show repetitive self-injurious or aggressive behavior, drug treatments that have a specific antiaggressive effect would be of great potential benefit. The same may be said for refractory aggression encountered following brain injury. But even in these cases, the effects of drugs and of social environments in causing or facilitating the expression of violence must be considered before drug treatments are begun.

DRUGS AND ENVIRONMENTS THAT FACILITATE AGGRESSIVE BEHAVIOR

Although the business of this chapter is with the pharmacotherapy of aggression and impulsivity, it should not be forgotten that drugs (both recreational and medicinal) can themselves be associated with aggression, and that certain social environments may promote aggressive behavior. The connections between aggression and such factors are not always direct, and there can be a complex interaction with personality and cultural variables. Addictive drugs, for example, may be associated with violence as part of a predatory aggression stimulated by withdrawal symptoms. Central nervous system stimulants, amphetamines, cocaine, and phencyclidine may be associated with aggression as a symptom of physiological arousal, as an aspect of a toxic psychosis in overdose, or as part of a paranoid psychosis precipitated by chronic use.

Alcohol and violence show a very strong association (Heather, 1994), but this too is not a simple relationship (Pihl & Peterson, 1995). The accepted rationale for the widely recognized association was that central nervous system depressants disrupt control over aggressive impulses as part of a general impairment of brain function. This concept of disinhibition ignores social and cultural cues to violence that may be only coincidentally related to alcohol consumption (Bogg & Ray, 1990; Pernanen, 1991); it also does not take account of the complex cognitive changes involved in the interpretation of potentially threatening environmental signals (Borrill, Rosen, & Summerfield, 1987). At the level of brain chemistry, alcohol is known to have a complex effect upon serotonin function (Editorial, 1987).

Other central nervous system depressants or tranquilizers, including benzodiazepines, may also give rise to a "paradoxical" violent reaction (Tobin & Lewis, 1960). Whereas benzodiazepines may tame isolated wild animals, allowing them to be handled safely, studies suggest that in crowded conditions they can promote spontaneous intraspecific aggression (Editorial, 1975). Along with a positive association between violent incidents and the use of benzodiazepines in a maximum-security penitentiary (Workman & Cunningham, 1975), this should justify caution in using sedating drugs in crowded institutional settings such as prisons (Conacher, 1996a).

Sedation is not the only effect of medication that may be the cause of impulsive aggression. Akathisia—a motor restlessness accompanied by an unpleasant subjective sensation—is a common side effect of the older neuroleptic drugs, and it too may be associated with assaultive behavior (Crowner et al., 1990). The high doses of anabolic steroids used by body builders and other athletes may be associated with a loss of control over violent impulses (Conacher & Workman, 1989; Pope & Katz, 1994). There is still controversy over whether testosterone in high levels is related to sexual aggression, and the effect upon aggression (especially aggression of a sexual nature) of manipulating hormone levels remains poorly understood (Prentky, 1985).

Prisons have already been mentioned as a milieu in which violence might be more commonly encountered. The same may be said of other environments where countercultural values are concentrated and socially repressed roles become unmasked (Bogg & Ray, 1990). Environments undergoing rapid social changes (Snyder, 1994), or in which unfamiliar faces appear (Fineberg, James, & Shah, 1988), can show an increase in violent incidents. Hospitals are still other sites where assaultive behavior is not uncommon (Yassi, 1994). Such factors require careful evaluation before drug treatment of impulsive aggression is considered, and drug treatment should be regarded as only one—and not necessarily the most important one—of a range of social (Carlile, 1993; Lion, 1975) and behavioral (Corrigan, Yudovsky, & Silver, 1993) interventions.

DRUGS THAT MAY HELP CONTROL AGGRESSION AND/OR IMPULSIVITY

The treatment of acutely disturbed behavior in the intoxicated, psychotic, or delirious patient is outside the scope of this chapter. Delirium should be regarded as a medical emergency (Adams, Fernandez, & Anderson, 1986), and the use of restraint or seclusion to contain violent behavior requires implementation of special policies and procedures by trained staff members (Fisher, 1994). What is sometimes referred to as "chemical restraint"—the forceful administration of psychotropic drugs to the uncooperative or violent patient (Rapp, 1987)—has been rendered considerably more effective and safe by the use of mixed regimens of injectable antipsychotics and benzodiazepines (Adams et al., 1986). Such combinations allow lower doses of both types of medications, reduce the risk of complications, and have thus been widely adopted.

Antipsychotic Agents

Tranquilizers, both major and minor, have not been considered an effective approach to the long-term control of pathological aggression (Goldstein, 1974); at the levels required to control aggression, side effects are also frequently problematic, particularly in the elderly (Yudofsky, Silver, & Hales, 1990). But the emergence of new antipsychotics has encouraged some to take a second look at these agents. Clozapine, an atypical neuroleptic effective in some previously non-treatment-responsive schizophrenic patients, has been shown in open, uncontrolled studies to have a beneficial effect on hostility and aggression (Ratey, Leveroni, Kilmer, Gutheil, & Swartz, 1993; Volavka, Zito, Vitrai, & Czobor, 1993).

Risperidone, another new antipsychotic with a different range of receptor effects and side effects, was found incidentally to have a possible selective effect on hostility compared with haloperidol and placebo in a double-blind study (Czobor, Volavka, & Meibach, 1995). Risperidone has a serotonergic effect and, like clozapine, is thought to cause fewer extrapyramidal side effects, including akathisia—the restlessness defined above and a potential cause of aggression (Crowner et al., 1990).

Beta-Blockers

The beta-adrenergic blockers, or beta-blockers, have been used in psychiatry since the 1970s (Tyrer, 1980) for the control of situational anxiety with accompanying peripheral symptoms, such as tremor and tachycardia. They have also been used for the relief of side effects of the neuroleptic drugs, such as akathisia (Ratey, Sorgi, & Polakoff, 1985). A number of studies have explored a possible antiaggressive effect for propranolol, and positive results have been reported for violent chronic schizophrenic patients (Sorgi, Ratey, & Polakoff, 1986), for aggressive and self-injurious mentally retarded patients (Luchins & Dojka, 1989), for those with organic brain disorders (Greendyke, Kanter, Schuster, Verstreate, & Wooton, 1986), and for elderly aggressive patients (Yudofsky et al., 1990).

Other beta-blockers have also been effective in reducing aggression (Ratey et al., 1992), but there is continuing debate on study design (Wong & Lee, 1993) and the drugs' mechanism of action (Whitman, Maier, & Eichelman, 1987). In many of the studies, the beta-blockers have been adjuncts to other medications, and it has been observed that beta-blockers can precipitate a marked rise in blood levels of concomitant antipsychotic drugs (Silver, Yudofsky, Kogan, & Katz, 1986). Their effectiveness in performance anxiety lies in their ability to inhibit signs of peripheral autonomic arousal, and it may be that a peripheral blockade can interrupt a positive feedback process in which sympathetic arousal leads to violent outbursts (Conacher, 1988). However, the effect of beta-blockers upon akathisia has already been mentioned, and other central nervous system effects, including an effect on serotonin, are recognized.

Anticonvulsants

The association between epilepsy and aggressive behavior has perhaps been exaggerated (Kligman & Goldberg, 1975), and violence between seizures is reported to be related to factors other than underlying epilepsy (Mendez, Doss, & Taylor, 1993). However, this association and a high incidence of electroencephalographic abnormalities in aggressors (Mattes, 1986) have encouraged researchers to investigate the use of anticonvulsants as a specific treatment for aggression. Carbamazepine has been studied most thoroughly in this respect, and the findings have recently been reviewed by Young and Hillbrand (1994). Phenytoin and valproic acid have also been reported to have an antiaggressive effect (Barratt, 1993). As with the other classes of drugs discussed here, the results are encouraging, but methodological problems limit the conclusions that can be drawn: The numbers involved are small, and important questions remain unanswered.

Lithium

Lithium salts have had a place in psychopharmacology for nearly 50 years (Cade, 1949), and their use in the stabilization of bipolar disorders is now familiar to most psychiatrists. Provided that certain well-defined guidelines are followed (Schou, 1986), the long-term safety of lithium is established. A possible action upon aggressive behavior was first reported in 1969 (Sheard, 1984), and a substantial literature has accumulated since then, with positive effects upon aggressive behavior on various groups: aggressive prisoners (Tupin et al., 1973); the chronically psychotic, the brain-damaged, and some mentally retarded patients (Tyrer, Walsh, Edwards, Berney, & Stephens, 1984; Worral, Moody, & Naylor, 1975); and even children with aggressive conduct disorder (Campbell, Kafantaris, & Cueva, 1995). Caution is necessary with patients suffering from epileptiform disorders, who may show an exacerbation of aggression (Schiff, Sabin, Geller, Alexander, & Mark, 1982).

In the face of this range of differing populations, Tupin (1978) has tried to define the common underlying features of lithium responsivity. He suggests that those who respond are likely to show a "hair-trigger" sensitivity, an inability to reflect, and a maximal, all-or-nothing response to perceived threat. These features are similar to those that Barratt (1993) believes to define impulsive aggression.

SSRIs and Other Serotonin Agonists

Like medications, neurotransmitters appear to go through phases of popularity in which they are postulated to be the cause of almost everything. This is currently true of serotonin. In the face of this interest, it should be noted that there is often overlap between transmitter systems, such as that between dopamine (formerly the most popular neurotransmitter) and serotonin, and that changes in one system will lead to secondary alterations in other systems (Bond, 1993). Changes in levels of neurotransmitters or their metabolites may be the effects as well as the causes of behavioral changes or environmental stresses. In captive vervet monkeys, blood serotonin levels are state-dependent and rise with social dominance (McGuire, Raleigh, & Brammer, 1984)—a potentially significant confounding factor in much of the research cited here. Some of these and other caveats are well recognized by responsible researchers (Golden et al., 1991), but are not always understood by clinicians or writers for a public readership.

As mentioned above, a finding of low levels of serotonin metabolites in the CSF of those who commit various impulsive and violent acts has been consistently replicated. Some reviewers believe that impulsivity rather than violence is likely to constitute the behavioral variable linked to these low levels (Brown & Linnoila, 1990), so it is necessary to bear in mind that serotonin agonist drugs may affect aggressive behavior indirectly through a favorable effect upon impulse control.

Fluoxetine was the first SSRI to be marketed as an antidepressant, and the profits have been enormous, but the drug has not been free of side effects (Editorial, 1990). There were early reports of suicidal preoccupation emerging during fluoxetine treatment (Teicher, Glod, & Cole, 1990). Open studies reporting a favorable effect upon violent behavior were quick to follow—in depressed outpatients (Fava et al., 1991), in five patients with borderline personality disorder (Cornelius, Soloff, Perel, & Ulrich, 1991), and in mentally retarded individuals with self-injurious behavior and aggression (Markowitz, 1992), among others. Controlled studies on small numbers of patients now support these early findings (Salzman et al., 1995), and case reports suggest a similar effect for the newer SSRIs (Buck, 1995).

A new class of specifically antiaggressive serotonin agonists, the "serenics," was announced in 1986 by Olivier, van Dalen, and Hartog, with application to human beings "within a couple of years" (Olivier et al., 1986, p. 491). The delay is presumably attributable to a proliferation of serotonin receptor subtypes and difficulties in classifying aggressive behavior in mice (Olivier, Mos, van der Heyden, & Hartog, 1989). Optimists might await the imminent discovery of the "nirvanics," or the impending development of "utopics"; however, clinicians must make do with hints in the literature about potential effects upon impulsive aggressive behavior, and with a recognition that we know almost nothing about the long-term effects of new psychotropic drugs (which young patients may have to take for a lifetime).

An interesting animal study supports the hypothesis that it is an effect upon impulsivity, rather than aggression, that explains the observed treatment responses. In adolescent male rhesus monkeys in a free-ranging wild population, low CSF concentrations of serotonin metabolites were correlated with more risky leaping behaviors within the forest canopy, as well as with greater aggression (Mehlman et al., 1994).

CASE VIGNETTE

The following vignette represents a fictionalized composite of a number of cases.

> Chuck, 28, was serving a 6-year sentence for offenses arising from an incident when he stabbed someone with a knife during a robbery. He claimed to have been intoxicated with alcohol and benzodiazepines at the time: "I have a blackout about it, but the guy came at me, and I just sort of tried to throw a scare into him. . . . I feel real bad about it." He was referred for a psychiatric opinion of his poorly controlled aggressive behavior in prison—fighting with fellow inmates and swearing at the guards.
>
> Adopted in infancy, Chuck had been noted to be clumsy as a child, and he had been a problem at school from an early age: "The teachers were always picking on me." He started shoplifting at the age of 8, began experimenting with drugs at the age of 13, and first used alcohol at 15. He was expelled from school for fighting: "I was bored, I guess." At the age of 16 he crashed a stolen car and was unconscious for some hours. He had an almost continuous adult criminal record, including arrests for impaired driving, car theft, breaking and entering, weapons offenses, and three previous assaults. Asked when he had stopped setting fires, he looked suspicious, then angry: "How did you know about that? I haven't done that since I was a kid." He had attempted suicide once in jail by slashing his wrists.
>
> Questioned about his strong history of violence (not all of which was associated with intoxication) Chuck replied, "Well, I've always had a bad temper." He described how, when he felt himself to be in a potentially threatening situation, he would just let himself go "all or nothing, like a hair-trigger. I would just explode, I couldn't control it." He seemed to take pride in this. The psychiatrist was not optimistic, but in view of Chuck's history of "soft" neurological signs and his possible head injury after his car crash, he was started on a course of Pacificin C. (*Note:* To the best of my knowledge, Pacificin C is not a real drug name.)
>
> Three months later, there had been no further violent incidents. Speaking before the parole board in an application for early release, Chuck enthused: "It's incredible, like I'm a new person. The doc—he's the first guy who's really listened to me. I mean, I've seen other psychiatrists and psychologists, but . . . this Pacificin C is amazing. . . . I get a little bit shaky, but I don't think I'll ever lose my temper again. I feel so . . . it's like I don't get worked up any more, no one's pushing my buttons. . . . I can walk away from it. I'm never coming back to jail. Just you make sure I keep getting the meds."
>
> In the event, Chuck was not given parole, but he left prison at his statutory release date. Nine months later, he was sentenced to life imprisonment for shooting an acquaintance through the neck with a handgun during a barroom brawl.

Chuck's case illustrates a number of problems with researching or treating "impulsive" violence. Any patient capable of giving informed consent, but particularly in a forensic context, might be able to see a certain advantage in showing a positive response to medication (Brown & Linnoila, 1990). The medications discussed in this chapter have distinctive side effect profiles that might place the "blindness" of both rater (Wong & Lee, 1993) and subject in question during any medication trial. Even in the most impulsive individuals, violent acts are relatively rare events induced by environmental variables in unpredictable ways, and prolonged periods without violence when such persons are under the observation of researchers may not be a treatment effect.

CONCLUSION

Although it is fair for Tardiff (1992) to claim that great progress has been made in research into the treatment of aggression over the past few decades, it has to be admitted that most of the progress has been in realizing just how complicated the subject is to study. Aggression is normal to the human being, and many different parts of the brain have been implicated in aggressive behavior or found to be damaged in abnormally aggressive individuals. Along with other classes of drugs, the SSRIs show promise in the treatment of impulsive aggression; however, the whole of this effect might still be explained by a beneficial effect purely on impulsivity, or, indeed, by behavioral changes related to perceived social status in subjects unused to the attentions of researchers.

It is a giant (impulsive) leap from these limited findings in small studies to the declaration of a "new day" in the treatment of aggression (Ratey & Gordon, 1993). We cannot yet advise psychiatrists to prescribe serenics, no matter how safe, to all who might harbor an aggressive impulse for the purpose of reducing "noise" in their heads. Optimism like this promises huge profits to members of the pharmaceutical industry, if only they can overcome the well-recognized association between violence and poverty. Still, even the limited state of our present knowledge is enough to support the assertion that pharmacological control of aggression (via serenics or any other class of drugs) is an unrealistic, and perhaps even irresponsible, claim.

Tranquilizers never did bring tranquility, and serenics are most unlikely to be a source of serenity. The "brave new world" of chemical happiness has already been examined in fiction (Huxley, 1932/1969). The complexity and plasticity of the human brain are such that it is likely to be a long time before Huxley's nightmare is realized. In the meantime, those who are required to treat aggressive behavior and who might be looking for possible indications for drug therapy, after treating any underlying psychiatric or medical disorder, might look for signs of impulsivity in the aggression and in other behaviors. Apart from differing side effects, there is as yet little evidence to support the choice of any particular class of drugs among those that have shown a positive result.

REFERENCES

Aarsland, D., Cummings, J. L., Yenner, G., & Miller, B. (1996). Relationship of aggressive behavior to other neuropsychiatric symptoms in patients with Alzheimer's disease. *American Journal of Psychiatry, 153*, 243–247.

Adams, F., Fernandez, F., & Anderson, B. S. (1986). Emergency pharmacotherapy of delirium in the critically ill cancer patient. *Psychosomatics, 27*(Suppl. 1), 33–37.

Barratt, E. S. (1993). The use of anticonvulsants in aggression and violence. *Psychopharmacology Bulletin, 29*, 75–81.

Bogg, R. A., & Ray, J. M. (1990). Male drinking and drunkenness in Middletown. *Advances in Alcohol and Substance Abuse, 9*(3–4), 13–29.

Bond, A. J. (1993). Prospects for antiaggressive drugs. In C. Thompson & P. Cowen (Eds.), *Violence: Basic and clinical science* (pp. 148–170). London: Heinemann.

Borrill, J. A., Rosen, B. K., & Summerfield, A. B. (1987). The influence of alcohol on judgement of facial expressions of emotion. *British Journal of Medical Psychology, 60*, 71–77.

Brown, G. L., & Linnoila, M. I. (1990). CSF serotonin metabolite (5-HIAA) studies in depression, impulsivity, and violence. *Journal of Clinical Psychiatry, 51*(4, Suppl.), 31–34.

Buck, O. D. (1995). Sertraline for reduction of violent behavior [Letter]. *American Journal of Psychiatry, 152*, 953.

Cade, J. F. J. (1949). Lithium salts in the treatment of psychotic excitement. *Medical Journal of Australia, 36*, 349–352.

Campbell, M., Kafantaris, V., & Cueva, J. E. (1995). An update in the use of lithium carbonate in aggressive children and adolescents with conduct disorder. *Psychopharmacology Bulletin, 31*, 93–102.

Carlile, J. B. (1993). The reduction of violence in a chronic psychiatric inpatient group: A social technique. *Canadian Journal of Psychiatry, 38*, 103–107.

Christoffel, K. K. (1994). Reducing violence: How do we proceed? *American Journal of Public Health, 84*, 539–541.

Coccaro, E. F. (1989). Central serotonin and impulsive aggression. *British Journal of Psychiatry, 155*(Suppl. 8), 52–62.

Conacher, G. N. (1988). Pharmacotherapy of the aggressive adult patient. *International Journal of Law and Psychiatry, 11*, 205–212.

Conacher, G. N. (1996a). *Management of th emntally disordered offender in prisons.* Montreal: McGill–Queen's University Press.

Conacher, G. N. (1996b). Psychiatric hospital downsizing and the Penrose Effect. *Journal of Nervous and Mental Disease, 184*, 708–710.

Conacher, G. N., & Workman, D. G. (1989). Violent crime possibly associated with anabolic steroid use [Letter]. *American Journal of Psychiatry, 146*, 679.

Conn, L. M., & Lion, J. R. (1984). Pharmacologic approaches to violence. *Psychiatric Clinics of North America, 7*, 879–886.

Cornelius, J. R., Soloff, P. H., Perel, J. M., & Ulrich, R. F. (1991). A preliminary trial of fluoxetine in refractory borderline patients. *Journal of Clinical Psychopharmacology, 11*, 116–120.

Corrigan, P. W., Yudofsky, S. C., & Silver, J. M. (1993). Pharmacological and behavioral treatments for aggressive psychiatric inpatients. *Hospital and Community Psychiatry, 44*, 125–133.

Crowner, M. L., Douyon, R., Convit, A., Gaztanaga, P., Volavka, J., & Bakall, R. (1990). Akathisia and violence. *Psychopharmacology Bulletin, 26*, 115–117.

Czobor, P., Volavka, J., & Meibach, R. C. (1995). Effect of risperidone on hostility in schizophrenia. *Journal of Clinical Psychopharmacology, 15*, 243–249.

Editorial. (1975). Tranquilizers causing aggression. *British Medical Journal, 5950*, 113–114.

Editorial. (1987). Serotonin, suicidal behaviour and impulsivity. *Lancet, ii*, 949–950.

Editorial. (1990). 5-HT blockers and all that. *Lancet, 336*, 345–346.

Eichelman, B. (1992). Aggressive behavior: From laboratory to clinic. *Quo vadit? Archives of General Psychiatry, 49*, 488–492.

Eichelman, B., & Hartwig, J. D. (1993). Toward a nosology of human aggressive behavior. *Psychopharmacology Bulletin, 29*, 57–63.

Fava, M., Rosenbaum, J. F., McCarthy, M., Pava, J., Steingard, R., & Bless, E. (1991). Anger attacks in depressed outpatients and their response to fluoxetine. *Psychopharmacology Bulletin, 27*, 275–278.

Fineberg, N. A., James, D. V., & Shah, A. K. (1988). Agency nurses and violence in a psychiatric ward [Letter]. *Lancet, i*, 474.

Fisher, W. A. (1994). Restraint and seclusion: A review of the literature. *American Journal of Psychiatry, 151*, 1584–1591.

Gil, D. G. (1996). Preventing violence in a structurally violent society: Mission impossible. *American Journal of Orthopsychiatry, 66*, 77–84.

Golden, R. N., Gilmore, J. H., Corrigan, M. H. N., Ekstrom, R. D., Knight, R. N., & Garbutt, J. C. (1991). Serotonin, suicide, and aggression: Clinical studies. *Journal of Clinical Psychiatry, 52*(12, Suppl.), 61–69.

Golding, A. M. B. (1995). Understanding and preventing violence: A review. *Public Health, 109*, 91–97.

Goldstein, M. (1974). Brain research and violent behavior. *Archives of Neurology, 30*, 1–35.

Greendyke, R. M., Kanter, D. R., Schuster, D. B., Verstreate, S., & Wooton, J. (1986). Propranolol treatment of assaultive patients with organic brain disease. *Journal of Nervous and Mental Disease, 174*, 290–294.

Gunn, J. (1977). Criminal behaviour and mental disorder. *British Journal of Psychiatry, 130*, 317–329.

Heather, N. (1994). Alcohol, accidents and aggression. *British Medical Journal, 308*, 1254.

Huxley, A. (1969). *Brave new world.* New York: Harper & Row. (Original work published 1932)

Kar, S. R., Wolkenfeld, F., & Murrill, L. M. (1988). Profiles of aggression among psychiatric patients. *Journal of Nervous and Mental Disease, 176*, 547–557.

Kligman, D., & Goldberg, D. A. (1975). Temporal lobe epilepsy and aggression. *Journal of Nervous and Mental Disease, 160*, 324–341.

Linnoila, M., Virkunnen, M., Scheinin, M., Nuutila, A., Rimon, R., & Goodwin, F. K. (1983). Low cerebrospinal fluid 5-hydroxyindoleacetic acid concentration differentiates impulsive from non-impulsive violent behavior. *Life Sciences, 33,* 2609–2614.

Lion, J. R. (1975). Conceptual issues in the use of drugs for the treatment of aggression in man. *Journal of Nervous and Mental Disease, 160,* 76–82.

Luchins, D. J., & Dojka, D. (1989). Lithium and propranolol in aggression and self-injurious behavior in the mentally retarded. *Psychopharmacology Bulletin, 25,* 372–375.

Mak, M., de Koning, P., Mos, J., & Olivier, B. (1995). Preclinical and Clinical Studies on the role of 5-HT$_1$ receptors in aggression. In E. Hollander & D. J. Stein (Eds.), *Impulsivity and aggression* (pp. 289–311). New York: Wiley.

Markowitz, P. I. (1992). Effect of fluoxetine in self-injurious behavior in the developmentally disabled: A preliminary study. *Journal of Clinical Psychopharmacology, 12,* 27–31.

Markowitz, P. (1995). Pharmacotherapy of impulsivity, aggression, and related disorders. In E. Hollander & D. J. Stein (Eds.), *Impulsivity and aggression* (pp. 263–287). New York: Wiley.

Mattes, J. A. (1986). Psychopharmacology of temper outbursts. *Journal of Nervous and Mental Disease, 174,* 464–470.

McGuire, M. T., Raleigh, M. J., & Brammer, G. L. (1984). Adaptation, selection, and benefit–cost balances: Implications of behavioral–physiological studies of social dominance in male vervet monkeys. *Ethology and Social Biology, 5,* 269–277.

Mehlman, P. T., Higley, J. D., Faucher, I., Lilly, A. A., Taub, D. M., Vickers, J., Suomi, S. J., & Linnoila, M. (1994). Low CSF 5-HIAA concentrations and severe aggression and impaired impulse control in nonhuman primates. *American Journal of Psychiatry, 151,* 1485–1491.

Mendez, M. F., Doss, R. C., & Taylor, J. L. (1993). Interictal violence in epilepsy: Relationship to behavior and seizure variables. *Journal of Nervous and Mental Disease, 181,* 566–569.

Mulvey, E. P. (1994). Assessing the evidence of a link between mental illness and violence. *Hospital and Community Psychiatry, 45,* 663–668.

Olivier, B., Mos, J., van der Heyden, J., & Hartog, J. (1989). Serotonergic modulation of social interactions in isolated male mice. *Psychopharmacology, 97,* 154–156.

Olivier, B., van Dalen, D., & Hartog, J. (1986). A new class of psychotropic drugs: Serenics. *Drugs of the Future, 11,* 473–494.

Penrose, L. S. (1939). Mental disease and crime: Outline of a comparative study of European statistics. *British Journal of Medical Psychology, 18,* 1–15.

Pernanen, K. (1991). *Alcohol in human violence.* New York: Guilford Press.

Pihl, R. O., & Peterson, J. (1995). Drugs and aggression: Correlations, crime and human manipulative studies and some proposed mechanisms. *Journal of Psychiatry and Neuroscience, 20,* 141–149.

Pope, H. G., & Katz, D. L. (1994). Psychiatric and medical effects of anabolic–androgenic steroid use. *Archives of General Psychiatry, 51,* 375–382.

Prentky, R. (1985). The neurochemistry and neuroendocrinology of sexual aggression. In J. Gunn & D. P. Farrington (Eds.), *Aggression and dangerousness* (pp. 7–55). Chichester, England: Wiley.

Quality Assurance Project. (1991). Treatment outlines for antisocial personality disorder. *Australian and New Zealand Journal of Psychiatry, 25,* 541–547.

Rapp, M. S. (1987). Chemical restraint. *Canadian Journal of Psychiatry, 32,* 20–21.

Ratey, J. J., & Gordon, A. (1993). The psychopharmacology of aggression: Toward a new day. *Psychopharmacology Bulletin, 29,* 65–73.

Ratey, J. J., Leveroni, C., Kilmer, D., Gutheil, C., & Swartz, B. (1993). The effects of clozapine on severely aggressive psychiatric inpatients in a state hospital. *Journal of Clinical Psychiatry, 54,* 219–223.

Ratey, J. J., Sorgi, P., O'Driscoll, G. A., Sands, S., Daehler, M. L., Fletcher, J. R., Kadish, W., Spruiell, G., Polakoff, S., Lindem, K. J., Bemporad, J. R., Richardson, L., & Rosenfeld. B. (1992). Nadolol to treat aggression and psychiatric symptomatology in chronic psychiatric inpatients: A double-blind, placebo controlled study. *Journal of Clinical Psychiatry, 53,* 41–46.

Ratey, J. J., Sorgi, P., & Polakoff, S. (1985). Nadolol as a treatment for akathisia. *American Journal of Psychiatry, 142,* 640–642.

Salzman, C., Wolfson, A. N., Schatzberg, A., Looper, J., Henke, R., Albanese, M., Schwartz, J., & Miyawaki, E. (1995). Effect of fluoxetine on anger in symptomatic volunteers with borderline personality disorder. *Journal of Clinical Psychopharmacology, 15,* 23–29.

Schiff, H. B., Sabin, T. D., Geller, A., Alexander, L., & Mark, V. (1982). Lithium in aggressive behavior. *American Journal of Psychiatry, 139,* 1346–1348.

Schou, M. (1986). Lithium treatment: A refresher course. *British Journal of Psychiatry, 149,* 541–547.

Serin, R. C. (1991). Psychopathy and violence in criminals. *Journal of Interpersonal Violence, 6,* 423–431.

Sheard, M. H. (1984). Clinical pharmacology of aggressive behavior. *Clinical Neuropharmacology, 7,* 173–183.

Silver, J. M., Yudofsky, S. C., Kogan, M., & Katz, B. L. (1986). Elevation of thioridazine plasma levels by propranolol. *American Journal of Psychiatry, 143,* 1290–1292.

Snyder, W. S. (1994). Hospital downsizing and increased frequency of assaults on staff. *Hospital and Community Psychiatry, 45,* 378–380.

Sorgi, P., Ratey, J. J., & Polakoff, S. (1986). Beta-adrenergic drugs for the control of aggressive behaviors in patients with chronic schizophrenia. *American Journal of Psychiatry, 143,* 775–776.

Storr, A. (1970). *Human aggression.* Baltimore: Penguin Books.

Tardiff, K. (1992). The current state of psychiatry in the treatment of violent patients. *Archives of General Psychiatry, 49,* 493–499.

Tardiff, K., & Sweillam, A. (1982). Assaultive behavior among chronic inpatients. *American Journal of Psychiatry, 139,* 212–215.

Teicher, M. H., Glod, C., & Cole, J. O. (1990). Emergence of intense suicidal preoccupation during fluoxetine treatment. *American Journal of Psychiatry, 147,* 207–210.

Teplin, L. A. (1985). The criminality of the mentally ill: A dangerous misconception. *American Journal of Psychiatry, 142,* 593–599.

Tobin, J., & Lewis, N. (1960). New psychotherapeutic agent, chlordiazepoxide: Use in treatment of anxiety states and related symptoms. *Journal of the American Medical Association, 174,* 1242–1249.

Tupin, J. P. (1978). Usefulness of lithium for aggressiveness [Letter]. *American Journal of Psychiatry, 135,* 1118.

Tupin, J. P., Smith, D. B., Clanon, T. L., Kim, L. I., Nugent, L. I., & Groupe, A. (1973). The long-term use of lithium in aggressive prisoners. *Comprehensive Psychiatry, 14,* 311–317.

Tyrer, P. (1980). Use of beta-blocking drugs in psychiatry and neurology. *Drugs, 20,* 300–308.

Tyrer, S. P., Walsh, A., Edwards, D. E., Berney, T. P., & Stephens, D. A. (1984). Factors associated with a good response to lithium in aggressive mentally handicapped subjects. *Progress in Neuro-Psychopharmacology and Biological Psychiatry, 8,* 751–755.

Virkkunen, M. (1993). Brain serotonin and violent behaviour. *Journal of Forensic Psychiatry, 3,* 171–174.

Virkkunen, M., De Jong, J., Bartko, J., Goodwin, F. K., & Linnoila, M. (1989). Relationship of psychobiological variables to recidivism in violent offenders and impulsive firesetters. *Archives of General Psychiatry, 46,* 600–603.

Volavka, J., Zito, J. M., Vitrai, J., & Czobor, P. (1993). Clozapine effects on hostility and aggression in schizophrenia [Letter]. *Journal of Clinical Psychopharmacology, 13,* 287–289.

Whitman, J. R., Maier, G. J., & Eichelman, B. (1987). Beta-adrenergic blockers for aggressive behavior in schizophrenia [Letter]. *American Journal of Psychiatry, 144,* 538.

Wong, M. K., & Lee, S. (1993). Nadolol in the treatment of aggression in chronic psychiatric inpatients [Letter]. *Journal of Clinical Psychiatry, 54,* 235.

Wooton, B. (1959). *Social science and social pathology.* London: Allen & Unwin.

Workman, D. G., & Cunningham, D. G. (1975, November). Effect of psychotropic drugs on aggression in a prison setting. *Canadian Family Physician,* pp. 63–66.

Worral, E. P., Moody, J. P., & Naylor, B. J. (1975). Lithium in non-manic depressives: Anti-aggressive effect and red blood cell lithium values. *British Journal of Psychiatry, 126,* 464–468.

Yassi, A. (1994). Assault and abuse of health care workers in a large teaching hospital. *Canadian Medical Association Journal, 151,* 1273–1279.

Young, J. L., & Hillbrand, M. (1994). Carbamazepine lowers aggression: A review. *Bulletin of the American Academy of Psychiatry and the Law, 22,* 53–61.

Yudofsky, S. C., Silver, J. M., & Hales, R. E. (1990). Pharmacologic management of aggression in the elderly. *Journal of Clinical Psychiatry, 51*(10, Suppl.), 22–28.

21

A Systems Approach to the Management of Impulsive Behavior

DEREK EAVES
GEORGE TIEN
DEREK WILSON

The concept of impulsivity is one that can be viewed from many different perspectives; as a consequence, it has been defined in a number of ways, not all of which are consistent with one another (Fink & McCown, 1993; McCown & VandenBos, 1994; Parker, Bagby, & Webster, 1993). Impulsivity is said to have many different etiologies, including both physiological and psychological factors. Instances of impulsivity, or the behaviors associated with impulsivity, have been identified as part of the constellation of symptoms in many psychiatric disorders. Impulsivity, in this sense, cannot be treated as a diagnostic category (see Coles, Chapter 10, this volume).

At its present stage of development, it would seem fair to observe that the concept of impulsivity has not been clearly or comprehensively defined, or perhaps even well understood. Furthermore, the utility of arranging a cluster of behavioral characteristics under the unifying framework of "impulsivity" has yet to be established. However, many mental health practitioners will attest to the fact that an appreciable portion of their time is consumed by clients with "impulsivity" problems. This is particularly true of those who work with certain subgroups of impulsive individuals, such as mentally disordered offenders and sex offenders. Therein lies the dilemma: How does the system mobilize to address a problem, when the problem has yet to be defined in a clear, convincing manner?

A PRACTICAL PERSPECTIVE ON IMPULSIVITY

The issues surrounding the concept of impulsivity, from mental health practitioners' point of view, differ according to the nature of the tasks they are expected to perform. For those on the front line who have to deal with the manifestations of impulsivity on a day-to-day basis, the finer points of distinction among the various conceptualizations of impulsivity are of little importance. They have to respond to the challenges of impulsive clients, whether a definitive scientific explanation exists or not. From this perspective, the task is immediate and the proposed solutions must be practical. It is of course not uncommon for solutions to be demanded before the scientific community is ready to declare the availability of a solution. The problem remains, however, for those who are charged with the responsibility of developing and providing services: It is difficult to devise coherent interventions and management strategies, as well as to allocate scarce resources, when the problem is inadequately defined.

Given these challenges, the approach taken in this chapter is therefore a practical one. This means that "impulsivity" is framed in a manner relevant to those working in mental health and correctional systems, including both practitioners and administrators. In this regard, it seems best not to view impulsivity as a specific disorder. Rather, those with manifestations of impulsivity should be seen as representing diverse but recognizable groups of individuals who have in common a particular set of dysfunctional behaviors. McCown and VandenBos (1994) have characterized such behaviors as "dysfunctional impulsivity." Individuals with dysfunctional impulsivity are said to be more likely to engage in destructive and disinhibited behaviors, such as excessive substance use, aggression, crime, and excessive unplanned sexual behavior. They form a heterogeneous group of individuals, in whom symptoms of mental illness are not uncommon. Some suffer from personality disorders, and many misuse alcohol and drugs. Another common characteristic of such individuals is that they tend to be in frequent conflict with the law. Many in this group have been variously labeled as "multiproblem individuals" or "system abusers," and are likely to be identified by front-line workers as individuals with impulsivity problems (Tien & Goresky, 1992).

From the perspective of the system, individuals with impulsivity problems are seen to cycle continually from the jurisdiction of one government agency, such as health, criminal justice, or social services, to another. They move from one caseworker to the next, often "burning their bridges" behind them. For most agencies, dealing with this instability and unpredictability is a major challenge. In a study conducted in British Columbia in 1989, the health and criminal justice records of 457 multiproblem individuals were examined (Tien & Lamb, 1989). As expected, the data indicated that all subjects had made numerous contacts with a number of community mental health centers, as well as with psychiatric wards of general hospitals, mental hospitals, and forensic psychiatric hospitals. All 457 had had dealings with the criminal justice system, and many had been involved in relatively serious offenses, such as assault or breaking and entering. As a result of this cycling, these individuals tended to experience discontinuity in services. This lack of continuity in care and services is yet another characteristic of those with impulsivity problems.

In brief, from the practical perspective, individuals who present with impulsivity problems are likely to belong to one of the following groups: (1) individuals with personality disorders, including borderline, antisocial, and histrionic; (2) sexual offenders; (3) individuals with attention-deficit/hyperactivity disorder (ADHD); and (4) individuals with *Diagnostic and Statistical Manual of Mental Disorders*, fourth edition (DSM-IV) Axis I disorders other than ADHD and paraphilias. In terms of characteristics, they tend to have a history of criminal justice problems, a history of psychiatric problems, and a high incidence of substance misuse. They tend to be noncompliant with interventions, to have a poor prognosis, to be at high risk for recidivism, and therefore to require close management and supervision. Some may even be dangerous to others as well to themselves. Most, however, are not certifiable under a mental health act at any given moment. In general, they are difficult to manage, and their problems tend to be long-standing. They are precisely the types of individuals whom conventional, generic health, and mental health services are not well equipped to handle.

CONVENTIONAL SYSTEMS OF CARE

Although there may be exceptions, conventional mental health systems in North America are not able to offer truly sustained services to the types of dysfunctional and violent individuals described above. A number of factors contribute to this state of affairs. For instance, the responsibility of generic mental health services for providing services to such individuals is not clearly delineated. Although many individuals with impulsivity problems are perceived as exceedingly troubled and troublesome, most are not certifiable under a provincial or state mental health act. Most do not have a current DSM-IV Axis I diagnosis; therefore, the conventional mental health system is not obliged to mobilize its resources to provide them with treatment or any other intervention measures. In fact, mental health services generally shy away from working with such individuals, often citing a lack of resources even for their "own" clients. This clearly suggests that individuals with impulsivity problems of the sorts described above are not considered to be part of the regular mental health system. In addition, since some of these individuals are seen as potentially disruptive or violent, agencies tend to consider themselves as justifiably concerned about the safety of their staff members and of their other clients. Indeed, such issues are often raised as reasons for their reluctance to extend their services.

Not only are conventional systems reluctant to provide services to individuals in this category, but most may not in fact be adequately prepared to assist them in ways that will be actually helpful. In general, programs and services provided by conventional systems are office-based. The patient or client has to assume much of the responsibility of making and keeping appointments, and of attending scheduled meetings and programs. Unfortunately, this kind of an arrangement is not suitable for individuals who tend to require a considerable amount of prodding, encouragement, and follow-up.

Experience indicates that such persons often require sustained efforts on the part of service providers, which include stepping out of their offices to meet clients on their "turf," if they are to keep their clients out of trouble. Most services, however, do not have the resources necessary to provide this level of care. This is an especially difficult problem when these individuals cross over agency boundaries, as they so often do. The tendency of individuals with impulsivity problems to cycle through various government agencies, and the inability of current systems to keep track of them, is a major shortcoming in conventional systems of service delivery. This is reflected by the fact that front-line staffers often find it difficult to refer clients to other agencies as these individuals move to the next phase of their cycle and cross the boundaries of responsibility of support agencies. In general, as they cross beyond the boundary and leave the responsibility of one agency, they do not necessarily land within the self-defined boundary of another agency. For example, in British Columbia, the responsibility for the provision of mental health services to legally defined "mentally disordered offenders" (MDOs) rests with the Forensic Psychiatric Services (FPS) Commission. This holds when the individual in question is under a court order with respect to specific sections of the *Criminal Code of Canada*, or under conditions set by the *Criminal Code* Review Board. For these individuals, the FPS Commission provides both in-custody and community-based services. Following the expiration of the terms imposed by the court or the Review Board, these individuals, when discharged, move beyond the responsibility of the FPS Commission. However, once they have been officially labeled as MDOs, other agencies are unlikely in some cases to extend their services to such individuals on a voluntary basis.

ELEMENTS OF A SUSTAINED MANAGEMENT SYSTEM

It can be concluded that the manner in which conventional systems deliver services is not well suited to individuals with impulsivity problems. There are undoubtedly many factors that account for the lack of fit between conventional systems and the needs of these individuals, and it seems appropriate at this point to examine at least some of them. The factor that is perhaps the most obvious, but at the same time the most difficult to address, is the changing makeup of those members of the population who are in need of intervention. During the past decade, the downsizing and closures of many mental health institutions have resulted in dramatic changes in the size and makeup of the mentally disordered population in the community. Along with this has come an increase in the number of homeless persons, as well as an increase in the number of mentally disordered persons in conflict with the law. Community mental health services, however, have not adapted quickly enough to these changes. Their focus, in general, continues to be on those who are seriously mentally ill; that is, they focus on psychotic persons or those with other DSM-IV Axis I diagnoses. Although the actual number of individuals with serious mental illness may not have declined, there is a sense that an appreciable number of those who now need intervention no longer fit in this category. Mental health services therefore need to reexamine their priorities to adjust to this new reality. This may be a difficult task to undertake; it may be particularly hard under the present circumstances, given the fact that in many cases, resources that have been promised as a result of the closing or downsizing of mental institutions have not been completely forthcoming, and most agencies are said to be already underresourced. Many agencies are therefore inclined to divert to other agencies the care of those with impulsivity problems. It must be recognized, however, that individuals with impulsivity problems are difficult for any single agency to manage, and that the responsibility for such individuals should not rest with a single government agency or department. Instead, it is argued, this responsibility should be shared by a number of agencies. That is, this responsibility should be jointly assumed by mental health agencies, forensic psychiatric services, corrections, mental hospitals, and even general hospitals with psychiatric wards, since persons with impulsivity problems are likely to come into contact with all these agencies and institutions. In addition, probation, police, and alcohol and drug agencies should have a role in managing such individuals.

Recognition of responsibility, however, is only a first step. Formal protocols for the joint management of individuals with impulsivity problems must be developed, so that as they cycle through the various systems, front-line staffers will have reasonably clear rules to guide their actions. This is a critical point. Agencies, particularly government agencies, operate strictly according to written policies and procedures. Thus, a formal written protocol is a necessary (though not always a sufficient) prerequisite. Not only must there be rules for one agency to hand clients over to other services, but agencies need to collaborate in order to provide the care and management necessary to sustain these persons in the community over extended periods of time. In this regard, coordination of the delivery of services is important, and some have suggested that this can take the form of a "case management system" (Dvoskin & Steadman, 1994; Marshall, Lockwood, & Gath, 1995). Such a system of coordination should possess a range of capabilities, including the ability to track a case across jurisdictional or agency boundaries; to make referrals to appropriate resources; to coordinate the services of one or more agencies; and, if called upon, to provide intensive case management. In this regard, the concept of "boundary spanners" (Steadman, 1992; Ogloff & Roesch, 1992) is relevant to this discussion. Clearly, even when protocols are in place, boundary spanners must be identified in order for a coordinated system of service delivery to function effectively, and such individuals need to be explicitly charged with the responsibility to interact and negotiate system interchanges.

CASE MANAGEMENT EFFORTS IN BRITISH COLUMBIA

Over the past decade in British Columbia, a number of initiatives have been undertaken with the aim of improving the performance of service systems with respect to difficult clients such as MDOs, as well as those described as multiproblem persons. One of the first efforts in this regard was the establishment of a small agency called the Multi-Service Network (MSN) in 1984. The MSN was a first attempt at bringing about a recognition that the problem of managing multiproblem individuals is a shared responsibility among a number of agencies. Spearheaded by a small group of individuals, MSN was successful in obtaining both support and funding from four organizations: the British Columbia Corrections Branch, the FPS Commission, the Alcohol and Drug Programs, and the Ministry of Social Services. The purposes of MSN were (1) to provide caseworkers with information regarding community resources, (2) to help caseworkers resolve difficult problems, and (3) to coordinate the services of agencies that deal concurrently with a client. In essence, MSN played a case coordination role. It assumed the responsibility of arranging case management conferences on behalf of its clients, and it invited the participation of agencies involved with the client. At these conferences, case management plans outlining the roles of the participating agencies would be developed.

The case of Sally illustrates the problems that service providers face, and also shows how an organization such as MSN can help by spanning the boundaries between service systems.

Sally was a single, developmentally delayed female. Although she had a friendly and likeable disposition, she could frequently behave in a disruptive, self-abusive, and demanding manner. Over the years, she was diagnosed as suffering from numerous mental disorders. Despite these numerous assessments, she refused mental health services. Sally had a long history of involvement with the correctional system, forensic psychiatric services, social services, the ambulance service, general hospitals, emergency departments in general hospitals, mental health services, and emergency mental health services, as well as countless community-based agencies. She had frequently appeared before the courts on a variety of charges, including assault, property damage, and theft. Sally manifested many of the dysfunctional behaviors associated with impulsivity, such as breaking windows; throwing items at passing vehicles, at windows, or at people; lying down in the middle of busy streets; and slashing her own wrists or neck. Sally would frequently demand help, but would as frequently refuse to be assisted.

Because of her dysfunctional behavior, Sally was refused services by many of the so-called "last-resort" agencies. She was considered to be unsuitable for boarding home placement, and she was refused admittance to or evicted from many of the city's rooming houses and hotels. Eventually Sally was referred to the MSN, and a case conference was arranged. At the first case conference—which was attended by representatives from corrections, social services, mental health, and emergency housing—a case management plan was developed. The plan included the provision of housing by an emergency housing agency, and then placement in a long-term housing unit. Since Sally had difficulty managing her finances, income assistance would be provided on a weekly basis by a financial assistance worker from social services. Therapy would be provided on a continuing basis, and the probation officer agreed to continue seeing Sally (at her own request) following the expiration of her probation order.

Sally was eventually placed in a long-term housing facility, according to the plan. With help to manage her finances and with ongoing therapy, her behavior stabilized; she continued to have episodes of self-slashing, but not to the same degree as previously. For a while she improved to such an extent that she was able to attend school, and she purchased a bicycle, which she enjoyed immensely.

Recently, a second case conference had to be convened. The reason was that Sally had disclosed a history of sexual abuse; and that the frequency of her self-slashing subsequently increased to the point where staff members at her long-term residence no longer felt they could guarantee her safety. The decision at the conference was to provide additional assistance to the long-term residence staff. This was a crucial decision, since Sally had nowhere else to go if she were to be evicted. Thus, social services agreed to provide additional one-on-one service, and funding was provided to have Sally visit a psychologist in order to address the issues related to her sexual abuse. At the last report, Sally's behavior had stabilized, and she was said to be doing well.

The MSN was successful in achieving a number of its stated purposes, the most important of which was bringing about the recognition that a collaborative approach can be successful, whereas individual agencies acting alone may fail. However, those who were involved in sponsoring MSN eventually came to realize that many of its difficult clients required a more intensive brand of case management than MSN was designed to offer. So, in 1987, 3 years after the establishment of MSN, a new pilot project was initiated. This project is named the Inter-Ministerial Project (IMP) because it is funded and managed by the FPS Commission, the Greater Vancouver Mental Health Services Society, and the British Columbia Corrections Branch. IMP is an assertive case management program that targets the most difficult cases, including cases that MSN could not effectively manage. More specifically, IMP provides intensive case management services to multiproblem MDOs. IMP can make long-term commitments to its clients if these are deemed necessary. It has the explicit focus of preventing reincarceration and/or rehospitalization. Because IMP is supported by a number of government agencies, its case managers have the capability of tracking their clients across jurisdictional and agency boundaries, to ensure that a sustained service is provided.

The following case illustrates the beneficial effects of the IMP on difficult-to-manage persons with impulsivity (and other) problems.

> Robert was a 46-year-old male who was diagnosed with bipolar I disorder and was also said to have a personality disorder. Given up by most service agencies as unmanageable, he was referred to IMP as a last resort. Over the years, Robert's dysfunctional and noncompliant behavior brought him into frequent contact with the criminal justice system, as well as numerous other agencies. These included forensic psychiatric services, mental health services, hospitals, and other community agencies. His criminal record dated back to 1978, and over a 7-year period prior to his involvement with IMP, Robert had received 84 criminal charges (including mischief, willful damage, fraud, theft to arson, extortion, harassing and threatening, assault, possession of a weapon, and indecent acts). During that same period, he served a total of 23 prison terms and four probation orders. Like many other mentally disordered, multiproblem persons, Robert's behavior made him an unwelcome guest at almost all agencies and residential facilities. He was unable to maintain housing for more than a short period of time and thus drifted from place to place.
>
> While serving one of his probation orders, Robert was referred to IMP. Over the course of the first year of supervision, the IMP workers spent a great deal of time "on the street" with Robert. Gradually, the workers were able to develop rapport with Robert, and he eventually began to respond to their efforts and to the efforts of community

social service workers. His progress was slow at first, but over time the IMP workers noticed that Robert was making significant progress. Over the first 3½ years that Robert was with IMP, he was placed at the forensic psychiatric facility on three occasions for brief periods of time. This represented a dramatic decrease in his admissions to mental health facilities, compared with those prior to his referral to IMP. During that same period of time, Robert was charged with a criminal offense a total of four times. This amounted to approximately one charge per year—a marked reduction, compared to approximately 10 charges per year prior to his IMP referral. Finally, when Robert was first assigned to IMP, it was almost impossible to find housing of any type for him. He had been evicted by every known housing agency in the area. After his placement with IMP, Robert's behavior began to stabilize, and he became much easier to place. Eventually Robert progressed from a supervised housing project to an apartment of his own.

As a service, IMP has proven itself to be quite successful. Compared to similar types of MDOs, clients of this assertive case management program had fewer contacts with the criminal justice system, spent less time in jails, and as a result spent more days in the community (Wilson, Tien, & Eaves, 1995). In other ways, however, IMP has not fared as well as might be hoped. First, IMP is, and continues to be, a victim of its own success. The services it provides have always been well regarded and sought after by a whole host of agencies who deal with the mentally ill. Since its establishment, the demand for services has always exceeded the capacity of the program. Unfortunately, this has led to a perception by the referring agencies that IMP is not easily accessible. This situation, however, may well be unavoidable, given the chronicity of the program's target population and the long-term commitment of the program to its clients. A second problem that IMP has had to face repeatedly relates to the interministerial makeup of the program. At the operational level, the functional relationships between IMP staff and management, as well as with those who sponsor the program, were not initially clearly defined. Despite the fact that these agencies have agreed to come together and work together, their individual priorities have not always coincided; on occasion, this has resulted in unclear directions to the IMP staff. On a different level, although the participating agencies recognized the need to collaborate, no formal agreements regarding their individual and joint responsibilities were negotiated. This meant that no clear guidelines regarding responsibilities could be given to front-line staffers. This, too, has occasionally led to difficulties for IMP staff and management. Nevertheless, IMP is generally considered a success, and it is successful only because the participating agencies have endeavored to work out their differences when these have arisen. At the present time, consideration is being given to using the IMP approach to manage persons found "not criminally responsible on account of mental disorder" (NCRMD) throughout the province of British Columbia. This will require the establishment of IMP teams in most larger communities.

In the spirit of moving toward a more coordinated, integrated system of services to multiproblem persons, the Ministry of the Attorney General, the Ministry of Health, and the Ministry of Social Services directed their next efforts to the development of protocols for the joint management of mentally disordered persons in conflict with the law. This important piece of work took a number of years to complete, but in 1992 the document entitled *Protocols for the Inter-Ministerial Coordination of Services for Persons with a Mental Disorder or Mental Handicap Involved in the Criminal Justice System* (hereafter referred to as the MDO Protocols; British Columbia Government, 1992) was signed by the deputy ministers of all three ministries. A total of seven groups of protocols were established; these are structured according to the key junctures in the processing of individuals through the criminal justice system, such as investigation and arrest, first court appearance, adjudication, release, and community supervision. Although the MDO Protocols were developed for the coordination of services for "persons with a mental disorder or mental handicap," they are relevant to the present text for two main reasons. First, the experience gained from MSN and IMP is clearly reflected in this difficult exercise, especially in the "guiding principles" that are part of the MDO Protocols document. A number of principles that are particularly relevant to persons with impulsivity problems are reproduced below:

> 3. It is acknowledged that the coordination of services for persons with a mental disorder or mental handicap is a shared inter-ministerial responsibility.
>
> 9. In the coordination of services for persons with a mental disorder or mental handicap, it is agreed that the tasks assumed by a ministry should be consistent with the ministry's strengths, and specific program expertise and allocated resources.
>
> 11. Nothing in these principles is to be viewed as precluding the desirability of different ministries pooling their resources in the development of specific responses to solving problems.
>
> 12. When offenders with a mental disorder or mental handicap are released from a correctional facility, all reasonable steps should be taken to ensure their reintegration into the community. Discharge planning should occur as early as possible.
>
> 13. Special attention will be paid to the provision of community support and services for persons with mental disorder or mental handicap. (British Columbia Government, 1992, pp. 3–4)

The MDO Protocols are also relevant because they operationalize the term "mental disorder." That is, the MDO Protocols are defined as applying to five categories of individuals, ranging from persons who are clearly certifiable under the Mental Health Act, to those with a situational disorder and those with a mental handicap. Of particular interest to the topic of this book is Category III, which is written with persons with impulsivity clearly in mind:

> Category III: This group comprises those who may show only borderline features of mental illness, but their behavior is frequently disturbing to others. They often present with multiple challenges which aggravate their situations: organic disorders, substance abuse, borderline mental handicap, and personality difficulties.
>
> Such persons are often described as "dysfunctional," in that they can be erratic and impulsive, show poor judgment, have low stress levels, be demanding, and require immediate gratification. Mood disorders, emotional lability, and poor anger control can result in suicidal ideation and render them victims or victimizers in the correctional system and outside.

Although this description may not encompass all those who might be identified as individuals with impulsivity problems, it certainly covers a large number of those persons with impulsivity problems who will be seen by front-line staff members.

The most recent project designed in the spirit of the MDO Protocols is the Surrey Pretrial Mental Health Project, a mental health program that operates in a pretrial facility. This project has brought together the Ministries of Social Services, Health, and the Attorney General, as well as such organizations as the FPS Commission, Mental Health Services, and Alcohol and Drug Programs. Each organization contributes both staff members and funding to the establishment and day-to-day operation of the project. The goals of the Surrey Project are to make mental health services accessible to inmates who require intervention, and, in the long term, to reduce recidivism.

The strategy adopted by the Surrey Project to achieve these goals involves (1) universal mental health screening of all inmate admissions (a feature that is unique to correctional facilities in Canada); (2) timely intervention for those who present with mental health problems; and (3) assertive case management and follow-up services upon release or transfer from the correctional facility. Services are delivered by an interdisciplinary team composed of staff members assigned to the project by the various participating organizations. In the designing of this project, the lessons learned from the previous projects were put to good use. Its key feature is the use of a collaborative, interministerial approach in both the management and the delivery of services to MDOs. This was intended to overcome a major difficulty of the conventional system in the provision of services to MDOs. Henceforth, for those who come into contact with the Surrey Project, it is expected that they should no longer experience discontinuity in services as they move from the jurisdiction of one ministry to another or when they cross agency boundaries.

Despite everyone's good intentions, however, sometimes even the best plans just do not work out, and early successes cannot always be sustained over time. In fact, this can be a real problem for collaborative, interministerial programs. Experience suggests that such projects will have to address at least one problem sooner or later: Although the participating organizations are undeniably drawn together to collaborate for their mutual benefit, there remain forces present that can push them apart at the slightest provocation. These divisive forces include unexpected budget constraints, changes in staffing, and particularly changes at the management level of the participating agencies. Such high-level administrative shifts can result in changes in philosophy or changes in priorities. This is, in fact, a problem that has been encountered by both the IMP and the Surrey Project. Over time, the participating organizations have begun to drift away from the principles of collaboration and to impose their individual regulations on the projects. This is a result of changes at the management level and of new managers' not being adequately briefed regarding the collaborative nature of the projects. Organizations must therefore be ever vigilant for these threats; more importantly, they must be willing to undertake decisive actions in a timely fashion. Following one particularly difficult episode in the Surrey Project, new guidelines for the collaborative management of multiagency projects were finally developed (Forensic Psychiatric Services Commission of British Columbia, 1993). These guidelines are reproduced in Table 21.1, in the hope that they may give some insight into the dynamics of collaborative multiagency programs.

Since the establishment of the Surrey Pretrial Mental Health Project, there have been other developments in British Columbia that have served to enhance the effectiveness of the case management of multiproblem persons. One of the most important of these developments relates to the sharing of information between ministries and between agencies. However well designed an interministerial or interagency program may be, it cannot help performing poorly if the information flow between agencies is impeded or blocked. If clients are to move freely between agencies, relevant client information must also be allowed to flow between agencies. In practice, client information is always closely guarded, and gaining access to this information even for legitimate purposes is no easy task. New efforts were made to overcome this difficulty, and in 1995 a memorandum was signed by the deputy ministers of the Ministries of Health, Social Services, and the Attorney General. This agreement established a protocol for the sharing and management of information. In this new protocol, the authority for the exchanging of information is derived from the Freedom of Information and Protection of Privacy Act of British Columbia, which sets out the conditions under which information can be released. The protocol addresses the need to transfer treatment information and case management information, as well as the need to make

TABLE 21.1. Guiding Principles for the Management of Inter-Ministerial Programs

1. The operation of the inter-ministerial program should be overseen by an inter-ministerial Management Committee. The members of the Management Committee represent the mutual, as well as the individual, interests of the ministries.
2. Members of the Management Committee should be selected so as to facilitate the shared governance of inter-ministerial projects. In order to provide a direct link between staff and parent ministries, immediate (line) supervisors of staff assigned to the inter-ministerial program should be appointed to the Management Committee. In this regard, it is important that they are well connected with decision makers within their own organization.
3. When ministries join together to establish a collaborative program, the responsibility for the day-to-day management of the program should be *delegated* to the on-site manager or coordinator.
4. When staff are assigned to an inter-ministerial program, the functional supervision of the staff should be *delegated* to the on-site manager or coordinator. The on-site manager serves as a liaison to the individual ministries, and all management and personnel issues which require the individual action of the ministries are referred by the on-site manager through the inter-ministerial Management Committee to the relevant ministries.
5. Inter-ministerial programs, by virtue of the task they have to perform, should *not* be made to operate in the exact same manner in which parent ministries operate their own programs.
6. Issues which impact on the inter-ministerial program should be brought to the Management Committee. Decisions should be arrived at by mutual consent and agreement. On matters which impact on the program, no unilateral actions should be undertaken by individual ministries or representatives of the individual ministries.
7. Details of the shared governance of each inter-ministerial project should be clearly and specifically documented.

Note. From Forensic Psychiatric Services Commission of British Columbia (1993, p. 2).

distinctions between the two information types. It is anticipated that the introduction of this protocol will further enhance the effectiveness of the case management of multiproblem persons. Thus, this is a process that other jurisdictions might follow.

CONCLUDING OBSERVATIONS

In British Columbia, we have been fortunate to have had the opportunity to begin putting into practice the elements of a case management system tailored to the needs of multiproblem persons. Since such individuals appear to share many of the characteristics of persons afflicted with impulse-driven problems, the programs and protocols discussed above would seem to have direct applicability to those persons with impulsivity problems as well.

Despite positive results, the use of case management approaches with the mentally ill has not gone without criticism. Marshall et al. (1995), for example, have criticized the increasing use of case management approaches that have not been tested in randomized trials. Their study pointed to the limited effectiveness of case management in terms of such indicators as quality of life, social behavior, employment status, and quality of accommodation. We would suggest, however, that access to resources is a critical factor in the success or failure of an impulsive person in the community, and that an intensive case management approach such as IMP facilitates the optimum use of existing community resources. Such case management efforts should be directed not only at impulsive persons living in the community, but at those leaving hospitals as well. Given that individuals with impulsivity problems are often discharged quickly, even precipitously, from the conventional hospital system, intensive case management teams attached to general hospital psychiatric units could target impulsive and hard-to-handle patients. The "bridging" role played by these teams would serve to reduce the inappropriate and inefficient contacts that such disorganized persons make upon discharge to the community.

The task of devising better service delivery systems can never be complete, however, since it appears that as soon as one innovation is introduced, other issues and requirements arise. In addition to the development of new service delivery approaches and new policies, it must not be overlooked that multiproblem persons—particularly persons with impulsivity problems—have a great range of needs, wishes, and expectations that are difficult to anticipate. Because of their dysfunctional behaviors, such individuals often do not have their social and security needs adequately met. Most, for example, may not even have adequate housing where they feel safe and secure. It is to these areas that those who develop social programs and those who conduct research should turn their attention next. A comprehensive system of support should not only involve service agencies and government facilities; it should also address the social and security needs of clients. This may involve helping clients to establish an adequate social support network and ensuring that they have adequate and appropriate housing. It is likely that gains in these areas may contribute to additional improvements in the conditions of multiproblem persons. Serious breakdowns can often be prevented if timely and appropriate interventions are available. Emergency services delivered by trained personnel working with the police on the street, where most incidents occur, may result in a reduction in unnecessary hospitalization or incarcerations. In Vancouver, for instance, the city police force and the local mental health service have jointly established the "Car 87" program. Using an unmarked police patrol vehicle, a mental health nurse and a plainclothes police officer respond to psychiatric emergencies in the community outside normal mental health service office hours. Supported by local hospitals, emergency residences, and on-call physicians, the service attempts to resolve emergencies in a timely, effective, and relatively unintrusive manner. A combination of such emergency interventions with ongoing case management support might result in a more humane and positive way of dealing with impulsive persons, who have historically been given meager attention by conventional mental health systems.

REFERENCES

British Columbia Government. (1992, November). *Protocols for the inter-ministerial coordination of services for persons with a mental disorder or mental handicap involved in the criminal justice system.* Victoria, BC: Author.

British Columbia Government. *Protocol for the sharing of information across ministries and agencies.* Victoria, BC: Author.

Dvoskin, J. A., & Steadman, H. J. (1994). Using intensive case management to reduce violence by mentally ill persons in the community. *Hospital and Community Psychiatry, 45*(7), 679–684.

Fink, A. D., & McCown, W. (1993). *Impulsivity in children and adolescents: Measurement, causes and treatment.* Washington, DC: American Psychological Association.

Forensic Psychiatric Services Commission of British Columbia. (1993, July). *Inter-ministerial projects/programs: A proposed framework for collaborative service delivery.* Burnaby, BC: Author

Marshall, M., Lockwood, A., & Gath, D. (1995). Social services case-management for long-term mental disorders: A randomized controlled trial. *Lancet, 345,* 409–412.

McCown, W., & VandenBos, G. R. (1994). Treating the impulsive patient. *Hospital and Community Psychiatry, 45*(11), 1075–1077.

Ogloff, J. R. P., & Roesch, R. (1992). Using community mental health centers to provide comprehensive mental health services to local jails. In J. R. P. Ogloff (Ed.), *Law and psychology: Broadening of the discipline* (pp. 141–260). Durham, NC: Carolina Academic Press.

Parker, J. D. A., Bagby, R. M., & Webster, C. D. (1993). Domains of the impulsivity construct: A factor analytic investigation. *Personality and Individual Differences, 15*(3), 267–274.

Steadman, H. J. (1992). Boundary spanners: A key component for the effective interactions of the justice and mental health systems. *Law and Human Behavior, 16*(1), 75–87.

Tien, G., & Goresky, W. (1992). Management of the multi-problem mentally disordered person: Deinstitutionalization and the B.C. Mental Health Initiative. *British Columbia Medical Journal, 34*(4), 219–222.

Tien, G., & Lamb, D. (1989). *Report on the Project to Determine the Impact of Deinstitutionalization on the Criminal Justice System.* Report to the Assistant Deputy Ministers Committee of British Columbia.

Wilson, D., Tien, G., & Eaves, D. (1995). Increasing the community tenure of mentally disordered offenders. *International Journal of Law and Psychiatry, 18*(1), 61–69.

22

Integrated Support: A Case Approach to the Management of Impulsive People

LEE RYAN

VLADIMIR: I get used to the muck as I go along. . . . Question of temperament.

ESTRAGON: Of character.

VLADIMIR: Nothing you can do about it.

ESTRAGON: No use struggling.

VLADIMIR: One is what one is.

ESTRAGON: No use wriggling.

VLADIMIR: The essential doesn't change.

ESTRAGON: Nothing to be done.

—SAMUEL BECKETT, *Waiting for Godot* (1954, Act I, p. 14)

A certain group of persons falls between the cracks of the criminal justice system and the mental health system: those who simultaneously pose disciplinary and psychological problems, and whose behavior is viewed as either socially disruptive or psychologically disturbed, depending largely upon which institution they happen to be housed within at a particular time. The careers of such persons follow a familiar and recurrent pattern. An individual is charged with a criminal offense and remanded for psychiatric assessment. Categorized as "personality-disordered" and channeled through the corrections system, he or she begins to act bizarrely, hallucinates, or becomes uncooperative, violent, and self-destructive. Now diagnosed as "schizophrenic," the person is trans-ferred to a psychiatric facility, where the psychotic symptoms begin to abate under the influence of medication. Once more the individual is most likely to be labeled a mere nuisance, and with the "personality disorder" diagnosis again in hand, he or she returns to jail. The cycle continues, with the person being shuffled back and forth between custodial institutions and mental health facilities, since there seems to be no single place where he or she belongs. This practice has been described succinctly by Toch (1982) as "bus therapy."

The institutional conditions and professional attitudes that influence the treatment of disturbed, disruptive individuals are complex, having as much to do with the political climate as with the theoretical orientation of a particular clinician. For present purposes, I focus less on the issue of why; rather, I address the essential question of whether there is, as Estragon contends, "Nothing to be done." In this chapter I describe the long and varied institutional career of one individual—here called Harry—and the treatment regimen that finally (at least for the moment) got him off the bus.

HARRY'S STORY

Harry's case history is very similar to other personal accounts reported in the professional literature (Menzies & Webster, 1987; Steadman & Co-cozza, 1974; Toch & Adams, 1989). From the ages of 8 to 26, Harry was institutionalized 24 times (9 of those within a 12-month period), oscillat-ing among a psychiatric hospital, a medium-security prison, a forensic psychiatric assessment unit, and an institute for the criminally insane.

Harry's parents died when he was 6 years of age. He first came into conflict with the law at the age of 8, when he was caught breaking into a department store. This deed brought Harry the dubious honor of being the first minor formally committed to the state psychiatric hospital (diag-nosis: adjustment reaction to childhood and chronic brain syndrome). Following foster home placements (four in 1 year) where he proved unmanageable, he was sent to a center for disturbed children, with several detours back to the psychiatric hospital (diagnosis: unsocialized regres-sive reaction to adolescence).

At age 16, Harry was arrested for burglary and placed in a juvenile detention center. At the detention center, it was determined that Harry's intellectual functioning was within the mildly retarded range. He was consequently transferred to a long-term care facility for the mentally retarded, where he remained until age 18, at which time he was released into the community. Hospital notes over this 2-year period described the adolescent Harry as "retarded," "behaviorally disturbed," "psychotic," "schizophrenic," "immature," "undisciplined," "unstable," "unmanageable," "lacking the ability to learn," "beyond self-control," "without conscience," and finally "of a criminal nature." Once he was released into the community, Harry's troubles escalated. Following two more admissions to a psychiatric hospital (diagnosis: antisocial personality disorder), Harry was sent to a federal penitentiary for two counts of burglary and for stealing a truck. During his incarceration, Harry had frequent violent outbursts, in which he destroyed government property and twice set fire to his cell. On several occasions he was severely beaten during fights with other inmates. He tried suicide by hanging, by electrocution, by cutting his wrists, and by drowning. Harry was sent to the forensic psychiatric unit during this period for several brief periods of assessment and treatment (diagnoses: acute psychotic episode, mental retardation, sociopathic personality disorder).

At the age of 26, Harry finally made the local newspapers. On being released after serving 9 months for car theft and breach of parole, he was arrested twice in a single day for trying to scale the outer perimeter fence of the prison. But Harry was not trying to break out of prison; he was trying to get back in.

WHAT'S TO BE DONE WITH PEOPLE LIKE HARRY?

Harry could be described as split into two distinct components—Harry the "mad" self, and Harry the "bad" self (Toch, 1982, p. 330). Since the standard response of the criminal justice system or the mental health system is geared to one component or the other, the combination of disturbed and disruptive behavior displayed by Harry is most often interpreted separately as indicating either underlying mental illness or sheer malevolence. Although lacking the skills to comply with the basic social obligations of living in the community, individuals like Harry are unwilling or unable to play the well-defined roles of "inmate" or "patient" (Jemelka, Trupin, & Chiles, 1989). Thus, they become sources of institutional dilemmas and professional frustration. Within the criminal justice system, the situation is exacerbated by massive overcrowding, which severely increases the stresses on both inmates and professionals. Pretrial waiting periods are long; forensic units are overcrowded; beds in prison psychiatric and hospital units are often unavailable; and treatment programs within the prison system are scarce, with long waiting lists. Often the only successful in-house control of severely disruptive behavior is complete isolation. On the other hand, psychiatric hospitals are reluctant to admit patients with a history of criminal behavior or violence, because of obvious concerns for the security of other patients and of staff members. Furthermore, since the deinstitutionalization movement, most psychiatric hospitals focus less on long-term care than on short-term therapies targeting psychological illnesses that are amenable to treatment. Personality disorders and antisocial behavior are most often considered inappropriate for traditional psychological treatments (e.g., Hare & Hart, 1993; Rice, Harris, & Cormier, 1992). Thus, psychiatric hospitals view themselves as having nothing to offer these individuals (Pogrebin & Poole, 1987). The dilemma faced by professionals in both mental health and criminal justice settings is evident in the following comments by individuals who had worked with Harry. These interviews were conducted by Harry's psychologist.

The Lawyer for the Defense

I defended [Harry] on a serious charge of misuse of private property, willful damage, and a dozen or so related charges. It was an effort in absolute futility. I'm embarrassed to go to the bar to plead a case when I know that I don't understand what my client is thinking and I don't understand the nature of his illness. You can't apply law to people who think that the world stops just a few steps beyond the "jab" that they will receive when they get back to the hospital.

The Social Worker

I dress them [the clients] up and tell them what to do and say, and then I wait and pray that we get a judge who will see the foolishness of it all and return the client to custody somewhere. But the community doesn't want our people. They would much rather not see them or know that they exist. They would much rather we took care of such matters quietly and privately.

The Psychiatrist

There are very few things that can be said to a 26-year-old man who has the mentality and intelligence of a 12-year-old. It is hard enough to deal with the patient of normal intelligence, but to try to explain very complex ideas and issues [to a patient] with a limited mind is impossible. Psychiatric medicine has to be directly linked to illness and to inabilities to cope with the world. Lifestyle and low intelligence are hardly the domain of the psychiatrist. I feel that my time is best spent in areas where I can be effective and where I have a good chance of correcting the problem or disorder.

The Probation Officer

The position that probation has to take is that we can be of no assistance to this young man. We don't have the resources to handle his needs, and we are having tremendous difficulty understanding what needs he has. Probation is a system, and it runs through a certain form or process. As soon as someone comes to us and needs special treatment or consideration, we are forced to begin to look at the system and make exceptions—and suddenly we find that everyone is an exception, and we can't accommodate a full clientele of exceptions.

The Counsel for the Crown (Prosecution)

I don't know what to do when these guys come up before me. I can't really think that the courts do them any good, because we see them time and time again, over years and years. They graduate from juvenile courts and come to adult courts; they are glad to see us. We are like country relatives that they visit from time to time. They come bounding through like playful great puppies. The Crown presents whatever we can and tries to make a case that isn't going to buy the guy hard time. We can't juggle all the things that come up—public interest, safety of the community, safety of the individual citizen, teaching the offender, justice for all men under the law—we go through all the arguments.

The Judge

I am bewildered by the people like this young man [Harry] that come before me. I can't be expected to know about psychology and areas of education that relate to deviant behavior, odd behavior. It is a very complex area, and when there are twists that complicate matters before the bench and crimes that are senseless, I have to ask myself about the application of the law as it applies to these cases.

Too often, the frustrations associated with people like Harry are dealt with by not dealing with them at all. Toch (1982) argues that despite the best professional intentions, the continually aversive nature of such a person's disruptive and incomprehensible behavior "reliably overwhelms decisions, and inspires caretakers to classify the person so as to make him primarily the client of other caretakers" (p. 332). The offending individual is repeatedly transferred through an ever-expanding "transcarceral system" (Menzies & Webster, 1987) consisting of a complex network of legal and medical institutions. Forensic psychiatrists act as the gatekeepers in the network, shuffling the individual through the system with the use of strategically chosen labels. The formulation of "mentally disordered offender" has blurred the once clearly separate concepts of "patient" and "prisoner," "treatment" and "punishment," "assessment" and "judgment." As a result, the labels available to describe an offender are numerous and interchangeable, dependent more upon the context in which the behavior occurs than upon the behavior itself (Webster, Menzies, Butler, & Turner, 1982). A typical example of this can be found in Harry's records. After a particularly violent bout of self-destructive behavior, the prison psychiatrist entered a diagnosis of schizophrenia, which resulted in Harry's being moved to a hospital for the criminally insane. Several weeks later the hospital psychiatrist rediagnosed him as having antisocial personality disorder, and Harry was returned to the prison. Menzies (1987) writes: "For their part, the subjects of forensic control are exposed to a circular process of stigmatization and enforcement, as they are recurrently held accountable to both judicial and psychiatric standards of normality" (p. 247).

Harry is not an exception; in recent years, "bus therapy" has been applied to a surprisingly large number of offenders. Menzies (1985) tracked 571 men and women after an initial court-ordered 1-day assessment at the Metropolitan Toronto Forensic Service (METFORS). At the conclusion of the 2-year follow-up period, only 35% of the patients were under no form of institutional or community control. During that period, fully 50% of the group were confined to multiple institutions, including remand centers, prisons, psychiatric hospitals, and forensic assessment units. Many of the METFORS patients had undergone repeated psychiatric assessments. Over the course of these assessments, diagnoses tended to shift from pathological to characterological as a history of disruptiveness was documented. Harry's diagnoses followed a similar pattern, moving from "adolescent adjustment reaction" to "adjustment disorder with psychotic episodes" to "chronic schizophrenia" and finally to "sociopathic personality disorder." The evolution from psychological distress to reified personality trait occurs because diagnoses including disruptiveness as a criterion highlight antisocial features that can be discounted as nonpathological (and hence untreatable). However, as Toch (1982) points out, a schizophrenic who assaults people is both psychotic and violence-prone. Both labels are equally applicable, yet one does not adequately explain or discount the other.

GETTING HARRY OFF THE BUS

Is there any hope of extrication, once a person like Harry is caught up in the system? The literature is far from optimistic. Menzies (1985) discouragingly reminds us that reforms directed at limiting the discretionary power of forensic psychiatry have no pragmatic effect, amounting to little more than "procedural band aids [*sic*] in an institutional forum where process and power are two facets of the same phenomenon" (p. 639). Toch (1982) has suggested creating new restorative institutional settings for the "walking wounded," but one suspects that these would only be subsumed into the transcarceral network. Indeed, it is difficult to conceive of a single rehabilitative program that could deal with the complex and often idiosyncratic mixture of problems within this group: psychotic disturbance; assaultiveness and self-destructiveness; mental retardation; poor social skills; depression; substance abuse and dependence; antisocial behaviors; and a lack of self-control, interpersonal skills, problem-solving skills, and vocational skills. Such a flexible and multifaceted program truly seems to be, as Harris and Rice (Chapter 19, this volume) have described it, "a kind of unattainable dream" (p. 385).

The ultimate irony of the situation is that the inmates themselves often understand the dilemma they face. Harry tried to break into the prison once he was released, realizing that he could not cope on the inside, yet knowing that he surely could not cope on the outside either. For Harry, at least, there was a (guardedly) happy ending. His notoriety in the local newspapers brought him to the attention of a psychologist who had worked for many years with juvenile offenders. Under her guidance, a detailed program plan was drawn up to provide Harry with the skills necessary to cope in the community. First, cognitive and psychological assessments identified key problem areas. Harry had minimal reading and writing skills, and his lack of even simple arithmetic made him unable to handle money and budgeting. He had difficulty with simple problem solving, planning, and organizing. He had trouble remembering new information and following through on daily tasks, which made self-medication and keeping appointments difficult. Harry also found it difficult to make decisions when faced with alternatives, and reacted violently to stressful situations or ones in which he was likely to fail. Finally, he had very low self-esteem and lacked even basic interpersonal skills.

In view of these findings, Harry's government assistance checks were sent directly to his psychologist in trust. Accommodation in a local rooming house was arranged, and his meals were prepaid at a nearby community club for the mentally retarded. A detailed daily plan was set up for the first few months. Harry reported briefly for 15–20 minutes every day to his psychologist, who gave him a daily allowance and his oral medications. During longer sessions held twice weekly, she counseled Harry in such basic skills as how to talk to people, how to deal with the police, how to cope with frustrating situations, how to count money, and generally how not to end up back in jail. A street worker from the local community college was assigned to be a companion to Harry, accompanying him to appointments and helping him to become familiar with the local area. Every 2 weeks Harry saw a general practitioner, who administered his injections of fluphenazine and counseled him in health and hygiene. A social worker monitored Harry's living situation and instructed him in general life skills such as housekeeping, dressing, cooking, shopping, and budgeting. Harry was assessed for vocational training, but it was decided that until he was more self-sufficient it would not be advisable to put him into a program in which he was likely to fail. Instead, Harry was given small jobs at community centers in the area for several hours per day; he also took on, with the help of his street worker, a paper route.

The primary goal of the program was to keep Harry in the community. Instead of placing him in an existing structured program—which would have called for enormous amounts of adapting on his part, and which might well have had little ecological relevance to his life in the community once he left the system—Harry was taught the basic skills that he needed in the society in which he would be living. For its part, the government paid only $60 (Canadian) per day for the first 2-year period to cover the costs of the entire support program. Given the ever-increasing costs of institutional care, and the untold monetary and professional resources already invested in Harry over the years, this seemed a small price indeed to keep Harry in the community. After the first 6 months of his program, the psychologist's report to the court read:

There has been a great deal of pressure on Harry to take on responsibilities that are new to him. He has been closely monitored and has been reporting to several different people. Harry has surpassed the prognosis of most of the professionals he has dealt with in the past—he may well be able to establish permanent lifestyle patterns if given the time to learn acceptable behaviors, but we must help him now while he is feeling appreciated and capable of accomplishing these tasks.

Two years after the implementation of the program, Harry had attained general self-sufficiency, although he still required a modest level of support and supervision. Importantly, the support program was successful in keeping Harry out of both the court system and the mental health system for nearly 7 years, when he was again charged with a misdemeanor and released into the care of his psychologist. Since that time, Harry has remained in the community without incident.

STOPPING THE BUS

Finding an answer to the question of how to help someone like Harry must begin with the basic assumption that treatment is possible. The well-established view that "nothing works" (Martinson, 1974) has been slowly replaced with the more encouraging view that, with careful planning and implementation, some rehabilitative programs do work. The question then becomes one of optimizing efficacy by identifying the components of treatment that will be most successful for a particular individual. Rice, Harris, Quinsey, and Cyr (1990) favor an individualized case management approach (much like the one described here) that targets an individual's needs in multiple areas: psychosocial functioning; psychotropic medications when appropriate; interpersonal skills; vocational skills; elimination of substance misuse; symptom management skills; and the development of prosocial skills, values, and attitudes. In such a treatment program, the clinician becomes as much a "director of operations" as a provider of treatment. Indeed, it is unlikely that all of Harry's problems could have been addressed by any one professional. Particularly in the early stages of his release, the key element provided by Harry's psychologist was a high level of coordination and management; this required hours of group planning, interviews, matching of client and counselors, financial organization, and family interactions. One cannot underestimate the importance of a determined and knowledgeable therapist who is willing to take on such a daunting task. Harry is over 6 feet tall and weighs over 220 pounds, whereas his psychologist is barely 5 feet tall. In the early months, Harry screamed at her, spat at her, threatened her, threw objects at her, and woke her up during the night on many occasions because he just wanted to talk. For such a client, caring is not enough; a case manager/therapist requires assertiveness, commitment, perseverence, enthusiasm, emotional stability, and perhaps, above all else, skill.

Alternative strategies for rehabilitation, both within the prison system and once the inmate has been released to the community, should be based on shared knowledge of treatment programs that have succeeded and those that have failed. If the circularity of an offender's career is to be halted, these programs must be geared toward providing the individual with the skills necessary to cope in society. "In society" must certainly be the primary focus for any successful rehabilitation program. Too often an offender is simply dumped back into the community, and is suddenly asked to contend with the complex world of parole obligations, boarding houses, recreational centers, and vocational training organizations. Menzies and Webster (1987) have written:

> Too much is demanded and too little offered, with the result that individuals recurrently fail and fall into the hands of the police. And once in their hands they do not have the knowledge or resources to free themselves. So round they go once more, with the result that all actors become inured and conditioned to a recurring script that is played out with little room for improvisation. (p. 290)

Criticism of the system is easy. The difficulty lies in the implementation of successful programs that effectively circumvent the pitfalls facing the released inmate. This is particularly true for people like Harry, whose behavioral and psychological problems interact in complex and poorly understood ways, so that no simple approach will suffice. The cautious reemergence of Harry as an acceptable member of the community is a reminder that it is possible (albeit difficult) to get off the bus. Harry will probably never win any personality awards, and it is more than likely that his criminal career is not over. His existence in the community is at best tenuous. This is something that Harry himself is very aware of, as a recent exchange with his psychologist indicates:

PSYCHOLOGIST: Harry, where are you going to be in 10 years?

HARRY: I don't know. Something will happen, and if I'm still on the outside I'll be okay, but if I'm in the can I'm dead. I can't do that again. They'll say "Harry, you're a goof," and then there'll be trouble. I go crazy and do wild stuff, like throw shit all over the place and start fires, and they'll kill me.

PSYCHOLOGIST: What will happen when I don't have as much time as I do now?

HARRY: I don't know. I guess I'll get into trouble if I can't get help to have my medication and someone to do my money with me. I couldn't do it all the other times I tried. I just can't seem to get it together—not without help—and the help has to be someone who cares about me and wants to talk to me and listen to me. I get really lonely sometimes.

PSYCHOLOGIST: I can't be here forever.

HARRY: I know. Maybe I'll just have to go back to the hospital or prison if I can't get help.

PSYCHOLOGIST: What do I do about that?

HARRY: Maybe if I get in trouble again, we can get a contract again? Do you think I could save enough for a color TV?

REFERENCES

Beckett, S. (1954). *Waiting for Godot.* New York: Grove Press.

Hare, R. D., & Hart, S. D. (1993). Psychopathy, mental disorder, and crime. In S. Hodgins (Ed.), *Mental disorder and crime* (pp. 104–115). Newbury Park, CA: Sage.

Jemelka, R. E., Trupin, E., & Chiles, J. A. (1989). The mentally ill in prisons: A review. *Hospital and Community Psychiatry, 40*, 481–491.

Martinson, R. (1974). What works?: Questions and answers about prison reform. *The Public Interest, 35*, 22–54.

Menzies, R. J. (1985). *Doing violence: Psychiatric discretion and the prediction of dangerousness.* Unpublished doctoral dissertations, University of Toronto.

Menzies, R. J. (1987). Cycles of control: The transcarceral careers of forensic patients. *International Journal of Law and Psychiatry, 10*, 233–249.

Menzies, R. J., & Webster, C. D. (1987). Where they go and what they do: The longitudinal careers of forensic patients in the medicolegal complex. *Canadian Journal of Criminology, 29*, 275–292.

Pogrebin, M. R., & Poole, E. D. (1987). Deinstitutionalization and increased arrest rates among the mentally disordered. *Journal of Psychiatry and Law, 15*, 117–127.

Rice, M. E., Harris, G. T., & Cormier, C. (1992). Evaluation of a maximum security therapeutic community for psychopaths and other mentally disordered offenders. *Law and Human Behavior, 16*, 399–412.

Rice, M. E., Harris, G. T., Quinsey, V. L., & Cyr, M. (1990). Planning treatment programs in secure psychiatric facilities. In D. N. Weisstub (Ed.), *Law and mental health: International perspectives* (Vol. 5, pp. 162–230). Elmsford, NY: Pergamon Press.

Steadman, H. J., & Cocozza, J. J. (1974). *Careers of the criminally insane,* Lexington, MA: Lexington Books.

Toch, H. (1982). The disturbed disruptive inmate: Where does the bus stop? *Journal of Psychiatry and Law, Fall, 10,* 327–349.

Toch, H., & Adams, K. (1989). *The disturbed violent offender.* New Haven, CT: Yale University Press.

Webster, C. D., Menzies, R. J., Butler, B., & Turner, R. (1982). Forensic psychiatric assessment in selected Canadian cities. *Canadian Journal of Psychiatry, 27,* 455–462.

23

A Guide for Creating Treatment Programs

CHRISTOPHER D. WEBSTER

In 1969, Jay Haley published an amusing article, "The Art of Being a Failure as a Psychotherapist." This was in part an attack on psychoanalytic approaches to psychotherapy, which to his mind were unduly prevalent at that time. But, as well as serving a humorous and polemical function, his paper had the curious effect of making even seasoned clinicians think about what they were doing. By standing the usual question "How do we succeed in psychotherapy?" on its head and instead wondering how best to set about failure, Haley was able to construct a set of principles likely to be of help in a wide range of clinical circumstances. His opening argument was that because the rate of spontaneous remission in many psychiatric disorders is high, it takes a certain skill and dogged persistence to prevent clients from recovering of their own accord. The wry suggestion was that although it is difficult to set back the recoveries of clients, it is a task that can, with effort, be accomplished. He then went on to point out how this might be done through refusing to address the presenting problem, unnecessarily confining persons to psychiatric facilities, avoiding evaluations of results, and so on.

The idea of inverting problems in order to obtain greater clarity of thinking is, of course, not original with Haley. Samuel Butler, for example, used the device in his utopian novel *Erewhon* (1872/1967), in which he put forward the idea that people with physical illnesses should be punished and people with mental problems should be endlessly indulged. I have previously taken this line to explain how to set about establishing bound-to-fail programs for autistic persons and their families (Webster, 1980), how to raise the level of mental disturbance in prisons (Webster, 1990), and how to fail in undertaking risk assessments (Webster, Chapter 18, this volume). In this chapter, with the indulgence of my readers, I invoke the device once more to try to show how persons with impulsivity problems can actually be assisted (see the Appendix for a positively worded version). In keeping with the tendency toward 20-item checklists in this book, the text that follows sets forth 20 tactics that, if used with determination and energy, ought to yield a massive rise in the rate of impulse-related conditions during the 21st century. This is particularly the case because, so far as my colleagues and I are aware, problems with impulsivity—unlike the neurotic conditions addressed by Haley—rarely remit of their own accord.

THE ART OF BEING A FAILURE AS A TREATMENT PROVIDER: TWENTY SUGGESTIONS

1. Ignore the "Psychoimpulsivity of Everyday Life"

Clinicians should take no account of the fact that millions of dollars are spent daily by advertisers selling habit-forming, self-destructive products aimed at inducing people to make expensive purchases on the basis of minimal reflection. Advertisements for liquor, cigarettes, sex, gambling, and the like are ubiquitous. It may be easy enough for the elderly and middle-aged to avoid exposure to a culture that frankly and openly promotes substance use, violence, and even suicide, but for young persons it is not perhaps so simple. The general point, then, is that it is a good idea for clinicians to pay as little attention as possible to what is going on around them, and to understand as little as possible about how hard it may be for some people to resist the assaultive force of advertising and, indeed, of popular culture. This step—particularly appealing, because for most therapists it requires only a small expenditure of energy—guarantees two things. First, a would-be helper remains in ignorance of how the world is turning and how staggering the dimensions of impulsivity-related problems are. Second, because the helper has no framework with which to explore the salient features of the client's world, it is possible to pursue the treatment path in almost complete ignorance of what might or might not be possible. Such ignorance is greatly to be prized. Clinicians should never ask impulsive persons what books they read or what TV programs and movies they watch. In seeking to understand impulsivity in the contemporary world, they should choose Mahler over Cobain.

2. Select a Single Cause to Explain Impulsive Conduct

The notion that impulsive behavior has a single, easily defined cause—a notion actually contained in Haley's "daily dozen" of the clinical field—can almost guarantee failure single-handedly. The idea is to latch on to some fairly simple explanation for all kinds of violent, impulsive behavior. Sugar in the diet might be a good contender (Rodale, 1968). A clinician might attribute impulsive behavior solely to alcohol or drugs, or form the idea that most paraphilic behavior results merely from an overabundance of testosterone. With a culprit isolated, it becomes easy to suggest a treatment plan. To give the sense of being on top of things, the clinician can invoke serotonin in a vague and general way.

3. Advocate for Dramatic Social and Political "One Stroke" Solutions

There is really not much point in tackling person after person on an individual basis. What is really needed is something that will get at the "root cause" of the problem and fix it. There comes a point in the life of any car when it no longer pays to tinker endlessly with the engine; the answer is to put in a new one. It is the same with people: Helpers can only fiddle about so much; after that, society needs to invest some money and solve the problem once and for all. The leaders of temperance movements and those responsible for Prohibition had the right idea. They may have failed to pull it off, but a new effort—aided perhaps by the results of the previous slight mishap—might stand a very good chance of success. It goes without saying that those convicted of violent sex offenses should be obliged to take treatment, should be detained for very long periods, and in some instances should be executed. These kinds of tough government-backed schemes would doubtless do well in North America, since it appears that they yield striking results elsewhere, at least in dealing with drug addiction (Webster, 1985). Clinicians should use the time they might have spent in the clinic to get themselves up to their necks in partisan politics.

4. Invest a Disproportionate Amount of Effort in Assessment and Diagnosis at the Outset

Once persons are referred to the unit, clinic, or service, they should receive the most thorough assessments ever attempted. It is best to use a standard package of personality and projective tests. Clinicians should not stint at this stage. It does not really matter if it takes clients 40 hours or more to complete the necessary tests. Some psychologists and psychometrists tell us that with such a bank of information, they will be able to pinpoint the clients' problems for sure. The same holds true for psychiatric diagnoses. It is imperative that each and every diagnosis in the current nosology be considered. Only when diagnoses are firmly established at the outset is it possible to get on with the job. As Haley (1969) pointed out in his use of this step, an emphasis on diagnosis at the expense of treatment can be an advantage because it elevates the status of clinicians. It gives them a chance to seem expert. And there is the additional point that an overemphasis on diagnosis will preclude the possibility of thinking about treatment solutions.

5. Make No Effort to Assess the Client's Strengths, Capabilities, and Assets

Impulsive people can often almost guarantee their own failure at the hands of mental health and correctional workers. They come "prewired," as it were, with long lists of liabilities, defects, and inadequacies. Indeed, so long are the lists are apt to be that it becomes hard to see any qualities that might enable them to reposition their lives. So the answer for those who would work to promote failure is perfectly clear and (like most of the points raised in this chapter) requires little or no effort. All that is needed is persistence with the prevailing drive to isolate inadequacies and to gloss over essentially positive characteristics.

6. Ignore the Client's Experience and Point of View

It is often hard to understand what points people with impulsive disorders are trying to make, or indeed what they are saying at all. Not infrequently, they have their own special language or argot (Anonymous, 1980), and it would take years to gain a knowledge of these various subcultures. It would be a waste of time anyway, since the prime purpose of the counseling or therapy is to get such a person to join the therapist's middle-class culture. Not knowing what the individual wants or expects almost guarantees failure. Yet there is room for a little perversity.

If the matter of success versus failure in therapy is considered in the broadest possible terms, there are two chances of success and two of failure. Success—not what is being aimed at here—is at least potentially possible if the client sees himself or herself as responsible for past actions and the therapist is of the same mind. The same holds true if the client, backed by the therapist, sees himself or herself largely in the role of patient—one who deserves to be excused past oddities or travesties on the grounds of sickness of some kind or other. Knowing these two points is helpful in promoting failure. If the person declares mental illness, the therapist adopts a strict model of personal responsibility; if the person opts for being held accountable, the therapist reaches for the prescription pad and the offer to languish in a clinic or hospital. Since success in treatment needs only to be feared when both the client and the therapist are working from the same basic premises and toward the same objective, it is fundamentally important to decide which tack the client is on and shift at the outset to the other.

7. Avoid Assessing Risks of Violence

Proceeding on the straight assumption that clients in the main will not act dangerously to others and themselves, perhaps despite oft-voiced threats, will go a long way toward ensuring failure of the worst possible kind. This strategy, so easy to apply, can yield even spectacular results. All that is required is the avoidance of systematic thought about risk. Once the notion of risk is abroad, it becomes almost impossible to avoid thinking about how it might be contained or reduced. This means that systematic evaluations should be eschewed, and that staff members should never consider the day-to-day risks they and other clients might run as a result of poor building design or bad policies and procedures.

8. Refuse to Set Any Realistic Objectives

The refusal to set realistic objectives is a point borrowed from Haley (1969), but it has of course been referred to constantly over the years (Rice, Harris, Quinsey, & Cyr, 1990; Webster, Hucker, & Grossman, 1993). If neither patient nor therapist has any clear idea of what might be achieved over a set period, failure is almost guaranteed. When the client does insist on establishing some link to the future, it is up to the therapist to head these efforts off at the pass or to fix on something that is all but impossible to attain. When in doubt, the therapist should encourage discussion of what it might mean to be a "whole person." If nothing else, time can be consumed in counting body parts, both within and without the therapeutic hour. Staff members should never consider writing a description of the program, and should also avoid the production of videotaped or filmed depictions.

9. Offer Well-Intentioned But Feeble Interventions

It is a really good idea to treat highly impulsive people for a set 50 minutes each week. This, after all, may be the only regularity in their lives. The very arrangement gives them something to look forward to. A calm atmosphere in the office, contrasting as it doubtless does with the chaos of their lives, is worth a great deal in itself. The chance for an impulse-driven person to be able to "ventilate" should not be underestimated. A passive effort on the therapist's part may result in remarkable effects throughout the remaining 167 hours of the week. The therapist should never vary the routine and should never see the person outside the hour, no matter how seemingly grave the circumstances.

10. Demand That Clients "Straighten Out" Their Problems with Impulsivity

Incredible though it may seem, a confirmed addict or gambler may not, to this very point, have thought that he or she needs to "get a grip." It is therefore a really good idea, using the bluntest and strongest terms possible, to let such an individual know that this weakness must stop. All it takes is a little strength of character to put aside the pill bottle; all that is required is a little determination. Effects of such "straight talking" can be profound. There is nothing like a bit of reality, a little confrontation. The therapist should make it clear that people who fritter away their lives taking drugs, pulling their hair out, or lifting stuff from stores are an unconscionable drain on the public purse. This approach is almost bound to create a sense of discouragement and despair so strong that clients will make no further attempts to deal with their problems.

11. Maintain a Strict Therapeutic Style

During the first meeting or two, it is a very good idea for the therapist to lay out to the client how the therapist intends to approach the issues over the next few months or years. The client deserves to know what the therapist stands for, and what he or she will not stand for. This approach should not be varied. It is a mistake for the therapist to wonder on the one hand whether anything is being accomplished (because issues are being avoided), and on the other whether the individual is being over-whelmed (through the introduction of ideas apt to evoke paralyzing emotional responses).

12. Have No Means of Evaluating Outcome

If there is no mechanism for bringing forward examples of cases that have succeeded, there is an evident likelihood that these will be submerged under the weight of failing cases. This penumbra of failure is very important in setting the scene for new adventures in defining the hope-lessness of the therapeutic enterprise. Such bias is most helpful in trying to promote failure. The aim is to keep the bulk of staff members more or less completely out of touch with what they are actually accomplishing. This occurs more or less automatically unless it is corrected periodically through the introduction of basic feedback information.

13. Do Not Enlist Multiple Measures of Successful Outcome

When a therapist or a program sticks to one central measure of outcome, and allows for no other, chances of failure are given a major boost. It is not usually difficult to find a problem to conquer; clients frequently arrive with at least one. It is important to stick with one and only one. Success is to be seen entirely in one-dimensional terms. If the problem is drug addiction, it is addiction that must be wrestled to the ground. For failure to be given its full chance and due, it is important not to be distracted by such irrelevancies as quality of life, improved social relations, vocational adaptation, or the like. Any lapse or relapse must be defined as irreparable failure.

14. Approach Symptoms One at a Time in Sequence

In the course of this text, the point is made many times that people with impulsive disorders tend to have problems in more than a single area. Concentrating exclusively on one set of symptoms—say, excessive drinking—will almost certainly assure failure. Even if together the client and therapist do eventually overcome this difficulty, the chances are that other symptoms will soon emerge with dramatic intensity. Indeed, a single focus of attention may mean that the therapist, in the quest for a solution to one problem, will have been suitably inattentive to other difficulties faced by the client. Tackling issues one at a time in a fixed, orderly sequence guarantees failure with impulsive people, and at the same time assures that each case will provide a lifetime of work for the therapist.

15. Treat Persons in Isolation from Family Members, Relatives, Friends, and Others

Without some actual knowledge of the individual's life except that glimpsed from his or her descriptions in the course of weekly appointments, the prospect of failure receives considerable enhancement. This was a point noted by Haley (1969) nearly 30 years ago, and it remains sound today. Unless some partnerships are formed and some agreements are forged with family members or others during times of relative quiet, there is little chance of garnering assistance for the individual during periods of chaos and disruption.

16. Refuse to Train Staff Members

After a therapist has spent some years encouraging failure in clients, their problems, whatever these might originally have been, will now have expanded greatly. The field of endeavor will now be very large, and, with the therapist's failure clear for all to behold, he or she will be promoted to some kind of directorship. Only rarely now will the new director's peace be disturbed by angry, anxious, and desperate people. Others, now employed by the director because of their training (or, in some cases, precisely because of their lack of it), will now take over the front-line role. Refusing to supervise and listen to these persons, who are usually quite young, will remarkably enhance failure potential. The staff members will form close relations with some of the clientele and will doubtless be of assistance in many cases. Yet, if they are left on their own, the burden will eventually get to be too large; sooner or later, they will abruptly buy the obligatory backpack and a one-way ticket to Europe. Able young people will become so discouraged about this kind of work, and about themselves, that they will give up. This means, of course, that such otherwise capable persons are permanently extruded from a field where they might have elevated treatment success rates.

17. Help Staff Members Become Co-Opted by Clients

Staff members who work with openly antisocial clients have a job on their hands. There may be talk of the "rehabilitation" of these persons, without a lot of consideration given to the fact that they were never "habilitated" in the first place. It becomes very easy in this kind of work—for example, in parole supervision, case management, and the like—for a counselor to become incorporated into a client's scheme of things. Moral boundaries are obscured and lost, and some therapists find themselves engaged in practices that are not only highly unethical and unprofessional, but in extreme cases on the wrong side of the law (Bolen, 1994).

18. Make Frequent Use of the Transfer List

Both at the level of the individual counselor, and at that of the agency as a whole, there comes a time when the energy for continuing with a particular client is seriously depleted. The tendency then is to try to find a solution by shifting the problem elsewhere. Since agencies not untypically work in relative isolation from one another, and since it is even possible to find arguments for a "fragmented" service delivery model (e.g., Bickman, 1996), there is ample opportunity for long-range failure through a "ship-out" procedure. On the books, it will look like just another referral matter and will seem like a sensible and acceptable solution. Yet, at bottom, everyone—most likely including the client—will see it for what it is. Some clients will feel justifiably injured and insulted; others will rest contented in the knowledge that they have manipulated the matter to their own ends. Either way, it spells trouble for the future.

19. Use the "Nothing Works in Therapy" Position as a Starting Point for Theory and Practice

A literature published in the not too distant past indicates that no approaches to treatment are likely to be effective (e.g., Martinson, 1974). These works need to be read and reread, for they inculcate an air of futility and hopelessness. Young staff members need to be sheltered from a more recent literature, which suggests that from time to time people do manage to overcome, or at least live with, problems of impulsivity (see Gendreau, Little, & Goggin, 1996; Harris & Rice, Chapter 19, this volume).

20. Avoid Any Attempt at Systematic Study

Every so often, some misguided survivor of a graduate course in statistics will appear on the scene anxious to examine the functioning of the organization. What will be proposed is that the current treatment program—which is well established and therefore in no need of testing—should be "verified." Under the plan will come random assignment of patients to various inane "control" and "contrast" conditions. These plans need to be nipped in the bud; they can most easily be set aside through reference to cost and, most especially, to ethical issues. The appeal to ethics is particularly compelling, as not only is it almost bound to win the day, but it identifies the would-be investigator as an evil force. It is particularly important to avoid establishing systematic longitudinal studies, for these invariably point up how impulsivity problems tend to surface at an early age (see Hodgins, 1996).

CONCLUSION

It is encouraging to think that as a result of rapidly accumulating knowledge about impulsivity and the disorders that involve impulsivity, there may soon arise solutions appreciably more potent than those presently available. Yet it is well at the same time to recognize that we already have information that can be of immense value, both practically at a clinical level and in terms of policy formation. We know from systematic longitudinal studies a good deal about how impulsivity-related problems tend to span the life cycle (point 20). These difficulties are not necessarily immutable (point 19), though it is usually an error to think that they can be resolved dramatically at a single stroke (point 3). The clinical and research evidence is strong that single-cause explanations usually turn out to be inadequate (point 2), and that the therapeutic ventures most likely to succeed are those that start out by determining the full extent of clients' particular difficulties (point 14), without at the time placing undue reliance on heavily "mechanical" approaches to assessment (point 4). This means being attentive to clients' capabilities (point 5) and establishing several markers of success that can be used simultaneously (point 13). Such markers need to be agreed upon with the client (point 8) and to be measurable in some definite way (point 12). Attitudes toward clients must be concordant with their expectations and points of view (point 6)—an observation that requires would-be helpers to vary their approaches and responses (point 11). Reliance on moral injunctions may exacerbate difficulties instead of resolving them (point 10); in any event, clients' problems are not likely to be overcome through cursory and ill-focused approaches to treatment (point 9). When clients give indications that they might harm themselves or other people, it is important that the matter be treated directly and seriously (point 7), and that efforts be made to minimize risk through understandings and agreements with family members, friends, relatives, employers, and the like (point 15). Staff members need encouragement and close supervision if they are to persist in their work with difficult clients (point 16), avoid taking easy ways out (point 18), and avert damage to themselves personally and professionally (point 17). Finally, we need to think long and hard about the way cultures and subcultures, including professional ones (see Menzies, Chapter 3, this volume), may wittingly or unwittingly add undue burden to already distressed and impulsive people (point 1).

REFERENCES

Anonymous. (1980). Arrest and trial: The bullpen. *International Journal of Offender Therapy and Comparative Criminology, 24,* 11–19.

Bickman, L. (1996). A continuum of care: More is not always better. *American Psychologist, 51,* 689–701.

Bolen, D. E. (1994). *Stupid crimes: A novel.* Toronto: Vintage Books.

Butler, S. (1967). *Erewhon.* New York: Airmont. (Original work published 1872)

Gendreau, P., Little, T., & Goggin, C. (1996). A meta-analysis of the predictors of adult recidivism: What works! *Criminology, 34,* 575–607.

Haley, J. (1969). The art of being a failure as a psychotherapist. *American Journal of Orthopsychiatry, 39,* 691–695.

Hodgins, S. (1996). The major mental disorders: New evidence requires new policy and practice. *Canadian Psychology, 37,* 95–111.

Martinson, R. (1974). What works? Questions and answers about prison reform. *The Public Interest, 35,* 22–54.

Rice, M. E., Harris, G. T., Quinsy, V. L., & Cyr, M. (1990). Planning treatment programs in secure psychiatric facilities. In D. N. Weisstub (Ed.), *Law and mental health: International perspectives* (Vol. 5, pp. 162–230). Elmsford, NY: Pergamon Press.

Rodale, J. I. (1968). *Natural health, sugar and the criminal mind.* New York: Pyramid Books.

Webster, C. D. (1980). How to fail as a director of programs for autistic children and their families. In C. D. Webster, M. M. Konstantareus, J. E. Mack, & J. Oxman (Eds.), *Autism: New directions in research and education* (pp. 125–134). Elmsford, NY: Pergamon Press.

Webster, C. D. (1985). Compulsory treatment of narcotic addiction. *International Journal of Law and Psychiatry, 8,* 1–27.

Webster, C. D. (1990). On the willful induction of mental disorder. *Forum on Corrections Research, 2,* 14–17.

Webster, C. D., Hucker, S. J., & Grossman, M. G. (1993). Treatment programmes for mentally ill offenders. In K. Howells & C. Hollin (Eds.), *Clinical approaches to the mentally disordered offender* (pp. 87–109). Chichester, England: Wiley.

Checklist for Evaluating Treatment Programs

Items	Deficiency		
	None	Some	Serious
	0	1	2
1. Recognition of sociocultural forces			
2. Recognition of multiple causation			
3. Advocacy of multiple approaches			
4. Focused assessment process			
5. Recognition of client's positive characteristics			
6. Incorporation of client's perspective			
7. Assessment of risks			
8. Definition of objectives			
9. Planning of robust interventions			
10. Avoidance of pejorative attitudes			
11. Varied therapeutic style			
12. Evaluation of outcomes			
13. Use of multiple outcome measures			
14. Efforts to attack problems concurrently			
15. Involvement of relatives and others			
16. Training and supervision of staff			
17. Avoidance of co-option by clients			
18. Planning for the long term			
19. Expectations of positive change			
20. Development of a research plan			
Totals			
Overall score			**/40**

Note. Copyright 1996 by Chrisopher D. Webster. Reprinted by permission.

Index